Duchenne Muscular Dystrophy
Animal Models and Genetic Manipulation

Duchenne Muscular Dystrophy
Animal Models and Genetic Manipulation

Editors

Byron A. Kakulas, M.D.
Medical Director
Australian Neuromuscular Research
Institute
Head, Department of Neuropathology
Royal Perth Hospital
Professor of Neuropathology
University of Western Australia
Nedlands, Western Australia

John McC. Howell, D.V.Sc.
Pro Vice-Chancellor (Research)
Professor of Pathology
School of Veterinary Studies
Murdoch University
Murdoch, Western Australia

Allen D. Roses, M.D.
Jefferson-Pilot Professor of Neurobiology and Neurology
Duke University Medical Center
Durham, North Carolina, USA

Raven Press New York

Raven Press, 1185 Avenue of the Americas, New York, New York 10036

Made in the United States of America

Library of Congress Cataloging-in-Publication Data

Duchenne muscular dystrophy : animal models and genetic manipulation /
   editors, Byron A. Kakulas, John McC. Howell, Allen D. Roses.
      p.   cm.
   Includes bibliographical references and index.
   ISBN 0-88167-938-0
   1. Duchenne muscular dystrophy—Animal models. 2. Duchenne
muscular dystrophy—Genetic aspects.   3. Gene therapy.   I. Kakulas,
Byron A. (Byron Arthur), 1932–   . II. Howell, J. McC. (John McC.)
III. Roses, Allen D.
   [DNLM: 1. Dystrophin—physiology—congresses. 2. Gene Therapy-
-congresses.   3. Muscles—transplantation—congresses.   4. Muscular
Dystrophy—pathology—congresses. 5. Muscular Dystrophy—therapy-
-congresses. WE 559 D828]
RJ482.D78D83 1992
616.7'48—dc20
DNLM/DLC
for Library of Congress   92-12210

Contents

Part I: Dystrophinopathies

Part II: Myoblast Transfer

Part III: Gene Therapy

Contributors

Eri Arikawa, M.D.
Division of Neuromuscular Research
National Institute of Neuroscience
NCNP 4-1-1 Ogawahigashi
Kodaira, Tokyo 187, Japan

Richard J. Bartlett, Ph.D.
Assistant Professor of Medicine
 and Cell Biology
Division of Neurology
Duke University Medical Center
Durham, North Carolina 27710, USA

Manfred W. Beilharz, B.Sc., M.Sc.,
 Ph.D.
Department of Microbiology
University of Western Australia
QEII Medical Centre
Nedlands, Western Australia 6009

Barry J. Cooper, Bvs., Ph.D.
Department of Pathology
Cornell University
New York State College of
 Veterinary Medicine
Ithaca, New York 14853, USA

Miranda D. Grounds, B.Sc.(Hons),
 Ph.D.
Senior Research Officer, NH & MRC
Department of Pathology
University of Western Australia
QEII Medical Centre
Nedlands, Western Australia 6009

Edna C. Hardeman, B.Sc.(Hons), Ph.D.
Senior Research Fellow
The Children's Medical Research
 Foundation, Children's Hospital
The University of Sydney
Camperdown, New South Wales 2050
Australia

John B. Harris, B.Pharm., Ph.D.,
 F.I. Biol.
Professor of Experimental Neurology
Head, School of Neurosciences
 University of Newcastle
Director, Muscular Dystrophy Group
 Research Laboratories
Newcastle General Hospital
Newcastle Upon Tyne NE4 6BE,
 United Kingdom

John McC. Howell, Ph.D., D.V.Sc.,
 F.R.C.Path.
Professor of Pathology
School of Veterinary Studies
Murdoch University
South Street
Murdoch, Western Australia 6150

Byron A. Kakulas, A.O., M.D.(Hon
 Athens), M.D. (WA), F.R.A.C.P.,
 F.R.C.Path., F.R.C.P.A.
Medical Director
Australian Neuromuscular Research
 Institute
Professor of Neuropathology
University of Western Australia
QEII Medical Centre
Nedlands, Western Australia 6009

George Karpati, M.D., F.R.C.P.(C)
Isaac Walton Killam Professor
Neuromuscular Research Group
Montreal Neurological Institute
3801 University Street
Montreal, Quebec H3A 2B4, Canada

Henry J. Klamut, Ph.D.
Hospital for Sick Children
Genetics Department
555 University Avenue
Toronto, Ontario M5G 1X8, Canada

Joe N. Kornegay, D.V.M., Ph.D.
*Department of Companion Animal and
Special Species Medicine
College of Veterinary Medicine
North Carolina State University
4700 Hillsborough Street
at William Moore Drive
Raleigh, North Carolina 27606, USA*

Nigel G. Laing, B.Sc.(Hons), Ph.D.
*Molecular Genetics Unit
Australian Neuromuscular Research
Institute
QEII Medical Centre
Nedlands, Western Australia 6009*

**Frank L. Mastaglia, M.D., F.R.C.P.,
F.R.A.C.P.**
*Deputy Medical Director
Australian Neuromuscular Research
Institute and
Professor of Neurology
University of Western Australia
QEII Medical Centre
Nedlands, Western Australia 6009*

**John K. McGeachie, B.D.Sc., Ph.D.,
F.D.S.R.C.S.**
*Department of Anatomy and Human
Biology
University of Western Australia
Nedlands, Western Australia 6009*

Anna E. Michalska, Ph.D.
*The Murdoch Institute for
Research into Birth Defects Limited
Royal Children's Hospital
Flemington Road
Parkville, Victoria 3052, Australia*

Terence A. Partridge, Ph.D.
*Reader in Experimental Pathology
Department of Histopathology
Charing Cross & Westminister
Medical School
Fulham Palace Road
London W6 8RF, United Kingdom*

Terry A. Robertson, B.Sc., M.Sc.
*Electron Microscopy Unit
Department of Pathology
University of Western Australia
QEII Medical Centre
Nedlands, Western Australia 6009*

Allen D. Roses, M.D.
*Jefferson-Pilot Professor of
Neurobiology and Neurology
Duke University Medical Center
Durham, North Carolina 27710, USA*

**Nicholas J. Sharp, B.Vet.Med.,
M.R.C.V.S.**
*Research Fellow
Department of Companion Animal and
Special Species Medicine
College of Veterinary Medicine
North Carolina State University
4700 Hillsborough Street
at William Moore Drive
Raleigh, North Carolina 27606, USA*

Corrado Spadafora, Ph.D.
*Department of Experimental Medicine
Institute of General Pathology
Policlinico Umberto 1
University La Sapienza-Viale Regina
Elena 324
00161 Rome, Italy*

Hideo Sugita, M.D.
*Director
National Institute of Neuroscience
National Center of Neurology and Psychiatry
Kodaira, Tokyo 187, Japan*

Preface

The cloning of the Duchenne gene and the discovery of dystrophin by Lou Kunkel and his group beginning in 1986 was followed by much hope that a curative treatment for Duchenne muscular dystrophy (DMD) would soon follow. Unfortunately this has not eventuated. The Duchenne gene has proved to be large and complex, being made up of 2.5 million base pairs, the largest in the human genome. Dystrophin, its product, is a fibrous protein of the cytoskeleton with a molecular mass of 427kD. Its role is suspected to be both physically and metabolically related to the regulation of intracellular calcium. However, the exact function of dystrophin has yet to be established. As an alternative to direct "gene therapy," myoblast transfer was recommended as an interim measure. This provides "gene complementation."

The purpose of this volume is to assess progress in both myoblast transfer and gene therapy in DMD. The underlying philosophy follows the tradition of the Australian Neuromuscular Research Institute (ANRI), which monitors advances in the basic sciences and applies them to the clinical problems of neuromuscular diseases. *Pathogenesis and Therapy of Duchenne and Becker Muscular Dystrophy* (edited by Byron A. Kakulas and Frank L. Mastaglia, New York: Raven Press, 1990) discussed the spectacular discoveries in the molecular genetics of DMD, relating them to the pathogenesis of the disease and to possible modes of treatment. It recommended that experiments be undertaken using myoblast transfer in *mdx* animals and in humans.

Our objective on this present occasion is to assess such progress in the human and in the *mdx* dog. Contemporaneously, advances have occurred in gene transfer in DMD and more widely in other contexts, so we broadened our focus to include these topics as well. As in the previous workshop, the "round table" format with free and open discussion, generated many ideas by cross fertilization of the disciplines with further stimulation of our cause.

This volume will be of interest to researchers, clinicians, and students in genetics, neuroscience, neurology, and medicine.

Acknowledgments

This monograph is a record of the proceedings of an international workshop held in the Australian Neuromuscular Research Institute (ANRI), Queen Elizabeth II Medical Centre, Perth, Western Australia, from August 7-9, 1991. The assistance of the workshop's sponsors, the Neuromuscular Foundation of Western Australia and the Australian Government Department of Industry, Technology, and Commerce is gratefully acknowledged.

It is a pleasure to acknowledge with gratitude 22 world experts who came to Perth for the purpose of this workshop. We are grateful that they gave their time generously for this purpose.

Grateful acknowledgment is also made of the assistance provided by Mr. Ian K. Passmore, Scientific and Executive Officer of the ANRI, his secretary Ms. Satu M. Brice, and Mr. Mark A. Robertshaw. The administrators of the Neuromuscular Foundation of Western Australia, Mr. John E. Hollingshead and the Muscular Dystrophy Research Association, Major (retired) Jeffrey P. Mackin, assisted in the organization of the workshop. Mrs. Lynn D. Cowe is thanked for the typing of the discussions.

Special gratitude is expressed to Mrs. Susan K. E. Lawless, Personal Assistant to the Medical Director of the ANRI, for completing the difficult task of producing the "camera ready" typescript including liaison with the publisher, proofreading, and many other activities most expertly undertaken.

Part I

Dystrophinopathies

DUCHENNE MUSCULAR DYSTROPHY: Animal Models and Genetic Manipulation, edited by Byron A. Kakulas, John McC. Howell, and Allen D. Roses.
Raven Press, Ltd., New York © 1992.

1

Status of Experimental Therapy for Duchenne Muscular Dystrophy

Allen D. Roses

Division of Neurology,
Duke University Medical Center,
Durham, North Carolina 27710, USA

Considerable progress over the past five years has allowed research to focus on specific treatments for Duchenne muscular dystrophy. The promise of the "reverse" molecular genetic strategy was that once the genetic defect was identified, rational therapies could be developed. DMD was one of the first diseases for which a new protein, dystrophin, was identified as the genetic defect by positional cloning (1-7). The discovery of dystrophin resulted from the identification of small deleted regions of the X chromosome (1,4). Coding regions for a previously unknown protein were then defined (7). The present contribution to the Workshop is not meant to review all the clinical manifestations of DMD, nor to detail the molecular genetic history. The purpose of this report is to focus on the current state of interaction between medical/basic science and the clinical situation, i.e., what has been done and what needs to be done to take care of patients and their families. As part of these comments, I would focus our attention to the factor of time: what aspects of research can shorten the time period for realistic therapy.

It is appropriate that we are meeting in Perth, at the Australian Neuromuscular Research Institute. One of the most astounding early results that underpins the hope for therapy was discovered and developed by Professor Byron Kakulas circa 1960 when he studied the muscle paralysis of the Rottnest Island Quokka *(Setonix brachyurus)* (8). The astonishing discovery was that vitamin E could not only correct the weakness but reverse the neuropathology from widespread degeneration and necrosis back to normal appearing muscle. Limited muscle regenerative capacity had been described in the late nineteenth century, so that the dramatic cure of the clinical and neuropathic dystrophic process in quokkas by administration of a vitamin has stood out as an example of

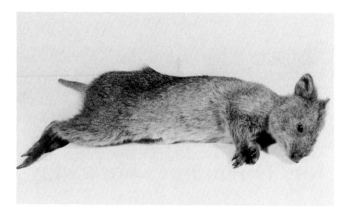

FIG. 1.   ROTTNEST ISLAND QUOKKA *(Setonix brachyurus)* with nutritional myopathy. Note the loss of muscle bulk especially of the hind limbs.

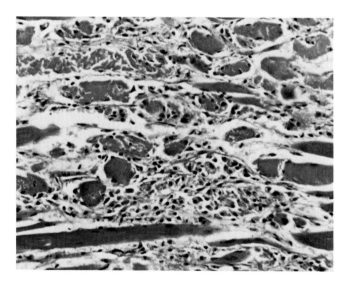

FIG. 2.   Muscle biopsy from the quokka in Fig. 1. showing widespread muscle fibre necroses.

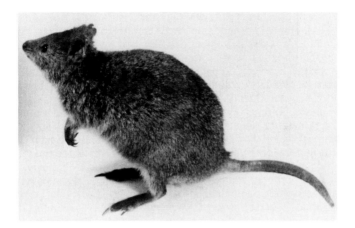

FIG. 3.   Same quokka as in Fig. 1. five months after treatment with oral tocopherol acetate (vitamin E) showing full recovery.

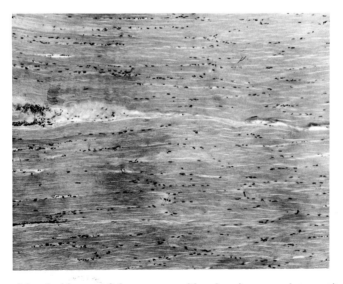

FIG. 4.   Muscle biopsy of the same quokka showing complete restitution of muscle architecture.

the unique possibilities for cure of other muscle dystrophies. The clinical disease, DMD, results when dystrophin is not made in humans, as well as in the golden retriever (9-11). It is not a problem of vitamin E deficiency. Yet the striking neuropathologic slides of quokka muscle regeneration prepared thirty years ago encourage research in experimental strategies designed to make dystrophin; or even convert the clinical situation to that of the mdx mouse, where dystrophin is lacking but the muscle functions well. The end point of our research is not the making of dystrophin, or even restoring normal muscle histology: it is the successful treatment of skeletal and cardiac muscle of affected boys so that they can live normal lives. With the high mutation rate creating new carriers and affected boys every generation, a treatment strategy must complement carrier detection and prenatal counselling since the disease will not disappear (12-14).

The first report concerning small deletions of the X chromosome that were not within the resolution of cytogenetics came in 1985 (1). Dr. Louis Kunkel's strategy was to test whether probes from the deleted area of a single DMD patient who had a large cytogenetic deletion could be found in other DMD patients (4). Our laboratory played an early role by supplying DNA (blinded samples) from 30 individuals from DMD families at a time when these samples were difficult for Kunkel's laboratory to obtain. When five affected individuals, including three from Duke, were identified, Kunkel's unusual experimental strategy (considered a "fishing expedition" by many at the time) was vindicated. Identification of the dystrophin message and protein proceeded directly (7).

Multiple laboratories have contributed to the rapid scientific and clinical efforts that identified dystrophin (2,15). The clinical impact of finding a deletion in a DMD family had immediate application to carrier diagnosis and prenatal testing. However, at a time when the accepted rate of deletions using genomic probes was 10-15%, our laboratory found approximately 50% by intensively screening each patient with every available probe (15,16). Once the cDNA was cloned and made available, approximately two years later, the proportion of patients with deletions was then accepted to be 60-70% (7). While this mini-historical point seems unimportant and trivial in retrospect, there is a significant point about timing. In the context of a large clinical population in the Duke University MDA Clinic, of which DNA from members of each pedigree was already available, we were able to effectively counsel 50% of those carriers and families at a time when this procedure was not generally applied because of the general acceptance of the 10-15% figure. When the cDNA became available, deletion diagnosis was made easier and quicker. During this window of time several affected fetuses were diagnosed at Duke but, even more importantly, several normal males were born from carrier pregnancies that would have been terminated previously. The simple time delay to the immediate application of known technology because of a scientific disagreement over the percentage of boys with deletions had an enormous potential impact for almost two years (1985-1987) before deletion testing based on the cDNA became available in 1988.

A comparable situation currently exists for support of development of an authentic animal model for therapeutic testing: golden retriever muscular dystrophy (GRMD). This authentic model of DMD is and will be of critical importance to experimental therapy strategies (10,11). The availability of the model for this purpose has been limited by lack of sufficient support for the breeding of this resource. Time has already been lost.

What is the clinical picture of DMD and how have recent discoveries changed it? As many textbooks can detail, DMD is a progressive proximal muscle weakness that interferes with normal gait in early childhood (16,17).

Most new cases from undetected families present in the third to fifth years. Earlier detection occurs when clinical signs are sought earlier because of known family histories, or by neonatal detection programs. The disease can occasionally be more serious, with neonatal deaths. In some uncommon cases, affected boys have difficulties in learning to walk. Becker muscular dystrophy (BMD) was the name applied to slower forms of the disease, including those families in whom the onset was later as well. For years BMD and DMD were incorrectly thought to be at distinct loci on the X chromosome but the situation has been clarified by the delineation of the multiple defects of dystrophin genetics and expression over the past several years (18,19).

The progressive dystrophy eventually leads to loss of ambulation, usually in the beginning of the second decade. The disease progresses to weaken the patient so that intercurrent illnesses hasten a bedridden state or death. The details of the clinical progression and deterioration have been documented for decades. What is the current state of treatment?

DMD can be treated but not cured. The treatments are ineffective in altering the progressive course of the dystrophic process. Mechanical or surgical palliations can prolong walking or provide improved postures for more effective breathing and wheelchair existence (20). There are no cures.

Unfortunately we are at that curious and painful stage in medical science where we seem to know so much and can do so little. This is not an uncommon phenomenon in medicine, but it invariably leads to potentially dangerous treatment efforts that can abuse the expectations of patients and their families. While there is a basis for the design of rational treatment, whether by cell mediated replacement therapy (myoblast transfer), direct genetic intervention, or some other expression manipulation, our current state of experimental therapeutics for DMD is comparatively undeveloped.

This Workshop underscores the nature of the problem. Several animal models exist. The real question is whether an animal model of dystrophin deficiency (mdx mouse) or one combining dystrophin mutation and skeletal muscular dystrophy (GRMD) are most appropriate to study (10,11,21-24). There is no question that each model has its own potential merits. On the other hand therapeutic experimentation with potentially dangerous strategies requires the use of a model in which not only is dystrophin addressed but the correction of muscular dystrophy is accomplished. While the mdx mouse offers a good system to study the effects of manipulations on dystrophin production, proportional support for GRMD has not been available. A direct leap to human experimentation with myoblast transplantation (supported with several US$ million) has occupied the field for the past two years. If it worked miraculously, perhaps the GRMD model would not have been needed. Parallel development would have been reasonable since, as less dramatic developments come from the human experiments, the GRMD model becomes more pertinent for therapeutic testing of strategies that cannot be worked out in boys. It takes time for carrier bitches to become fertile and for litters to be raised.

It is my view that the scientific excitement and experimentation concerning the biology of dystrophin and the jump to human myoblast experimentation have obscured a focused, scientific commitment to the needs of the patients. The loss of years until therapy has a terrible human cost. The example provided earlier: e.g., the loss of almost two years in applying genomic deletion screening to carrier detection and prenatal diagnosis under after the cDNA probes were available; affected many families who could have received valuable counselling. In fact, viewed world-wide, a significant population could have been aided by screening in the interim period. Certainly there was valuable time lost for those families.

In order to produce pharmacologic, genetic, or cellular therapies, the best substrate for experimentation is the clinical disease. Two years ago at a Conference on Myoblast Therapy in New York, several of the investigators at this Workshop took a strong but less than enthusiastically supported position that the GRMD model should receive adequate development funds to be available for therapeutic testing (25). For two years, the human myoblast experiments have received very strong support, even though they have been limited by multiple factors inherent in human experimentation. Almost no programmatic funding has supported the development of the GRMD model so that it could be made more generally available for experimental studies. Other than the isolated efforts of the participants of this Workshop, little investment in this valuable resource has been made for the past two years.

This Conference will emphasize several facts. GRMD is a genetic defect in dystrophin that leads to the canine clinical analogue of DMD. The defect has been characterized clinically, pathologically, and genetically. The model should be developed and made available for therapeutic research before more time is lost. The expense of developing large colonies for testing protocols is a small fraction of what has already been spent on human myoblast transfer alone over the past two years.

If a group of committed researchers meeting in Perth, Australia, can have an effect, I would hope it would be to catalyze a balance of experimental therapeutic options that can provide the necessary substrate for modelling therapies for DMD. It is relatively ineffective to continue talking to ourselves; by publishing these proceedings perhaps we can influence those international private foundations and associations, as well as government agencies, that the model of GRMD must be exploited for DMD therapy development that cures dystrophy, not simply expresses dystrophin. Certainly when the publication of the data presented at this Workshop, including the genetic basis of the GRMD model, reach the general scientific public, the rationale for experimental therapeutic research using the GRMD model will be very obvious. Unfortunately, before it is obvious, more time will pass, more boys will stop walking and many will die. Molecular genetics has provided the efficient tools to race with the destructive effects of disease. This is a race, and passing time is on the side of the disease.

REFERENCES

1.　Monaco, A.P., Bertelson, C.J., Middlesworth, W., Colletti, C.A., Aldridge, J., Fischbeck, K.H., Bartlett, R., Pericak-Vance, M.A., Roses, A.D., Kunkel, L.M. (1985): *Nature,* 316:842-845.
2.　Monaco, A.P. Kunkel, L.M. (1987): *Trends Genet.,* 3:33-37.
3.　Ray, P.N., Belfall, B., Duff, C., Logan, C., Kean, V., Thompson, M.W., Sylvester, J.E., Gorski, J.L., Schmickel, R.D., Worton, R.G. *Nature,* 318:671-675.
4.　Kunkel, L.M., Monaco, A.P., Middlesworth, W., Ochs, H.D., Latt, (1985): *S.A. Prc. Natl. Acad. Sci. USA,* 82:4778-4782.
5.　Monaco, A.P., Neve, R.L., Colletti-Feener, C., Bertelson, C.J., Kurnit, D.M., Kunkel, L.M. (1986): *Nature,* 323:646-650.
6.　Burghes, A.H.M., Logan, C., Hu, X., Belfall, B., Edwards, Y., Worton, R.G., Ray, P.N. (1987): *Nature,* 328:434-437.

7. Koenig, M., Hoffman, E.P., Bertelson, C.J., Monaco, A.P., Feener, C., Kunkel, L.M. *Cell,* 50:509-517.
8. Kakulas, B.A. (1982): Man, Marsupials and Muscle. University of Western Australia Press 422 pp.
9. Hoffman, E.P., Brown, R.H., Kunkel, L.M. (1987): *Cell,* 51:919-928.
10. Cooper, B.J., Winand, N.J., Stedman, H., Valentine, B.A., Hoffman, E.F., Kunkel, L.M., Oronzi-Scott, M., Fischbeck, K.H., Kornegay, J.N., Avery, R.J., Williams, J.R., Schmickel, R.D., Sylvester, J.E. (1988): *Nature,* 334:154-156.
11. Sharp, N., Kornegay, J., Van Camp, S., Dykstra, M., Roses, A., Bartlett, R. (1991): In: Gage, F. and Christen, Y. (eds.), Gene Transfer Therapy in the Nervous System, Springer-Verlag (Paris) in press.
12. Emery, A.E.H. (1987): Duchenne Muscular Dystrophy, Oxford University Press (New York), 315 pp.
13. Lane, R.J.M., Robinow, M., Roses, A.D. (1983): *J. Med. Genet.,* 20:1-11.
14. Lanman, J., Pericak-Vance, M.A., Bartlett, R.J., Chen, J.C., Speer, M., Hung, W.-Y., Roses, A.D (1987): *Am. J. Human Genet.,* 41:138-144.
15. Worton, R.G. Burghes, A.H.M. (1988): *Int. Rev. Neurobiol.,* 29:1-76.
16. Bartlett, R.J., Pericak-Vance, M.A., Koh, J., Yamaoka, L.H., Chen, J.C., Hung, W.Y., Speer, M.C., Wapenaar, M.C., VanOmmen, G.J.B., Bakker, E., Pearson, P.L., Kandt, R.S., Siddique, T., Gilbert, J.R., Lee, J.E., Roses, A.D. (1988): *Neurology,* 38:1-4.
17. Walton, J.N. (ed.) Disorders of Voluntary Muscle, Churchill-Livingstone (Edinburgh), 5th edn.
18. Mabry, C.C., Roeckel, I.E., Munich, R.L., Robertson, D. (1965): *New Engl. J. Med.,* 273:1062-1070.
19. Becker, P.E., Kiener, F. (1955): *Psychiat. Zeitsch. Neurol.,* 193:427-448.
20. Roses, A.D. (1990): Duchenne muscular dystrophy. In: Current Therapy in Neurologic Disease. R.T. Johnson, ed., B.C. Decker (Philadelphia), 399-402.
21. Bulfield, G., Siller, W,G., Wight, P.A.L., Moore, K.J. (1984): *Proc. Natl. Acad. Sci. USA,* 81:1189-1192.
22. Kornegay, J.N. (1986): In: Kirk, R.W. (ed.), Current Veterinary Therapy IX, Saunders (Philadelphia).
23. Kornegay, J.N., Tuler, S.M., Miller, D.M., Van Camp, S.E. (1988): *Muscle and Nerve,* 1:1056-1064.
24. Hoffman, E.P., Monaco, A.P., Feener, C.C., Kunkel, L.M. (1987): *Science,* 238:347-350.
25. Griggs, R.C., Karpati, G. (1990): (eds.) Adv. Exper. Med. Biol., 280, Plenum (New York), 316pp.

DUCHENNE MUSCULAR DYSTROPHY: Animal Models
and Genetic Manipulation, edited by Byron A. Kakulas,
John McC. Howell, and Allen D. Roses.
Raven Press, Ltd., New York © 1992.

2

Pathological Features of Duchenne and Becker Muscular Dystrophy

Byron A. Kakulas

*Australian Neuromuscular Research Institute,
Department of Pathology, University of Western Australia.
Department of Neuropathology, Royal Perth Hospital.*

Since the discovery of dystrophin it has been possible to formulate a hypothesis which relates the underlying molecular lesion to the pathogenesis of the disease (12). Dystrophin is a 3685 amino acid cytoskeleton protein weighing 427kD. It is a member of the greater spectrin family. It accounts for .001% of all mRNA and .002% muscle protein. It is mainly localised to the sarcolemma of which it forms 2-3%. It shows strong homology to actin and spectrin. There are several other very similar proteins under investigation (2). Dystrophin is an oligomeric protein associated with four glycoproteins, one of which is either totally absent or found only in very low concentrations in Duchenne muscular dystrophy (DMD). The DMD gene is the largest yet recognised making up 0.05% of the human genome consisting of 2.5 million base pairs with 75 exons.

The exact role of dystrophin remains to be established. However from its size and location it seems that at least one function is the provision of mechanical stability to the membrane. Another suggested role is related to regulation of intracellular calcium. The membrane glycoproteins to which it is attached may be important in that respect.

Nevertheless, concerning the pathogenesis of DMD or Becker MD it is reasonable to postulate that breaks occur in the membrane under conditions of hypercontraction. This results in focal necrosis. It is possible that eccentric contractions, ie force generation while the muscle is lengthening, are more damaging than concentric or shortening contractions. This factor may contribute to the topographic distribution of the more affected muscles in the proximal limb girdle groups in DMD. Focal necrosis is followed by regeneration. Regeneration has been shown to be incomplete or abortive (14) so that the cycle of necrosis and regeneration rapidly proceeds to exhaustion of regeneration (10). At the end stage of the disease there is passive replacement of muscle by fat and fibrous tissue. This concisely expressed mechanism is now the standard explanation of the pathogenesis of the disease. These concepts were derived from the original experimental work on the necrobiotic vitamin E responsive myopathy of the Rottnest Island Quokka (9).

It is still not known when the DMD lesions first manifest in life. It is evident that muscle development and maturation are compatible with the absence of dystrophin. "At risk" Duchenne foetuses with deletions show no morphological lesions, even by electron microscopy. It has been reported that calcium levels are increased (6).

Although data for the neonatal period is sketchy sufficient evidence exists to suggest that immediately after birth skeletal muscles are intact, although serum creatine kinase levels are moderately elevated (10).

A two and a half week "at risk" DMD newborn male was biopsied by Bradley et al (3) and the muscle was found to be normal. The same patient was biopsied again at the age of 2 years at which time polyfocal necrosis was well developed. Another DMD infant had well established lesions at 2 months (7). Thus it is with the acquisition of voluntary motor activity in the infant that necrosis begins. When the boy becomes ambulant following a slightly delayed onset, the infant "Hercules" appearance with large muscles and exaggerated lumbar lordosis presents the classic clinical appearance. Later the waddling gait reflects the severe involvement of the proximal muscles of the lower limb girdle especially the glutei. The gastrocnemius muscles are enlarged and firm and Gower's sign becomes positive at 5 or 6 years of age. The disorder is relentlessly progressive until death occurs somewhere between 15-25 years of age or later depending upon the degree of specialised care available (15). In the final stages the respiratory muscles are involved and the patient dies of anoxia.

The topographic distribution of muscle involvement was quantified in a series of 19 Duchenne autopies by Dr. Guo Yu Pu (11). In this work the very consistent pattern of selective vulnerability of the bodily musculature was fully documented. The extraocular muscles escape. The muscles innervated by cranial nerves are only slightly involved and show active necrosis eg. the temporalis is only just affected at the time of death. The intercostal muscles and diaphragm also show very early lesions, mainly polyfocal necrosis in the terminal period. In contrast the large proximal muscles of the upper and lower limb girdles are at the end stages with very little intact muscle being identified by the age of 12 to 14 years. The pectoral muscles are early and are severely affected as is the quadriceps femoris before the age of 10 years. The gastrocnemius also shows advanced changes early in the disease but is associated firstly with true hypertrophy and later with pseudohypertrophy with fat and fibrous tissue accumulation. The underlying reasons for this consistent pattern of involvement remains enigmatic.

The myopathology of DMD and BMD can be divided into early, middle and late changes (10). In the established lesion the overall picture is one of total disorganisation of muscle architecture. Muscle fibres are irregular in size and shape. There are many internal nuclei and others are irregularly placed. Muscle fibre splitting as a feature of incomplete regeneration becomes prominent. Polyfocal necrosis is present at all stages followed by regeneration which becomes abortive.

By light microscopy, nuclei become pyknotic and the myofibrillar structure of regenerating myotubes ill defined. By electron microscopy there is prominent exo and endocytosis and homogenised sarcomeres occur in the cytoplasm. Groups of small fibres frequently found in cross-sections are believed to represent regeneration by budding. There is much redundant basement membrane. Endomysium is condensed. It is believed but not fully established that the regeneration originates from satellite cells which are increased in number in DMD (10).

A milestone was reached in the neuropathology of DMD when Mokri and Engel (16) discovered electron microscopic breaks in the sarcolemma. Careful work on the earliest changes lead to the coining of the term "delta lesion" (4). A detailed study of the ultrastructural lesions in DMD has been reported by Schmalbruch (18).

Dystrophin is expressed in the heart and the consequent myocardial lesions are well known. It seems that this takes the form of a progressive outfall of myocardial fibres with fibrous tissue replacement. Necessarily, only the end stage of the myocardial lesions are available for study at necropsy. It is not known whether polyfocal necrosis is a feature of the early lesions. From work on the Rottnest Island Quokka it is evident that necrosis and regeneration may be found in the heart of necrobiotic myopathies (8).

Dystrophin is also expressed in smooth muscle but to date reports of abnormalities in smooth muscle have not been convincing.

It is known that approximately 2/3 of patients with DMD have borderline mental retardation. The neuropathological basis for this disorder is unknown. It was discovered that dystrophin was expressed in the foetal brain (10). It is not exactly known with certainty in which cells this dystrophin occurs. It may be at synapses or in astrocytes. Early reports by Rosman and Kakulas (17) suggested that minor degrees of migrational arrest of neurons with resultant microscopic heterotopias and pachygyria was the basis for the static mental retardation. If dystrophin is found to be expressed in the radial glial this may give support to the migrational arrest this explanation for the mental defect but this remains to be confirmed (5).

In a series of Duchenne and Becker "at risk" male foetuses, independent DNA deletion diagnosis and immunohistochemical dystrophin studies were undertaken. Of six male foetuses "at risk" for DMD, two showed absent or reduced dystrophin and one of these had a DNA deletion. The other four, which did not have deletions, showed normal dystrophin immunohistochemistry. Of 11 BMD "at risk" male foetuses seven had dystrophin deficiencies by immunochemistry of which five showed microdeletions of DNA. Four did not have deletions and showed normal amounts of dystrophin. There were five normal controls, all of which showed the presence of dystrophin. Therefore of the total of 17 "at risk" DMD or BMD foetuses, nine were abnormal. This retrospective verification of the disease in such foetuses gives comfort to the genetic counsellor and is reassuring to all concerned.

In recent times it has become evident that abnormalities of the dystrophin gene are present in neuromuscular syndromes other than "classic" Duchenne or

Becker stereotyped clinical picture. Even patients with disorders consistent with denervation and with normal creatine kinase levels in the serum (Kugelberg Welander sydrome) have been shown to have deletions of the DMD gene by our group. We have also found dystrophin deficiency or deletions in three male patients, one with scapulo-humeral dystrophy, one with limb girdle MD and a boy with the 'stick-man' type of congenital MD. Dr. Arikawa (2) has also shown abnormalities of dystrophin to be present in patients with fascioscapulohumeral syndrome, quadriceps myopathy, the Fukuyama type of congenital muscular dystrophy and limb girdle muscular dystrophy, thus widely extending the range of phenotypic expression of the dystrophin gene.

Remarkably another male patient, 26 years of age with proximal limb girdle and axial muscle weakness of 6 years duration has shown an excess of dystrophin evident in the centre of the muscle fibre. His creatine kinase was 302 (N 200 u/l).

Therefore contrary to standard teaching in genetics, both the genotype and phenotype for the dystrophinopathies is now shown to be quite variable. As experience accumulates in this regard it may be possible to reclassify these disorders according to molecular criteria. More importantly this variability presents a challenge to those concerned with the pathogenesis of these diseases to provide an explanation for this.

Given the variability of manifestation of the dystrophinopathies in different patients together with the nature of the lesions and the topographic distribution of severity, the task of the gene therapist is considerable. Myoblast transfer is only capable of correcting local defects, while the Duchenne gene, being so large, is not amenable to viral transfection and other avenues need to be explored.In this regard a recent report of dystrophin expression, *in vivo* in mdx mice and *in vitro*, by direct injections of DNA constructs is most exciting (1).

In conclusion the above comments on the myopathology and pathogenesis of DMD provides essential information for those seeking to arrest the changes, the topic of this Workshop.

ACKNOWLEDGMENTS

Gratitude is expressed to Dr. N.G. Laing, Mr. David Chandler and Mr. Russell Johnsen for the laboratory data.

REFERENCES

1. Acsadi, G., Dickson, G., Love, D.R., Jani, A., Walsh, F.S., Gurusinghe, A., Wolff, J.A., Davies, K.E. (1991): Human Dystrophin Expression in mdx Mice After Intramuscular Injection of DNA Constructs. *Nature*, 352:815-818.
2. Arikawa, E., Arahata K., Sunohara, N., Ishiura, S., Nonka I., Sugita H. (1992): Immunocytochemical Analysis of Dystrophin in Muscular Dystrophy. This volume.
3. Bradley, W.G., Hudgson, P., Larson, P.E., Papapetropoulos, T.A., Jenkinson, M. (1972): Structural changes in the early stages of Duchenne Muscular Dystrophy. *J. Neurol. Neurosurg. Psychiatry,* 35:451-455.
4. Cullen, M.J., Fulthorpe J.J. (1975): Stages in Fibre Breakdown in Duchenne Muscular Dystrophy; An Electron Microscopic Study. J *Neurol., Sci* 24:179-200.

5. Dubowitz, V., Crome, L. (1969): The Central Nervous System in Duchenne Muscular Dystrophy. *Brain,* 92:805-808.
6. Emery, A.E.H. (1988): Duchenne Muscular Dystrophy. Oxford University Press pp 139-44.
7. Hudgson, P., Pearce, G.W., Walton, J.N. (1967): Preclinical muscular dystrophy: Histopathological changes observed on muscle biopsy. *Brain,* 90:565-576.
8. Kakulas, B.A., Owen, C.G., Papadimitriou, J.M., Durack D.T. (1968): The myocardial lesions in the Rottnest quokka with nutritional myopathy. Proceedings of the Australian Association of Neurologists 5:565-571.
9. Kakulas, B.A. (1982): Man, Marsupial and Muscle; The Invesigation of Muscular Paralysis Occurring in the Rottnest Island Quokka (Setonix Brachyurus). University of Western Australia Press, Nedlands.
10. Kakulas, B.A., Adams R.D. (1985): Diseases of Muscle; Pathological Foundations of Clinical Myology. Harper and Row, IVth Edition, Philadelphia.
11. Kakulas, B.A., Guo Yu Pu.(1986): Quantitative Assessment of Muscle Lesions in 19 Duchenne Necropsies. *Muscle and Nerve,* (Supp 1986) 9 No.55:206. Abstract 39.23.
12. Kakulas, B.A., Mastaglia, F.M. (1990): Pathogenesis and Therapy of Duchenne and Becker Muscular Dystrophy. Raven Press NY, NY.
13. Koenig, M., Hoffman, E.P., Bertelson, C.J., Monaco A.P., Feener, C., Kunkel, L.M.(1987): Complete Cloning of the Duchenne Muscular Dystrophy (DMD) cDNA and preliminary Genomic Organization of the DMD Gene in Normal and Affected Individuals. *Cell,* 50:509-517.
14. Mastaglia, F.L., Kakulas, B.A.(1969): Regeneration in Duchenne Muscular Dystrophy; a Histological Study. *Brain,* Vol 92:809-818.
15. Miller, G., Kakulas, B.A.(1986): Management of Muscular Dystrophy in Western Australia. In: Recent Achievements in Restorative Neurology 2, Progressive Neuromuscular Diseases. Edited M.R. Dimitrijevic, B.A. Kakulas and G. Vbrova. Kruger, Basal 15-27.
16. Mokri, B., Engel, A.G. (1975): Duchenne Dystrophy: Electron Microscopic Findings Pointing to a Basic or Dearly abnormality in the Plasma Membrane of the Muscle Fibre. *Neurology,* (Minn) 25:1111-1120.
17. Rosman, N.P., Kakulas, B.A.(1966): Mental Deficiency Associated with Muscular Dystrophy; A Neuropathological Study. *Brain,* 89:769-788.
18. Schmalbruch, H.L.(1982): Ch 6 The Muscular Dystrophies. In: Skeletal Muscle Pathology. Edited F.L. Mastaglia, J.N. Walton. Churchill Livingstone, London.

DISCUSSION

Professor Allen D. Roses:
Does anybody have any comments, questions or additions?

Dr Terence A. Partridge:
Byron, you spoke of the intellectual deficit associated with dystrophin deficiency. If there is a direct effect of dystrophin on neural development and function we could expect to pick this up in the Becker's and more interestingly possibly in the carrier mothers in whom half the neurons would lack dystrophin.

Professor John B Harris:
If I may comment first. Most would concede that there is a tendency for patients with Xp21 dystrophy to have a reduced IQ. It is also generally felt that the more severe the disability the greater the deficit. The association between the two aspects of Xp21 dystrophy, however, is rather loose. We have found no relationship between any pattern of deletion and the level of IQ or between protein expression and IQ. I think it is most improbable that a detailed study of IQ will allow us to make any comment on the role of dystrophin in central neurons in general or on the level of 'intelligence' in particular.

Dr Terence A. Partridge:
But even so some intermediate effect on intellectual function should be evident.

Professor Byron A. Kakulas:
Well, yes, Terry, in general your premise is correct. However, there is a difficulty with BMD because one does not know whether a particular IQ is reduced or not if it is in the normal range when tested. For example, if a Becker patient has an IQ of 120 perhaps it should have been 140 if he did not have BMD.

Dr. Terence A. Partridge:
Family IQ studies might supply this information.

Professor Byron A. Kakulas:
I think that probably it would be a valuable thing, to review the question in BMD. On the other hand, perhaps it would be more productive to learn about the role of dystrophin in the CNS and pursue the I.Q. question neurobiologically.

Dr. Terence A. Partridge:
It might prove difficult because the brain is not an easy organ in which to study cellular function.

Professor John B. Harris:
I wish to enlarge on my previous comments. We do not know how to properly define intelligence, or what intelligence in man means in terms of neuronal function and integrative activity. We do not even know which population of neurons we might study with the greatest potential profit. In terms of the expression of dystrophin in the CNS, I find it puzzling that the highest levels of dystrophin appear to be present in cerebellar Purkinje cells and the cells of the dorsal root ganglia. Patients with dystrophin-deficient diseases do not appear to suffer a cerebellar ataxia or a ganglionopathy, so the deficit must lead only to subtle changes in cellular function that have little bearing on the ability of the cells to operate within a neuronal system. We have never been able to identify dystrophin in spinal neurons, but I have to admit that our expertise on spinal cord is limited. It is also possible that for one reason or another our antibodies cannot detect a neuronal-form of dystrophin (if such exists).

Professor Hideo Sugita:
The localisation of dystrophin related protein (DRP) in the central nervous system (CNS) is very controversial. We have obtained a cross reactive band of a 400kDa protein in brain and spinal cord in mdx mice. Immunofluorescent micrography revealed that the outside of the small arteries and the pia mater of the brain strongly reacted with the antibody. This result suggests the presence of a cross

reactive protein other than dystrophin, possibly a DRP in the *pia mater*.

Professor George Karpati:
In relation to the mental subnormality that occurs in about one third of Duchenne boys, there has been another suggestion made recently by David Yaffe's group in Israel. According to their suggestion the problem may not be in the deficiency of the brain type of dystrophin but it may be due to a new isoform which they call the "liver type", which is a much smaller molecule. It is not expressed in skeletal muscle but it is expressed in many cell types including glia and neurons. It has only about a 6 kB cDNA and presumably it has its own promoter. Thus, it is conceivable that if one wants to look for the answer for the mental subnormality in DMD, it may be necessary to focus on this isoform rather than the brain isoform.

Professor Joe N. Kornegay:
I would like to go back to the question of whether there are pathologic changes in neonates or foetuses with DMD. Dogs with golden retriever muscular dystrophy (GRMD) certainly have dramatic, early pathological changes. The sartorius muscle, for example, at one day of age, has evidence of not just myofiber necrosis, but also mineralization. This would suggest that there are changes *in utero*, as well.

Dr. Miranda D.Grounds:
I am also curious to know when the earliest pathological changes are identified in foetuses with DMD.

Professor Byron A. Kakulas:
Apart from immunocytochemistry, I do not think anybody has a means of accurately answering the question in the foetus. Large nuclei and hyaline fibres are reported in the DMD foetus with increased levels of calcium also being found as I described in my paper. Betty Banker in a detailed study of one DMD foetus stated that there was necrosis in the deltoid but not in the vastus lateralis muscle so that whether focal necrosis occurs remains somewhat of an open question. Nevertheless the bulk of the data suggests that the destructive aspects of DMD begin after birth.

DUCHENNE MUSCULAR DYSTROPHY: Animal Models
and Genetic Manipulation, edited by Byron A. Kakulas,
John McC. Howell, and Allen D. Roses.
Raven Press, Ltd., New York © 1992.

3

Ultrastructural Localization and the Possible Role of Dystrophin

J. B. Harris and M. J. Cullen

*Muscular Dystrophy Group Research Laboratories,
Regional Neurosciences Centre,
Newcastle General Hospital,
Newcastle upon Tyne NE4 6BE, England*

INTRODUCTION

Dystrophin is a large cytoskeletal protein with a calculated molecular mass of 427 kD. Immunocytochemical studies have identified dystrophin or closely related proteins in the skeletal muscles of all vertebrates thus far examined (24). It is also found in a range of other tissues including cardiac and smooth muscle, the plexiform layer of the retina, the corneal epithelia, central neurones, tactile nerve endings and the myoepithelial layers of sweat and salivary glands (see for example 22, 26). In some cases the level of immunoreactivity is low, but it is important to note that non-contractile as well as contractile cells contain dystrophin. It is of additional interest that in skeletal muscle, dystrophin or a related protein is concentrated at the myotendinous and neuromuscular junctions (see for example 18, 36, 37). At least some of the dystrophin-related proteins are probably encoded by a gene located on an autosome rather than on the X-chromosome (25), and they may be involved in non-X-linked muscular dystrophy.

Dystrophin is virtually absent from the muscles of patients with severe Xp-21 muscular dystrophy and is present in an abnormal form or in reduced abundance in patients with less severe Xp-21 muscular dystrophy. The protein is also absent from the muscles of dogs, cats and mice with X-linked muscular dystrophy.

The consequences of the lack of dystrophin from skeletal muscles of dog and man are devastating, and give rise directly or indirectly to the progressive degeneration of skeletal muscle fibres and possibly to the malfunction and/or degeneration of cardiac and smooth muscle as well. The early stages of regeneration of the muscles of dystrophic patients do not appear to be affected by the absence of dystrophin, but the growth and maturation of the newly regenerated fibres is clearly impaired, and it is generally accepted that the muscle fibres enter repeated cycles of degeneration and regeneration until the regenerative capacity of the tissue is exhausted (see for example, 43). In contrast, the dystrophin-deficient muscles of mice compensate well for the loss of dystrophin, go through a limited cycle of degeneration and regeneration, grow to maturity and have apparently normal functional capacity.

Clearly the widespread occurrence of dystrophin between species and in numerous cell types, both contractile and non- contractile, indicates that it is a protein of considerable importance to the architecture, development, survival and function of the cell. Its precise role in the life-cycle of the cell is, however, less clear. For example, although it is generally accepted that the lack of dystrophin is causally related to the dystrophic process, causation has not been proven beyond reasonable doubt. It is easy to overlook the fact, for example, that many children who go on to develop rather severe Xp-21 muscular dystrophy are difficult to diagnose on clinical/behaviourial grounds when very young, despite the fact that their muscle fibres are dystrophin-deficient (41). Similarly, it is extremely difficult to understand how the well established regional differentiation between severely affected and less severely affected muscles in boys with severe Xp-21 muscular dystrophy can arise when all fibres should be dystrophin deficient. Moreover, within even severely affected muscles there are fibres that are able to contract and relax in the absence of dystrophin.

An adequate description of the role of dystrophin in both contractile and non-contractile cells, is needed but determining the role of the protein requires above all a complete understanding of its localization within the cell. In this paper we describe briefly some of our observations on the localization of dystrophin in skeletal muscle and we then evaluate critically the techniques we have used in our work on the distribution of dystrophin. We conclude by discussing some of the proposed roles of the protein in skeletal muscle.

METHODS

Selection of Technique

During the last ten years many new techniques have been developed to aid the generation of reliable, reproducible information on the localization of antigens at the ultrastructural level. Innovations have been introduced at each stage of tissue processing so there is now considerable variety in the approaches available to the investigator. It is not appropriate to list here all the different protocols that have been used, but pertinent nevertheless to consider the guiding principles for selection of the most appropriate technique.

The most important requirements for any EM immunocytochemical technique are that:

(1) The antibodies must be highly specific.
(2) The target antigen must still bind the antibody after chemical fixation (if this is used).
(3) The cell morphology must be well preserved.
(4) The marker or probe must be distinct and visible.
    In addition if quantitation is to be carried out;
(5) Particulate markers which can be easily seen and counted must be used.

The requirement that the antibodies should be specific is self-evident in that an antibody which cross-reacts with more than one protein in the tissue could produce highly misleading results. Thus, by preference, monoclonal antibodies should be used although affinity-purified polyclonal antibodies are often suitable.

The second and third requirements are to some extent mutually exclusive in that the procedure of fixation, normally used to preserve fine structure, acts by cross-linking amino acids thereby destroying the tertiary structure of the protein. If the antigenic determinant is cross-linked the reaction with the antibody will often be prevented. It is therefore sometimes inevitable that a degree of morphological preservation is sacrificed in order to preserve antigenicity. Dystrophin unfortunately appears to be particularly 'sensitive' to glutaraldehyde fixation so only very low concentrations (0.001 or 0.01%) of this primary fixative are used. The glutaraldehyde is however used in conjunction with 2% formaldehyde which is a weaker and partially reversible fixative. Intimately related to the question of the preservation of antigenicity versus the preservation of morphology is the type of embedding that is used. The combination of dehydration and heating involved in embedding in resins such as Araldite or Epon destroys all but the most robust antigens and even these will only be exposed on the cut surface of resin sections. 'Cryofixation' and cryosectioning have therefore become the techniques of choice for EM immunolabelling. Freezing does not denature proteins and so antigenicity is preserved. At the same time, freezing physically hardens the specimen so it may be sectioned without infiltration with extraneous materials. Ideally freezing would also obviate any necessity for chemical fixation but unfortunately thin sections of completely unfixed tissue tend to dissolve when thawed and incubated with labelling solutions. In the case of muscle, little can be seen under the electron microscope apart from a few disorganised myofilaments if the tissue is unfixed. (This of course is not the case at the light microscope level where unfixed frozen tissue sections are considerably thicker and more stable). The low concentrations of fixative described above are probably close to the maximum that is compatible with good antigenicity and the minimum that is compatible with an acceptable level of preservation of cell structure. Even so, we observe some slight osmotic damage.

After the tissue has been lightly fixed, and before it is frozen, it should be exposed to a cryoprotectant to minimise ice crystal damage. Cryoprotectants are compounds that bind water to the extent that no water molecules are available for nucleation, the first step in ice-crystal formation. Short chain sugars such as sucrose make ideal cryoprotectants. Sucrose would normally be excluded from intact cells but the light chemical fixation renders the plasma membrane permeable. We therefore infuse our material overnight with high concentrations of sucrose (2.3 M) to protect it from freezing damage.

An alternative to cryofixation and cryosection is offered by the use of water soluble or low temperature resin-based embedding media, such as Lowicryl or L.R. White, which give good fine-structural preservation. Unlike cryosections, however, low temperature resin sections can only be labelled on their surface. This is not a problem when the antigen is densely concentrated but for dystrophin, the molecules of which are relatively widely spaced (see below), it would probably result in a very low signal density, and would be quite inadequate for quantitative analysis.

Cryosectioning also has the advantage over other techniques in that it allows semithin section (approximately 1 um) to be cut from the same frozen block for high-resolution immunofluorescent studies.

The fourth requirement, that the probe must be distinct, becomes especially important if quantitation is to be carried out. Labelling procedures can be divided into two classes (a) those using diffuse labels (autoradiography, fluorescent or peroxidase conjugates); and (b) those using particulate labels (ferritin, colloidal gold). For quantitation a particulate marker is necessary. Colloidal gold is preferable to ferritin because it is more distinct under the electron microscope. It is also extremely versatile and be produced in a wide range of diameters (5 nm to 150 nm), and, as undecagold, down to 0.8 nm (15). Moreover, whilst in this laboratory we largely concentrate on gold conjugated to antibodies, it can also be conjugated to a variety of different macromolecules such as enzymes, lectins, streptavidin and proteins A and G.

Protocol

While muscle is the tissue with which we are most familiar, the processing and labelling protocol that we use should be equally suitable for most other tissues.

The human and experimental animal material is processed in the same way. Small pieces of muscle are held slightly stretched (approximately 1.2 x resting length) while being fixed for one hour in 2% formaldehyde with 0.001% glutaraldehyde. They are then cut into small blocks (1.0 x 0.5 x 0.5 mm) and fixed for a further hour. After washing with phosphate-buffered saline of composition 0.02 M NaH_2PO_4 $2H_2O$; 0.08M Na_2HPO_4; 0.15 M NaCl; pH 7.2 (PBS) the muscle blocks are placed in 2.3 M sucrose (cryoprotectant) for at least 2 hours or preferably overnight. The blocks are then mounted on stubs and plunge-frozen in liquid nitrogen. Sections, 100 nm thick, are cut on a cryoultramicrotome (Reichert FC4D) at a knife temperature of -100°C and a block temperature of -90°C.

Longitudinal sections are cut with the knife edge at 90° to the fibre axis because when cut conventionally, with the knife-edge parallel with the fibre axis, the cryosections tend to fragment. Good transverse sections are technically more difficult to obtain than longitudinal ones.

After collection on carbon and formvar-coated grids the sections are quenched with 80 mM ammonium chloride for 10 min, then washed in 0.1 M PBS containing 0.5% bovine serum albumin (BSA) and 0.15% glycine, followed by normal goat serum diluted 1:20 PBS/BSA.

After further washing the sections are incubated for one hour with the primary antibody at an appropriate dilution (if it is polyclonal) or in culture supernatant containing 10% foetal calf serum (if it is monoclonal). The sections are washed again and then incubated for one hour with an appropriate gold-conjugated secondary antibody.

After a further six washes in PBS/BSA and four with distilled water the sections are stabilized in 2% methyl cellulose containing 0.2% uranyl acetate and allowed to dry in air. The sections are then ready for examination under the electron microscope.

In every case immunofluorescence observations are made on 1 um sections from the same blocks used for immunogold labelling. The sections are collected on gelatin-coated slides, immersed in PBS and washed in 50 mM ammonium chloride in PBS. After incubation in the primary antibody and washing, the sections are incubated in an appropriate rhodamine-conjugated anti-serum for one hour at room temperature. The slides are washed twice in PBS, once in distilled water, dried around the sections and mounted with Uvinert before examination under a fluorescence-optics microscope.

As controls, sections from the same blocks are processed in an identical way to that described above for both immunogold labelling and immunofluorescence except that pre-immune serum or virgin tissue culture medium is substituted for that containing the antibody.

Antibodies

We have used the following antibodies to dystrophin for immunogold labelling and immunofluorescence:

Code	Monoclonal (M) or Polyclonal (P)	Raised Against	Source
Dy4/66D3	M	Fusion protein, amino acids 1181-1388	L. Nicholson Newcastle
Dy8/6C5	M	Peptide, last 17 amino acids at C-terminus	L. Nicholson Newcastle
Dy10/12B2	M	Fusion protein, amino acids 67-713	L. Nicholson Newcastle
2-5E2	M	Peptide, amino acids 440-489	K. Arahata Tokyo
3-4C4	M	Peptide, amino acids 2359-2408	K. Arahata Tokyo
P1460	P	Peptide, last 17 amino acids at C-terminus	E. Zubrzycka-Gaarn, Toronto

RESULTS

Non-Dystrophic Muscle

With every antibody to dystrophin that we have used to date, the labelling has been close to the plasma membrane of the muscle fibres (Figs. 1-3). It has not been found on the T-tubules, triads or any other component or constituent of the fibres.

For the reasons to be discussed later, the position of the gold probe seldom corresponds exactly to the position of the epitope, but should lie within a radius of approximately 20 nm from it. Within any one fibre, therefore, there was inevitable variation in the exact positioning of the gold particles but with each of the antibodies, the majority of the gold particles lay within 50 um of the plasma membrane.

When histograms of the distance of the gold probe from the plasma membrane were constructed, differences in the position of the mode could be detected dependent on which antibody was used. When Dy4/6D3 (raised against a segment - amino acids 1181-1388 - of the rod domain) was used, the mode was approximately 15 nm internal to the cytoplasmic face of the plasma membrane (Figs. 4, 5). Similarly when Dy10/12B2 or 2-5E2 (both raised against peptides corresponding to sequences close to the N-terminus end of the rod domain) or 3-4C4 (raised against a peptide corresponding to amino acids 2359-2408) were used, the label was most commonly located internal to the plasma membrane,

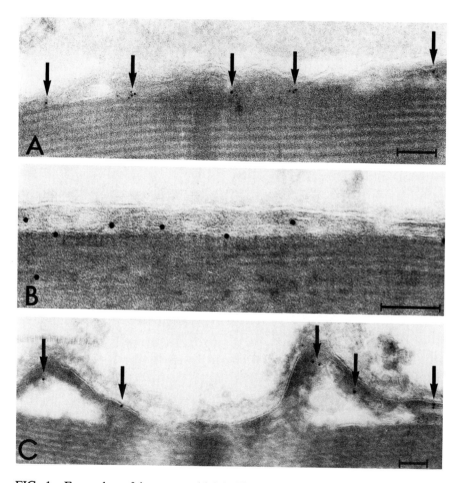

FIG. 1. Examples of immunogold labelling using antibodies raised against different segments of the rod-like domain of dystrophin. A. Dy4/6D3, 5 nm gold. B. Dy10/12B2, 10 nm gold. C. 2-5E2, 10 nm gold. Bar = 100 nm in each figure. (We are grateful to Dr. K. Arahata for the gift of 2-5E2).

(Figs. 1B, 1C). When P1460 or Dy8/6C5 (polyclonal and monoclonal antibodies, respectively, raised against a peptide containing the last 17 amino acids at the C-terminus) were used, the label was frequently located over the membrane itself and the mode of the distributions was shifted 20-25 nm peripherally (Figs. 2, 3, 5). It is known that dystrophin forms a complex with four glycoproteins, at least one of which is an integral membrane protein (2, 11). One interpretation of our own results is that the C-terminus of dystrophin, as well as being tightly associated with the glycoproteins, is inserted along with them into the plasma membrane.

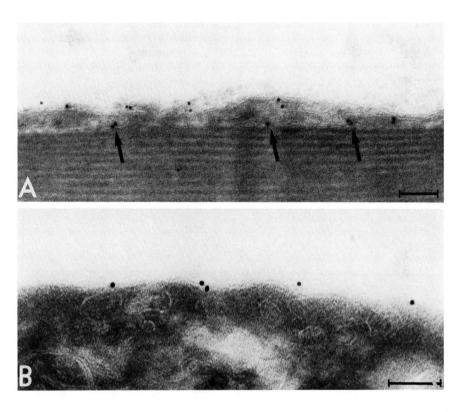

FIG. 2. Examples of immunogold labelling using the polyclonal antibody P1460 raised against the C-terminus of dystrophin. A. Longitudinal section, 10 nm gold. Note that where the gold is internal to the plasma membrane it is often associated with another membrane (arrows). B. Transverse section, 10 nm gold. (Antibody P1460 was a generous gift from the late Elizabeth Zubrzycka-Gaarn.)

The proposal that the C-terminus of dystrophin is inserted in the membrane is given some support by some recent preliminary experiments in which small blocks of biopsied muscle were first bathed with the C-terminus antibody, then with the gold-conjugated secondary antibody and before being processed for normal resin embedding and sectioning. In a few areas gold particles were found bound to the plasma membrane [Fig 6]. This suggests that the C-terminus epitope, the last 17 amino acids, was accessible to antibodies which were bathing the external surface of the fibres.

The measurement of distances between adjacent labelling sites allowed the construction of appropriate distribution histograms. Histograms derived from labelling patterns obtained with a C-terminus antibody (P1460) were compared with those obtained with a rod domain antibody (Dy4/6D3). The histograms showed the same mode (100-140 nm) (Fig 7). This similarity suggests that there is an underlying periodicity to the sites of 100-140 nm. This distance is close to the predicted rod domain length of 100-125 nm (4, 21) and to the length of 100-120 nm measured from rotary-shadowed images of dystrophin purified from rabbit skeletal muscle (29) (but less than 175 nm measured from rotary-shadowed images of dystrophin isolated from chicken gizzard smooth muscle, 33). A repeat of approximately 125 nm has been reported in mouse (42) and an occasional repeat of 100-120 nm was observed in rat muscle after immunoperoxidase labelling (36).

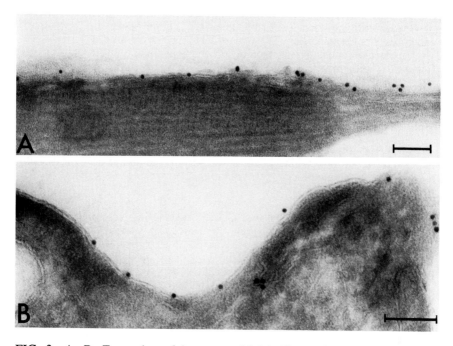

FIG. 3. A, B. Examples of immunogold labelling using the monoclonal antibody Dy8/6C5 raised against the C-terminus of dystrophin. 10 nm gold. Bar = 10nm.

Comparison of the spacing of the labelling sites in longitudinal and transverse sections from the same muscle showed no differences in the periodicity (Fig 7 Case 2). As the length of the sarcomeres in longitudinal section (2.6 μm) corresponded to those in a relaxed state, this implies there is no strong axial component to the arrangement of the dystrophin at the plasma membrane in relaxed muscle. It is our intention to examine muscles at different degrees of contraction and stretch to investigate in what way the spacing of the binding site changes with sarcomere length.

A triangular, square or hexagonal lattice of molecules could each, in theory, give a spacing distribution which was the same in both longitudinal and transverse section. Koenig and Kunkel (20) have proposed a hexagonal arrangement for dystrophin, although in their model the sides of the hexagons are not composed of single molecules but of two hinged (and partially dimeric) molecules. We hope, by obtaining *en face* views of labelled membranes, to get a two dimensional view of the labelled epitopes and thus be able to describe a structural model of the molecular lattice. This will be rendered more accurate by using double labelling techniques so that the location of one epitopic site relative to that of another on the same molecule can be identified.

Dystrophic Muscle

We have never obtained any labelling of fibres from Duchenne muscular dystrophy biopsies although immunofluorescence and immunoperoxidase labelling at the light level, has shown that a variable proportion of revertant fibres can be found in the majority of samples of Duchenne muscle (31). The numbers of fibres with 'normal' levels of labelling are probably too small to be encountered in the small samples taken for EM immunolabelling.

In Becker muscular dystrophy, on the other hand, dystrophin-positive fibres are frequently found. The example shown in figure 8 is particularly interesting because it is from a patient with a deletion which removes a central part of the dystrophin gene encompassing 5,106 base pairs of coding sequence, i.e. nearly half the coding information (10). This mutation results in the production of a severely truncated molecule yet the molecule is located, as shown, in the normal position at the plasma membrane. Moreover nearest neighbour measurements show that there is no reduction in the side to side spacing thus implying that the positioning is not controlled by the length of the dystrophin molecule but by another factor; perhaps the spacing of the glycoprotein complex.

Rat Muscle

We have recently been monitoring the loss and re-expression of dystrophin during the breakdown and regeneration of rat skeletal muscle following exposure of the muscle to the venom of the Australian tiger snake, *Notechis scutatus* (Vater et al, unpublished results). Normally in rat muscle, dystrophin is arranged at the plasma membrane in a way similar to, or the same as, that in man. Three to six hours after venom inoculation dystrophin begins to break down, giving a discontinuous labelling pattern, and at 12 hours it is absent from the plasma membrane. It is first seen again on Western blots three days after inoculation (approximately 24h after regeneration can be detected) but is not seen in sections until 4 days after inoculation when regeneration is well advanced (Fig 9). Experiments are now in progress to determine whether the reincorporation of dystrophin is influenced by innervation (functional reinnervation occurs at 4-5 days post inoculation) or by some other critical factor in the fibre's maturation.

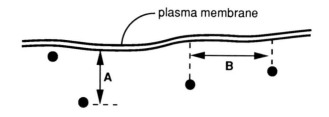

A Gold particle to cytoplasmic face of membrane

B Nearest neighbour

FIG. 4. Diagrammatic representation of the dimensions measured in constructing the histograms shown in Figs. 5 and 7 respectively.

DISCUSSION

Our work on the localization of dystrophin has involved a considerable amount of quantitative analysis, and our experience in this field - as applied to the examination of pathological tissue -is probably unique. We encountered numerous problems in the course of the work most of which are either ignored or only infrequently acknowledged in comparable literature. We address some of the more significant (see also 14).

Labelling density
The quantitative assessment of labelling at a binding site in any tissue should be based on an estimate of the density of labelling. Such estimates are, in turn, based on the assumption that all available antigenic sites are labelled selectively by the primary antibody, and that all bound primary antibody molecules in turn bind the secondary antibody. In the case of gold decorated secondary antibody, it is a further requirement that all secondary antibody molecules are decorated.

Labelling noise
If it is possible to make an accurate assessment of the number of binding sites in a tissue or tissue section, the distribution of those binding sites should be studied. This introduces a second problem - 'noise'. A typical IgG molecule is 8-10 nm in length, and so a gold particle carried on the Fc region of the secondary antibody could be between 15 and 20 nm away from the primary binding site. Thus a study of the distribution of binding sites, and particularly one involving inter particle distances must take into account the noise generated by the experimental technique.

Antibody stacking
While it is attractive to suppose that each binding site is occupied by a single primary Ab molecule, and that each primary Ab molecule is recognised by a single secondary Ab molecule decorated with a single gold particle, it is well known that clusters of up to 4 or 5 gold particles may be seen in all labelled

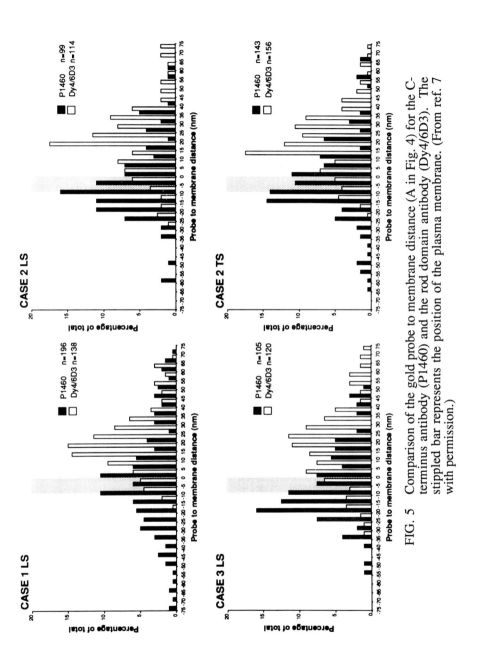

FIG. 5 Comparison of the gold probe to membrane distance (A in Fig. 4) for the C-terminus antibody (P1460) and the rod domain antibody (Dy4/6D3). The stippled bar represents the position of the plasma membrane. (From ref. 7 with permission.)

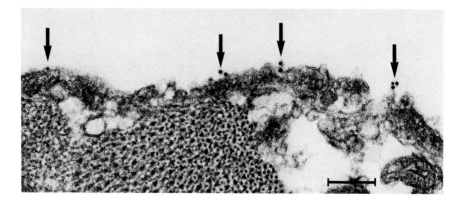

FIG. 6   Part of a muscle fibre which had been incubated with the primary antibody, Dy8/6C5, followed by a 10 nm gold conjugated secondary antibody before being resin-embedded and conventionally sectioned and stained. Some gold particles (arrows) are seen labelling the outside of the fibre. Bar = 100 nm.

sections. There are two explanations for clustering - the first is that a given Fc region of the secondary antibody may be decorated with more than one gold particle and the second that each Fc region of the primary antibody can bind up to 10 secondary IgG molecules. In practice, gold conjugation by experienced manufacturers usually ensures that >80% of labelled IgG carries a single particle, and steric hindrance limits the number of secondary IgG molecules bound to the Fc fragment of a primary IgG molecule. Nonetheless, clusters need to be interpreted with caution. It is particularly important not to be misled into believing that one particle represents one labelled antigenic molecule.

Depth of penetration
IgG molecules are large molecules of a molecular mass of approximately 150 kD. They are, however, theoretically capable of penetrating a typical ultracryosection. The limitations usually occur when the binding is to large, dense organelles such as Golgi bodies or mitochondria or in situations where cross-linking or steric hindrance due to very dense binding occurs. This does not arise in the study of the labelling of molecules of low abundance and with a limited density of binding sites.

The application of quantitative analysis to dystrophin
The analysis of the distribution of dystrophin described in this article and in detail by Cullen et al (6) avoided several of the problems identified above. Thus, the study was made on thin frozen sections so penetration was not a problem. The primary antibodies used were either monoclonal or affinity purified polyclonal antibodies, recognising defined epitopes. The secondary antibody (goat anti-mouse IgG) was labelled with 5 nm colloidal gold, and >85% of antibody molecules were decorated by a single particle. Dystrophin is, overall, of low abundance in skeletal muscle (0.01-0.02% overall; 5% of membrane related proteins) and so steric hindrance was unlikely to be a major problem in determining labelling.

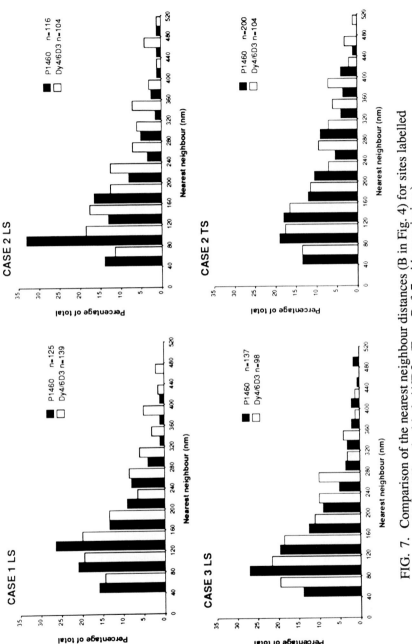

FIG. 7. Comparison of the nearest neighbour distances (B in Fig. 4) for sites labelled with P1460 and with dy4/6D3. (From Ref. 7 with permission.)

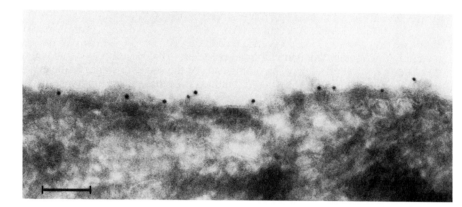

FIG. 8. Immunogold labelling of the muscle of a Becker patient lacking 5,106 base pairs of coding sequence with the C-terminus. Dy8/6C5 as primary antibody. The labelling is normal. 10 nm gold. Bar = 100 nm.

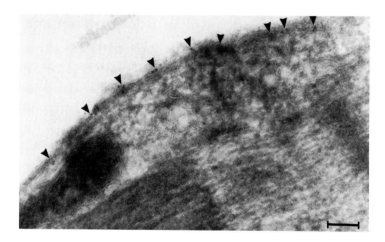

FIG. 9. Immunogold labelling (Dy4/6D3 as primary antibody) of rat soleus muscle 4 days ater snake venom inoculation, by when myofibre regeneration is under way. Gold particles (arrow heads) can be seen at the fibre periphery. 10 nm gold. Bar = 10 nm.

If we consider, now, labelling with Dy4 6D3, it will be noted that the labelling was almost entirely confined to a rim of 50 nm around the periphery of the fibres, and within that rim the distance between gold probe and plasma membrane was approximately 15 nm. It seemed reasonable to assume that dystrophin could be considered a membrane-associated protein, and we were, therefore, able to make two estimates of labelling efficiency. In the first we attempted to determine the proportion of binding sites in a fixed area of muscle membrane ultimately labelled with gold particles. This would provide us with a measure of overall efficiency, involving each of the separate stages in the entire protocol. We made the following assumptions: 1) there is no hindrance to the complete penetrance of antibody, 2) each molecule exists as a monomer and carries a single binding site, 3) dystrophin forms a regular square lattice, 4) binding sites are 125 nm apart. If the epitopes are 125 nm apart in a regular square lattice, we would expect 64 binding sites per um^2. Thus in a section 0.1 μm thick, we would expect to identify 6.4 sites per 1 um (length) of membrane. Measurements were made on sections cut from 6 different biopsies and we identified, on average, 2.1 ($\pm$ 0.3) sites per μm (6), giving an overall labelling efficiency of 33%.

The efficiency of binding of secondary (i.e. gold-labelled) antibody to primary antibody was then calculated. For this calculation we assumed: 1) that all molecules of secondary antibody were decorated with gold and 2) that any clustering of particles around a single site arose as a result of the binding of multiple copies of decorated secondary antibody by a single primary antibody molecule. This allowed us to test whether the number of sites labelled respectively with 1, 2, 3, 4 etc. gold particles formed part of a Poisson series.

Having shown that was the case (Table 1) we could calculate the number of unlabelled sites (38% of the total) and hence calculate labelling efficiency (62%). Knowing overall efficiency (35%) and the efficiency of binding of secondary to primary antibody (62%) we calculated the efficiency of binding of primary antibody to antigen (53%). This is higher than might be expected (14) and allows us to be reasonably confident that our statistical data are as good as any available.

The analysis of inter-particle distances is rather more problematic. The strict application of spatial statistics to data such as ours requires primarily that the reference points are fixed and that any one distance between reference points should not be influenced by any adjacent distance.

This criterion may be met if the binding epitope on the molecule of dystrophin is considered, but it is certainly not met measuring the distribution of gold particles in which the noise around any binding site can be as large as $\pm$ 20 nm. The fact that our measured inter-particle distances corresponded closely to the length of the dystrophin molecule appeared to justify our rather loose use of a formal statistical procedure, but it required validation using antibodies to other domains of dystrophin. This was completed by Cullen et al, (7) who have used both an affinity purified polyclonal antibody and a monoclonal antibody to the last 17 amino acids of the C-terminus. The inter-particle distance again averaged 120-125 nm.

TABLE 1.   Observed and expected distribution of gold particles assuming that the number of particles labelling a particular site formed part of a Poisson series. The correspondence between the observed and expected distribution was such that the series was confirmed and we could calculate the number of unlabelled sites (123). Since we counted 198 labelled sites, we could calculate that the efficiency of labelling was 62%.

Number of Particles	Observed Distribution	Expected Distribution
0	-	123
1	122	118
2	50	57
3	18	18
4	4	4
5	4	1

How might the quantitative analysis of dystrophin localization be improved? The most important single improvement would be to conjugate colloidal gold to the primary antibody. Provided all antibody molecules were decorated the 'noise' in the system would be halved, the precision of our methods would be greatly enhanced, and overall efficiency would be increased. A further refinement would be achieved by the application of double labelling technique, using primary antibodies to difference domains, each antibody being decorated with gold particles of a different size.

THE FUNCTION OF DYSTROPHIN

Since dystrophin was first identified, there have been numerous suggestions as to its function. The various suggestions are considered in turn.

Dystrophin is concerned with excitation/contraction coupling

Fractionation studies by Knudson et al (19) and Salviati et al (35) were interpreted as showing that dystrophin was enriched on the T-tubule at the triadic junctions of skeletal muscle. Knudson et al (1988) suggested that dystrophin might have one of two possible roles at such a location - a functional role in excitation/contraction coupling and/or a structural role in stabilising the triad. The structural role was preferred on the basis that the muscles of mdx mice and patients with Xp-21 dystrophy are quite clearly capable of excitation-contraction coupling; but this reasoning could also apply to a consideration of the structural role since there is no evidence of changes in the structure of the T-tubule in dystrophic muscle prior to necrosis (Cullen, unpublished). Salviati et al (35) were much more specific, suggesting that dystrophin preserves the crucial alignment of plasma-membrane and T-tubule with the myofibrils. In support of their argument they cited the work of Nunzi and Franzini-Armstrong (32) in which intermediate filaments were said to connect the Z-discs to the triads in amphibian muscle. Salviati et al (35) were possibly not aware that in mammalian muscle, the triad is opposite the A-I junction not the Z disc, and that no filaments have ever been seen to bind triads to the A-I junction in mammalian skeletal muscle. Moreover, during contraction, the plasma membrane is thrown into deep folds and remains closely apposed to the sarcomere only at the Z and M lines where desmin and skelemin respectively act as linking filaments (23, 34). Detailed studies on the localization of dystrophin using immunocytochemical and immunogold labelling techniques have consistently failed to confirm that dystrophin is localized to any part of the triad (see for example 3, 6) and a detailed and sophisticated biophysical study of excitation contraction coupling in the muscle fibres of the mdx-mouse by Hollingworth et al (16) identified no differences whatever between the dystrophic fibres and those of phenotypically normal littermates.

It seems, in retrospect, that the earlier fractionation studies that localised dystrophin to the triads were technically flawed in that triad junctions were contaminated by fragments of plasma membrane.

Dystrophin is involved in the regulation of Ca2+ movement

It is generally accepted that an increase in $[Ca^{2+}]_i$ is responsible for many pathological features of dystrophic muscle and for the activation of a number of proteases and phospholipases in degenerating muscle fibres (see for example 1, 5, 45). It is not clear whether the increase in $[Ca^{2+}]_i$ is necessarily primary - it may be secondary to a relatively non-specific lesion in the plasma membrane - but it has been shown that the increase in proteolytic activity in the muscles of mdx-mice is associated with the increase in $[Ca^{2+}]_i$ (Turner et al., 1988). The possibility that dystrophin directly or indirectly plays a role in stabilising the resting permeability of the muscle fibre to Ca2+ has been considered by several authors.

Fong et al (12) hypothesized that 'the underlying pathology of muscular dystrophy could involve the modulation of Ca2+ leak channels whose properties are altered by the absence of dystrophin'. They compared free resting $[Ca^{2+}]_i$ levels in cultured myotubes derived from normal human and murine muscle. At rest, $[Ca^{2+}]_i$ in human and murine myotubes was 55 nM and 82 nM respectively. Analogous values for dystrophic myotubes were 76 and 110 nM. The $[Ca^{2+}]_i$ in both human and murine dystrophic myotubes increased with increases in $[Ca^{2+}]_o$. In normal myotubes of the mouse, there was no change in $[Ca^{2+}]_i$, when $[Ca^{2+}]_o$ was increased and in normal human myotubes the increase was smaller than in dystrophic human myotubes. Thus, it appeared that $[Ca^{2+}]_i$ is poorly controlled in dystrophic cells. Fong et al (12) went on to identify a population of Ca2+ leak channels (channels that admit Ca2+ but that are unaffected by membrane potential, or mechanical stretch). If these channels were open at rest, it could result in the ingress of Ca2+ and would possibly contribute to the elevated $[Ca^{2+}]_i$. They showed that the channels continually fluctuated between an open and a closed state. Fong et al found that the mean leak-channel open times in normal and dystrophic myotubes were similar but that the time the channels were closed in mdx- and human dystrophic myotubes, was approximately 1/3rd of that of normal muscle. The authors argued that the increase in the probability that the channels were open, would be sufficient to ensure that $[Ca^{2+}]_i$ remained elevated. Fong et al (12) did not explain how the absence of dystrophin altered the function of the Ca2+ leak channels. Curiously, the dystrophin-deficient myoblasts of both mdx and human dystrophic muscle behaved in a manner indistinguishable from normal.

At about the same time as Fong et al were working on the Ca^{2+} leak channels, Franco and Lansman (13) reported that single channel recordings from normal myotubes in culture were dominated by Ca^{2+} channels that are normally closed at rest but that are opened when the membrane is stretched. In myotubes derived from mdx muscle, similar Ca^{2+} channels were predominant, but there appeared a second population of channels that were opened at rest and that closed when the membrane was stretched. It was suggested that these latter channels could act as a pathway for Ca^{2+} to enter the cell under resting conditions. Franco and Lansman (13) suggested that one explanation of their results was that dystrophin was normally bound to the stretch inactivated channels and balanced a stretching force maintained by resting membrane tension. In dystrophin deficiency, the resting membrane tension was sufficient to keep the channels in the open state allowing the continuing influx of Ca^{2+}.

It is not clear whether the Ca^{2+} channels identified by Franco and Lansman (13) and Fong et al (12) are the same or whether they represent two different populations; in some ways it is irrelevant to the underlying reasoning that both groups identified Ca^{2+} channels that are open at rest and that could cause the elevation of $[Ca^{2+}]_i$.

The questions that arise are firstly how is the behaviour of Ca^{2+} channels affected by the absence of dystrophin - for which there is no satisfactory answer - and could the elevated $[Ca^{2+}]_i$, calculated to be only 2-3 times above resting levels, activate the proteolytic enzymes and result in muscle fibre breakdown?

The obvious candidate enzymes are the calpains - calcium activated neutral proteases present in the majority of cells. They have been shown in laboratory exercises to hydrolyse a number of cytoskeletal and other proteins and have often been considered to be crucially important in cellular pathology. Typically two forms of calpains co-exist - calpain I, activated by Ca^{2+} in the μM range and calpain II activated by Ca^{2+} in the mM range. The enzymes are dimers, and the first stage of activation appears to be the Ca^{2+}-dependent autolysis of one subunit of the dimer. The 'liberated' subunit is activated in turn by lower Ca^{2+} concentrations (typically 10 - 20x lower than that required for autolysis). The activity of the enzymes can be further enhanced by the presence of a number of other agents such as phospholipids, and their close association with internal cell membranes may be of physiological significance. The autolysed forms of the calpains are not normally present in cells (9) and the enzymes are so closely regulated that it is not clear whether they could be activated by $[Ca^{2+}]_i$ in the range of 100 nm. There is a related problem. Turner et al (40) measured protein degradation in terms of tyrosine release. The calpains break down large proteins to rather large polypeptides. Other enzymes continue the process to release single amino acids. The enzymes have not been formally identified in terms of cellular pathology. If, then, the activation of Ca^{2+} channels in dystrophic muscles does result in $[Ca^{2+}]_i$ levels reaching levels of only 100 nm or thereabouts, it is reasonable to ask which enzymes are activated and what are their substrates. There is, as yet, no answer to these questions.

Dystrophin confers flexibility and stability on the plasma membrane

Dystrophin is believed to form a lattice on the internal face of the plasma membrane. The precise form of the lattice and whether it consists of dystrophin molecules arranged as monomers or dimers is not clear (6, 20). It is a common working hypothesis (derived from an analogy with spectrin and -actinin) that the molecule is inherently flexible (20), that the C-terminus is bound tightly to the plasma membrane by intrinsic glycoproteins (2, 7) and that the amino terminus is attached to other cytoskeletal proteins.

This hypothesis has given rise in turn to several suggestions that the lack of dystrophin would remove an element that was important in conferring both flexibility and protection against overstretching to the plasma membrane. To test this, Menke and Jockusch (27) used hypo-osmotic shock to determine stress-resistance in cultured myotubes and intact muscle fibres of the mdx-mouse. The muscle fibres and myotubes of mdx-mice appeared to be more easily damaged by osmotic shock than those of normal mice. For example, 50% of normal fibres were destroyed by exposure for 10 min to about 105 mOsm, whereas 50% of mdx-fibres were destroyed by exposure to 130 mOsm. This is however a modest difference against a normal extracellular osmolarity of 300 - 320 mOsm.

Weller et al (44) tried to determine whether the muscle fibres of mdx-mice were more susceptible than normal to damage caused by eccentric contractions. Although mdx-muscles contained more necrotic fibres than normal both at rest and after the imposition of the contractions, the increase in the number of necrotic fibres after the imposition of a series of eccentric contractions was 12-fold in normal muscles and only 4-fold in dystrophic muscles. The authors' claim therefore, that 'dystrophin-deficient mdx-muscle fibres are particularly vulnerable to eccentric contractions' seems exaggerated.

Franco and Lansman (13) applied suction pressure via micro-electrodes to normal and mdx-myotubes. They detected no differences at all in the pressure needed to rupture the cell membrane.

In summary, it would appear that if the absence of dystrophin does make plasma-membranes more susceptible to stress-induced damage the differences are marginal at best. It is difficult to believe that those differences that have been identified are of significance to the overall pathogenesis of X-linked muscular dystrophy.

A particular variant of the suggestion that dystrophin confers both flexibility and strengthening on the plasma membrane is that it is intimately involved with the binding of actin filaments to plasma membrane at the myotendinous junction. The myotendinous junction is highly folded, and the thin filaments are formed into bundles as they approach the junction. These features allow the generation of considerable force over the plasma membrane at this region. Dystrophin is heavily concentrated at the myotendinous junction (36). In murine dystrophin-deficient muscle, the folding is reduced and there is a deficiency in the lateral association between thin filaments (39). It has been speculated that dystrophin is associated with the bundling of the thin filaments and their attachment to the folds of the myotendinous junction. The loss of dystrophin, it is argued, would lead to weakening of the structure and the inability of the junction to bear the force of muscular contractions. There is no experimental evidence for or against this hypothesis but it is worthy of note that the muscles of mdx-mice may actually be more powerful than controls (8).

Miscellaneous

Various other suggestions of a role for dystrophin have been made, but none, in our opinion, are yet convincing. They include, for example, the suggestion that dystrophin may link plasma membrane to basal lamina (3); that dystrophin is involved in the interaction between the cytoskeleton and the extracellular matrix (22); and that dystrophin is involved with the stabilisation of junctional receptors (24).

At present, it can be safely said that there are almost as many views on the role of dystrophin as there are investigators searching for a role. We doubt that the role will be determined until we know exactly how dystrophin and its related proteins are organised within the cell, how its expression is regulated and how some cells survive without dystrophin while others degenerate rapidly and apparently irreversibly.

ACKNOWLEDGEMENTS

We acknowledge our principal collaborator Dr. L. V. B. Nicholson, Mrs. R. Vater, Mrs. C. Young, Mr. J. Fulthorpe and Mr. J. Walsh and those who have generously provided antibodies. The work was supported by the MDGGB, MRC, Wellcome Trust, the University of Newcastle Research Committee and Newcastle Health Authority. We thank Carol Atkinson for secretarial assistance.

REFERENCES

1. Bodensteiner, J.B., Engel, A.G. (1978): Intracellular calcium accumulation in Duchenne dystrophy and other myopathies: a study of 567,000 fibers in 114 biopsies. *Neurology* (Minneapolis), 28:439-446.

2. Campbell, K.P., Kahl, S.D. (1989): Association of dystrophin and an integral membrane glycoprotein. *Nature* (Lond.), 338:259-262.

3. Carpenter, S., Karpati, G., Zubrzycka-Gaarn, E., Bulman, D.E., Ray, P.N., Worton, R.G. (1990): Dystrophin is localised to the plasma membrane of human skeletal muscle fibres by electron-microscopic cytochemical study. *Muscle and Nerve*, 13:376-380.

4. Cross, R.A., Stewart, M., Kendrick-Jones, J. (1990): Structural predictions for the central domain of dystrophin. *FEBS Lett.*, 262:87-92.

5. Cullen, M.J., Fulthorpe, M.J. (1975): Stages in fibre breakdown in Duchenne muscular dystrophy. An electron microscopic study. *J. Neurol. Sci.*, 24:179-200.

6. Cullen, M.J., Walsh, J., Nicholson, L.V.B., Harris, J.B. (1990): Ultrastructural localization of dystrophin in human muscle by gold immunolabelling. *Proc. Roy. Soc., B.* 240:197-210.

7. Cullen, M.J., Walsh, J., Nicholson, L.V.B., Harris, J.B., Zubrzycka-Gaarn, E.E., Ray, P.N., Worton, R.G. (1991): Immunogold labelling of dystrophin in human muscle, using an antibody to the last 17 amino acids of the C-terminus. *Neuromusc. Dis.,* (in press).

8. Dangain, J., Vrbova, G. (1984): Muscle development in mdx mutant mice. *Muscle and Nerve*, 7:700-704.

9. Edmunds, T., Nagainis, P.A., Sathe, S.K., Thompson, V.F., Goll, D.E. (1991): Comparison of the autolyzed and unautolyzed forms of μ- and m-calpain from bovine skeletal muscle. *Biochim. Biophys. Acta.*, 1077:197-208.

10. England, S.B., Nicholson, L.V.B., Johnson, M.A., Forrest, S.M., Love, D.R., Zubrzycka-Gaarn, E.E., Bulman, D.E., Harris, J.B., Davies, K.E. (1990): Very mild muscular dystrophy associated with the deletion of 46% of dystrophin. *Nature* (Lond.), 343:180-182.

11. Ervasti, J.M., Ohlendieck, K., Kahl, S.D., Gaver, M.G., Campbell, K.P. (1990): Deficiency of a glycoprotein component of the dystrophin complex

12. Fong, P., Turner, P.R., Denetclaw, W.F., Steinhardt, R.A. (1990): Increased activity of calcium leak channels in myotubes of Duchenne human and mdx mouse origin. *Science*, 250:673-676.
13. Franco, A., Lansman, J.B., (1990): Calcium entry through stretch-inactivated ion channels in mdx myotubes. *Nature* (Lond.), 344:670-673.
14. Griffiths, G., Hoppeler, H. (1986): Quantitation in immuno-cytochemistry:correlation of immunogold labelling to absolute number of membrane antigens. *J. Histochem. Cytochem.*, 34:1389-1398.
15. Hainfield, J.F., (1987): A small gold-conjugated antibody label: improved resolution for electron microscopy. *Science*, 236:450-453.
16. Hollingworth, S., Marshall, M.W., Robson, E. (1990): Excitation-contraction coupling in normal and mdx mice. *Muscle and Nerve*, 13:16-20.
17. Jackson, M.J., Brooke, M.H., Kaiser, B.S., Edwards, R.H.T. (1991): Creatine kinase and prostaglandin E_2 *Neurology*, 41:101-104.
18. Jasmin, B.J., Cartaud, A., Ludosky, M.A., Changeux, J.P., Cartand, J. (1990): Asymmetric distribution of dystrophin in developing and adult *Torpedo marmorata* electrocyte: evidence for its association with the acetylcholine receptor-rich membrane. *Proc. Natl. Acad. Sci. U.S.A.*, 87:3938-3941.
19. Knudson, C.M., Hoffman, E.P., Kahl, S.d., Kunkel, M., Campbell, K.P. (1988): Characterization of dystrophin in skeletal muscle triads. *J. Biol. Chem.* 263:8480-8484.
20. Koenig, M., Kunkel, L.M. (1990): Detailed analysis of the repeat domain of dystrophin reveals four potential hinge segments that may confer flexibility. *J. Biol. Chem.*, 265:4560-4566.
21. Koenig, M., Monaco, A.P., Kunkel, L.M. (1988): The complete sequence of dystrophin predicts a rod shaped cytoskeletal protein. *Cell*, 53:219-228.
22. Kramarcy, N.R., Sealock, R. (1990): Dystrophin as a focal adhesion protein: Colocalization with talin and the $M_r48,000$ sarcolemmal protein in cultured Xenopus muscle. *FEBS Letters*, 274:171-174.
23. Lazarides, E. (1980): Intermediate filaments as mechanical integrators of cellular space. *Nature* (Lond.), 283:249-256.
24. Lidov, H.G.W., Byers, T.J., Watkins, S.C., Kunkel, L.M. (1990): Localization of dystrophin to post-synaptic regions of central nervous system cortical neurons. *Nature* (Lond): 348:725-728.
25. Love, D.R., Hill, D.F., Dickson, G., Spurr, N.K., Byth, B.c., Marsden, R.F., Walsh, F.S., Edwards, Y.H., Davies, K.E. (1989): An autosomal transcript in skeletal muscle with homology to dystrophin. *Nature* (Lond.), 339:55-58.
26. Meng, G., Kress, W., Scherpf, S., Bettecken, T., Feichtinger, W., Schempp, W., Schmid, M., Muller, C.R. (1981): A comparison of the dystrophin gene structure in primate and lower vertebrates. In: *Muscular Dystrophy Research: From Molecular Diagnosis Toward Therapy.* edited by C. Angelini, G. A. Danieli, and D. Fontanari. pp. 23-30, Excerpta Medica, Amsterdam.
27. Menke, A., Jockusch, H. (1991): Decreased osmotic stability of dystrophin-less muscle cells from the mdx mouse. *Nature* (Lond.), 349:69-71.
28. Miyatake, M., Miike, T., Zhao, J.-E., Yoshioka, K., Uchino, M., Usuku, G. (1991): Dystrophin: localization and presumed function. *Muscle and Nerve,* 14:113-119.
29. Murayama, T., Sato, O., Kimura, S., Shimizu, T., Sawada, H.,

Maruyama, K. (1990): Molecular shape of dystrophin purified from rabbit skeletal muscle myofibrils. *Proc. Jap. Acad.*, 66:96-99.

30. Nicholson, L.V.B., Davison, K., Falkous, G., Harwood, C., O'Donnell, E., Slater, C.R., Harris, J.B. (1989a): Dystrophin in skeletal muscle. I. Western blot analysis using a monoclonal antibody. *J. Neurol. Sci.*, 94:125-136.

31. Nicholson, L.V.B., Davison, K., Johnson, M.A., Slater, C.R., Young, C., Bhattacharya, S., Gardner-Medwin, D., Harris, J.B. (1989b): Dystrophin in skeletal muscle II. Immunoreactivity in patients with Xp21 muscular dystrophy. *J. Neurol. Sci.*, 94:137-146.

32. Nunzi, M.G., Franzini-Armstrong, C. (1980): Trabecular network in adult skeletal muscle. *J. Ultrastruct. Res.* 73:21-26.

33. Pons, F., Angier, N., Heilig, R., Leger, J., Mornet, D., Leger, J.J. (1990): Purification of dystrophin and visualization by rotary-shadowing in electron microscopy, and deletion detection using domain-specific antibodies. *Proc. Nat. Acad. Sci. U.S.A.*, 87:7851-7855.

34. Price, M.G. (1987): Skelemins: cytoskeletal proteins located at the periphery of M-discs in mammalian striated muscle. *J. Cell. Biol.*, 104:1325-1336.

35. Salviati, G., Betto, R., Ceoldo, S., Biasia, E., Bonilla, E., Miranda, A.F., Di Mauro, S. (1989): Cell fractionation studies indicate that dystrophin is a protein of surface membranes of skeletal muscle. *Biochem. J.*, 258:837-841.

36. Samitt, C.E., Bonilla, E. (1990): Immunocytochemical study of dystrophin at the myotendinous junction. *Muscle and Nerve*, 13:493-500.

37. Sealock, R., Butler, M.H., Kramarcy, N.R., Gao, K.X., Murnane, A.A., Donville, K., and Froehner, S.C. (1991): *J. Cell Biol.*, 113:1133-1144.

38. Shoeman, R.L., Traub, P. (1990): Calpains and the cytoskeleton. In: *Intracellular Calcium-Dependent Proteolysis.* Edited by R. L. Mellgren and T. Murachi. pp. 191-224. CRC Press, Boca Raton, Florida.

39. Tidball, J.G., Law, D.J. (1991): Dystrophin is required for normal thin filament-membrane associations at myotendinous junctions. *Amer. J. Pathol.*, 138:17-21.

40. Turner, P.R., Westwood, T., Regen, C.M., Steinhardt, R.A. (1988): Increased protein degradation results from elevated free calcium levels found in muscles from mdx mice. *Nature* (Lond.). 335:735-738.

41. Walton, J.N., Gardner-Medwin, D. (1988): The muscular dystrophies. In: *Disorders of Voluntary Muscle.* edited by J. N. Walton. pp. 519-568. Churchill Livingstone, Edinburgh.

42. Watkins, S.C., Hoffman, E.P., Slayter, H.S., Kunkel, L.M. (1988): Immunoelectron microscopic localization of dystrophin in myofibres. *Nature,* 333:863-866.

43. Webster, C., Blau, H.M. (1990): Accelerated age-related decline in replicative life-span of Duchenne muscular dystrophy myoblasts: implications for cell and gene therapy. *Som. Cell. Molec. Gen.*, 16:557-565.

44. Weller, B., Karpati, G., Carpenter, S. (1990): Dystrophin-deficient mdx muscle fibres are preferentially vulnerable to necrosis induced by experimental lengthening contractions. *J. Neurol. Sci.*, 100:9-13.

45. Wrogemann, K., Penna, S.D.J. (1976): Mitochondrial calcium overload: A general mechanism for cell-necrosis in muscle disease. *Lancet i*, 672-674.

DUCHENNE MUSCULAR DYSTROPHY: Animal Models
and Genetic Manipulation, edited by Byron A. Kakulas,
John McC. Howell, and Allen D. Roses.
Raven Press, Ltd., New York © 1992.

4

Normal and Abnormal Dystrophin Gene Expression

Richard J. Bartlett*#, Nicholas J.H. Sharp*#,
Joe N. Kornegay#, Allen D. Roses*

*Department of Medicine, Division of Neurology,
Duke University Medical Center,
Durham, N.C. 27710, USA
#Department of Companion Animals and Special Species,
College of Veterinary Medicine,
North Carolina State University,
Raleigh, N.C. 27606

The genes associated with Duchenne and Becker muscular dystrophy are inherited mutations in a normal gene which codes for a protein termed dystrophin. Application of the techniques of molecular biology to the study of the genes which cause Duchenne and Becker muscular dystrophy have produced an explosive increase in our understanding of the normal and abnormal expression of the dystrophin gene. Herein is a brief chronicle of some of the discoveries which have led to our current level of understanding and how the use of these discoveries has been applied to the study of the canine dystrophin gene in golden retriever muscular dystrophy. The delineation of the defect in golden retriever muscular dystrophy (see Sharp et al, this volume) confirms the homology of this defect with DMD and underscores the value of this model for studies of potential therapy.

The discovery of the gene that is affected in DMD was hailed as a triumph of "reverse" genetics (103). In "traditional" or "forward" genetics, the gene product is known before investigators begin to seek the gene. Hemoglobin is a good example, the gene being discovered following the use of relatively straightforward recombinant DNA techniques. It is more difficult to identify the gene if the gene product is unknown. The first gene discovered using reverse genetics was that belonging to the rare disorder, chronic granulomatous disease (104). Even then the gene product turned out to be a recognized protein, a component of cytochrome C in granulocytes.

The discovery of the DMD gene proved the theory of Botstein et al (19) that it would be possible to find a disease gene whose product was previously unknown, by using nucleic acid markers known as restriction fragment length polymorphisms (RFLP's). These are variations in the DNA of individuals that can be identified after the DNA is fragmented by the action of restriction endonuclease enzymes. These differences are identified by electrophoresis and can sometimes be linked to chromosomal loci for a particular disease. Botstein et al (19) also designed a scheme for isolation of random DNA probes, whereby human genomic DNA fragments were cloned and selected against repetitive DNA sequences in order to isolate unique fragments representing the entire genome.

In 1983, a group at St. Mary's Hospital in London found flanking markers, for the DMD gene located within the proximal half of Xp (41). The use of these probes also showed that BMD mutations map to the same region of the X-chromosome as DMD (63). This work using RFLP's was in agreement with the results of cytogenetic analysis of a series of young girls with muscle disease who also possessed balanced X:autosomal translocations. The exchange point was shown to consistently reside on the short arm of the X-chromosome at a locus designated Xp21. There have been more than 20 examples reported in the literature (103). The final evidence to support this potential localization of the DMD locus was the presence of microscopic deletions in some DMD boys with complex phenotypes. The first such patient had five different X-linked conditions including DMD, chronic granulomatous disease, retinitis pigmentosa, the McLeod syndrome, and mental retardation (53). High resolution cytogenetic analysis of DNA from a similar patient mapped the locus to within sub-bands Xp21.2-Xp21.3 (14).

The DMD patient described by Francke et al (53), also known as patient BB, played a crucial role in further defining the DMD gene. Kunkel et al (74) used a method (phenol enhanced reassociation technique or PERT) to enrich for DNA sequences that lay within the deleted region of this patient. The method involved the hybridization of sheared DNA from the BB patient with trace amounts of restriction-enzyme digested DNA from a male with four X-chromosomes. The conditions of annealing were such as to enhance the reassociation of unique sequences. Seven clones were isolated, which mapped within the BB deletion. Only one clone of 200 bp, called pERT87, was a candidate for the DMD locus because it failed to hybridize in five of 57 unrelated DMD males (84). One of the five also had a brother with the same deletion. Analysis of this pedigree demonstrated that the DMD deletion had been inherited from the maternal great grandmother, to the mother of the affected boy (9).

A second, independent approach was used to isolate sequences within the DMD locus by isolating a DNA fragment from a female with DMD that had a balanced X:21 translocation (112). The site of the translocation in the autosome was found to be within genes encoding for ribosomal RNA (122). The identification of ribosomal DNA sequences on both translocation-derived chromosomes led to the isolation of an 11 kb DNA fragment, XJ1, which contained the translocation junction from the X-derived chromosome (100).

Bi-directional chromosomal walks expanded the loci identified by each method and led to the joining of the DXS164 (pERT87) and DXS206 (XJ1) loci to give approximately 380 kb of contiguous genomic DNA (84). Subclones were then used to analyze the DNA of DMD and BMD patients. A pattern of non-overlapping deletions were found in these patients, extending in both directions. The chromosomal loci identified also failed to segregate with the DMD/BMD mutations in approximately 5% of meioses (75,85). These two observations suggested that the gene itself was very large. This was in agreement with the large cytogenetic heterogeneity of chromosomal breakpoints in DMD females with translocations, which implied that the DMD locus might be as large as 3-4 Mb (20). A macro-restriction map of the DMD region suggested that the gene region was in the 2-3 million base-pair range (24,111). By using DNA fragments containing the breakpoints of four large deletions originating in the DXS164 locus, sequences were obtained from regions proximal and distal to this locus (24,86,87). Studies with these cloned sequences have supported the conclusion that the DMD locus is 2.3 Mb in length.

The next step was to isolate the complete DMD cDNA. Monaco et al (85) screened subclones of DSX164 for cross-species homology, on the assumption that any expressed sequences within this region would be conserved. One such conserved clone, called pERT87-25, identified a transcript of 16 kb in a Northern blot of human fetal skeletal muscle RNA. Burghes et al (23) also identified a 16 kb transcript in adult skeletal muscle using fragments from the DXS206 locus. The DMD transcript was eventually characterized as being 14 kb in length, formed by a minimum of 60 exons, and gave a deduced mean size for exons as 200 bp and introns as 35 kb (64).

The full length cDNA allowed for a considerable improvement in the ability to diagnose and characterize defects in patients with DMD and BMD. In 1986, Kunkel et al (75) reported that 6.5% of DMD or Becker patients showed deletions at the DXS164 locus. The frequency increased to 11-17% when probes in the DXS206 locus were also used (43). The use of further genomic probes detected rearrangements in 38% of patients (10), and together with field inversion gel electrophoresis (FIGET) and subsequent Southern analysis, up to 50% of DMD patients could be defined (43). The use of genomic probes may detect occasional individuals who demonstrate deletions, presumably to intronic DNA alone, yet do not show any clinical signs of DMD (11,67). This suggested that the diagnostic accuracy in prenatal screening of fetuses using such intronic probes might not be 100%. Diagnostic accuracy should be higher using cDNA probes, but one normal male was identified in this manner having inherited deletion of one exon within the DMD gene (94). By using cDNA probes covering the whole DMD locus, it has been possible to detect deletions in 67% of DMD/BMD patients (52,116). Duplications have also been detected at a low frequency (2,61), but the basis of the other one third of mutations (10,64,66,115,116) is unknown. There is no correlation between the size of deletion and the resultant phenotype (42,48), although deletion prone regions of the DMD gene have been identified.

Two deletion prone regions, corresponding to cDNA probe 2a (approximate location between nucleotides 400-1200 of the DMD cDNA) and probes 7 and 8 (nucleotides 6400-7800) have now been confirmed by several independent groups (16,34,64,116). The majority of these deletions are clustered in the region identified by probes 7 and 8. Combined use of probes from these two areas detects from 86-99% of deletion mutations (16,34,64). This has had considerable impact on the development of screening strategies for pre-natal diagnosis (80,116). A recent technique proposed for diagnosis of DMD/BMD is multiplex PCR amplification of genomic DNA (30). An alternative approach is PCR amplification of first strand cDNA generated from mRNA of muscle (51, and see Sharp et al, this volume), which can detect deletions in up to 98% of DMD patients (15).

This deletion prone region corresponding to probes 7 and 8 is defined by a single intron of approximately 170 kb and the deletion end-points within this region have now been mapped for over 200 patients (16). The distal 80 kb of this intron has been cloned in contiguous cosmids, mapped with HindIII, and has been used to screen HindIII digests of patient DNA to detect the extent of the deletions for each of the patients. Analysis of the proportion of deletion end=points and fragment size suggested that there was no difference between the observed and expected values for this intron (16). Despite repeated attempts, the proximal 90 kb of this intron resisted cloning in contiguous cosmids (16). This, coupled with the origin of the original P20 probe (43), a spontaneous deletion in a cosmid during propagation, suggested that this region of the genome was unstable in bacteria and human chromosomes.

The complete sequence for the DMD transcript was reported by Koenig et al (65). It contained a single open reading frame (ORF) of approximately 11 kb, the deduced amino acid sequence of which predicted a protein of 3685 residues with a relative molecular mass of 427 kD. Smaller molecular weights of 360 kD (25) and 400 kD (57) were suggested by Western analysis. This discrepancy is related in part to the difficulty in accurately estimating the size of extremely large protein molecules (90).

The protein product of the DMD gene was termed dystrophin and on the basis of homology to previously recognized proteins, it could be divided into four distinct domains (65). The amino-terminal 240 residues showed similarity to the highly conserved actin binding domain of alpha-actinin, suggesting that dystrophin may interact with the actin filaments in myofibers. A large domain of 26 spectrin-like repeats, each repeat being 88-126 residues long and organized in tandem, was predicted to give dystrophin a rod-shaped structure having a length of 125 nm. The repeat domain was followed by a cysteine-rich domain of 165 residues that was similar to the carboxy-terminal domain of Dictyostelium discoideum alpha-actinin, with 24% identity over 142 aligned amino acids. This region contains two potential calcium binding sites (93), although it does not appear that dystrophin is involved in calcium trafficing (58). The fourth, carboxy-terminal domain comprised 420 residues that do not exhibit any significant similarity to other published sequences (65).

During the initial stages of the search for the DMD gene, it had been ascertained that there was at least 90% homology between the human and mouse cDNA's (55,57,64). Polyclonal antibodies were raised against fusion proteins encoded by two distinct regions of the mouse CDNA (57). Both antibodies recognized a protein of approximately 400 kD in normal human and mouse skeletal and cardiac muscle (57). The abundance of dystrophin was estimated to be approximately 0.002% of total skeletal muscle protein, which correlated well with the abundance of its mRNA (32,52,55). It has subsequently been shown that dystrophin makes up 2% of the total protein in rabbit sarcolemma (96).

Initial studies by subcellular fractionation suggested that dystrophin was associated with the triad region (56), but subsequent immunohistochemical evaluation disproved this and showed dystrophin to be localized in subsarcolemmal regions (4,17,117,123). Immunoreactivity was absent in DMD patients using the same techniques. Female carriers of the gene for DMD showed normal, mosaic and dystrophin deficient fibers (5). The proportion of deficient fibers was found to be higher (18-32%) in manifesting carriers than in asymptomatic carriers, where the proportion of deficient fibers was 0-4.3% (18).

Immuno-gold electron microscopy confirmed the major distribution of dystrophin to be on the cytoplasmic face of the sarcolemma (117). This work was subsequently extended using a monoclonal antibody directed to the rod portion of dystrophin. Labelling was confined to a narrow 75 nm rim at the periphery of myofibers. The distance between the gold probe and the cytoplasmic face of the plasma membrane was approximately 15 nm, and the distance between the gold probes (nearest neighbor in a plane parallel with the plasma membrane) was approximately 120 nm, which is in close agreement with the predicted size of dystrophin. These observations suggested that the rod portion of the dystrophin molecule is normally arranged close to the cytoplasmic face of the membrane and that molecules form an interconnecting network (38).

The precise function of dystrophin is not known, but the predicted homologies and localization suggest that it may exist as an antiparallel homodimer (60), linked in some manner to form a subsarcolemmal lattice. The amino-terminal domain of dystrophin probably interacts with myofibrillar actin filaments (80). This assertion is supported by the finding of increased binding of anti-dystrophin antibody at the myotendinous junction, where it is proposed that dystrophin is one of the components linking terminal actin filaments to the subplasmalemmal surface of the junctional folds of the myotendon (105). It has been speculated that the carboxy-terminus may mediate attachment to membranes (80).

Dystrophin has also been shown to exist in a large oligomeric complex with four glycoproteins, at least one of which is an integral membrane protein (25). One of these glycoproteins is also markedly deficient in DMD patients and in dystrophin deficient mdx mice. It has been suggested that absence of dystrophin may lead to a loss of dystrophin-associated glycoprotein, and the reduction in this glycoprotein may be one of the first stages of the molecular pathogenesis of muscular dystrophy (49).

Overall it seems likely that dystrophin functions as a cytoskeletal protein that maintains the mechanical stability of the sarcolemma so that it can withstand the normal strains imposed by the contraction-relaxation cycle (29,105). Support for this theory has been provided by Mencke and Jockusch (82), who showed a decrease in osmotic stability of mdx mouse muscle, compared to normal mouse muscle. This proposed function is also in agreement with the long held view that there was a biochemical abnormality of cell membranes in DMD (102) and by the finding of sarcolemma defects, or so called delta lesions, in DMD myofibers (83).

A number of potential models could be proposed for the putative structure of a complex between dystrophin and the membrane bound glycoprotein complex that has been described by Campbell and Kahl (25). One suggestion (M. Koenig, personal communication) was that of a simple hexagonal array derived from an assembledge of anti-parallel dystrophin diamers (See Figures 1 and 2). Examination of this model in more detail suggests that these structures would have the capacity to flex with the membrane as indicated (Figures 3 and 4). Two different square arrays have been presented elsewhere in this volume (See Harris et al and Klamut et al, this volume). Finally, the structure in Figure 5 would combine both a hexagonal and rectangular arrays to produce a structure with some interesting periodicities for the membrane bound glycoprotein complex which binds to dystrophin (25). Each of these different geometries will lend themselves to proper testing when enough useful mono-specific, monoclonal antibodies (90, and see Harris et al, and Sugita et al, this volume) are available.

The distribution of dystrophin in tissue is restricted to muscle and brain. The very small amounts of dystrophin detected in other tissues may correlate with the myogenic cell population as represented by smooth muscle cells of associated vascular tissue (59). Dystrophin in the brain appears to be produced predominantly by neurons (8,59). This has led to speculation that the mental retardation found in 30% of DMD boys is causally related to dystrophin deficiency. Given the variable penetrance and nonprogressive nature of mental

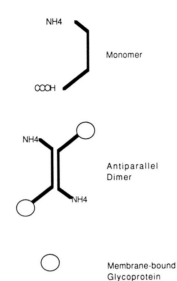

FIG. 1.   Theoretical dystrophin monomer and dimer configurations.

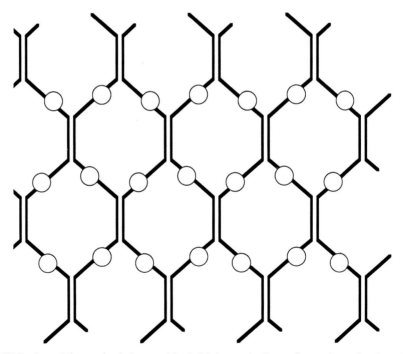

FIG. 2.   Theoretical dystrophin "chicken-wire" configuration of relaxed
           muscle.

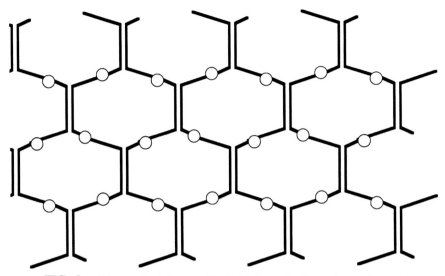

FIG. 3.   Theoretical dystrophin "chicken-wire" configuration of contracted muscle.

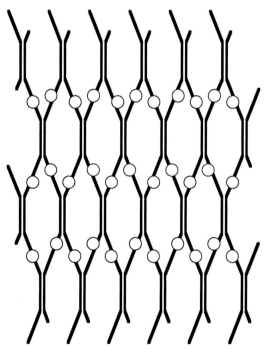

FIG. 4.   Theoretical dystrophin "chicken-wire" configuration of extended muscle.

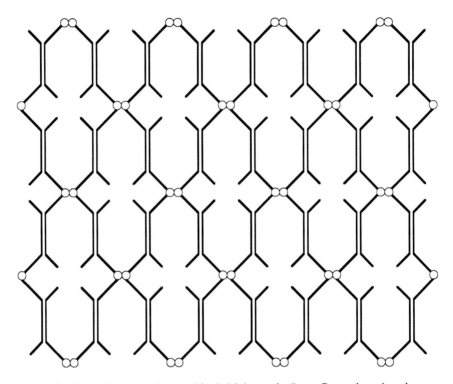

FIG. 5.   Alternate dystrophin "chicken-wire" configuration showing
mixed hexagonal and square lattice structures.

retardation in DMD, neurons must be relatively insensitive to the effects of dystrophin deficiency. An alternative hypothesis is that mild defects of the vascular smooth muscle cells may result in vascular insufficiency to the fetal brain (59). More recently, discrete localization of dystrophin has been demonstrated in Purkinje cells of the cerebellum and in some populations of pyramidal neurons in the cerebral cortex. The dystrophin appeared to be restricted to specialized regions of the post-synaptic membrane of these cells (78). It was speculated that the finding of dystrophin in the cerebellum might relate to the mild ataxia and tremor reported in some mdx mice (20). A dystrophin-like protein has also been demonstrated at the neuromuscular junction of muscle from both normal humans and DMD patients (50). This protein may be the same as that termed Dystrophin-related Protein (DRP), which has the same size and relative abundance as dystrophin but is found in DMD muscle as well as in a wide range of other tissues (62).

There does not appear to be a specific association of dystrophin with any particular type of skeletal muscle fiber (59), although type IIB (fast, glycolytic) myofibers may be more sensitive to the effects of dystrophin deficiency than other fibers (118). Dystrophin in skeletal muscle normally resolves as a doublet by Western blotting, with a prominent high molecular weight form and a much less abundant, slightly smaller additional form. The smaller form was originally thought to co-migrate with the smooth muscle isoform of dystrophin, and it was suggested that it may represent dystrophin produced by vascular tissue (59). More recent evidence has shown that the lower band does not, in fact, co-migrate with the smooth muscle isoform of dystrophin (90). There is an apparent transition in size from the largest skeletal muscle isoform, through that found in the smooth muscle of visceral and sexual organs to that of vascular smooth muscle. The species found in brain is also slightly smaller than the larger band of skeletal muscle (90). This work is in agreement with the demonstration of alternate splicing of dystrophin mRNA that produces distinct transcripts in brain (32,51,95), smooth muscle (32,51), and embryonic skeletal muscle (44), all of which are smaller than the original adult skeletal muscle isoform. A 6.5 kb mRNA is also found in a number of tissues, in equal abundance to the 14 kb dystrophin transcript. It shares the same 3' untranslated region, cysteine-rich and carboxy-terminal domains as dystrophin, but lacks the amino-terminal and spectrin-repeat domains (7).

One tremendous advantage of the ability to demonstrate dystrophin on Western blot analysis of skeletal muscle is that diagnosis of DMD can be performed very early in the course of the disease, before clinical manifestations of myopathy are evident. A small muscle biopsy is able to reveal the typical absence of dystrophin in DMD patients. In addition, it has been found that BMD patients also show abnormalities of dystrophin on immunoblot, usually relating to an altered molecular weight and/or decreased abundance of this protein (58,60,92). Although a faint pattern of minor dystrophin bands is also found on Western analysis of normal skeletal muscle, the dystrophin bands seen in BMD patients appear distinct from these minor bands in normal muscle. These bands are likely to represent partially functional proteins, and are not thought to be degradation products of dystrophin. Rather, they may be either less abundant isoforms of dystrophin, or synthetic intermediates which accumulate during pauses at precise points during translation of this huge protein (33,90,91).

The apparent correlation between the clinical and dystrophin phenotypes has also been confirmed at the genomic DNA level. In a selection of DMD and BMD patients, deletions in the DMD patients were shown to produce a frameshift in the reading frames of the mRNA, with stop codons immediately downstream of the deletion end-points in the cDNA sequences. The predicted premature termination of translation was thought to result in severely truncated dystrophin molecules. In contrast to the situation in DMD patients, BMD patients were shown to maintain an open reading frame across the deletion such that a low molecular weight dystrophin would be expected to be produced (88). The hypothesis that disruption of an ORF correlates with the DMD phenotype, whereas preservation of the ORF correlates with BMD seems to hold true in general, and is in agreement with the results of dystrophin analysis by Western blot in these conditions (58). There are, however, important exceptions to this reading frame hypothesis, which are of particular relevance to GRMD and will be discussed later (33,66,81,91).

Of the several characterized, and potential, animal models for dystrophin deficiency now known, the best described is the mdx mouse (20). The mdx mouse lacks dystrophin protein and shows levels of its transcript some 16-21% that of normal mice (31). This dystrophin deficiency results from a single, $C > T$ base transition at nucleotide 3185 which causes a premature termination codon at 27% the length of the dystrophin molecule (106). Despite its lack of dystrophin immunoreactivity, the mdx mouse shows no obvious muscle weakness at any point in its normal life span and, due to mild muscle hypertrophy, is actually slightly larger than its normal counterpart. There is histopathologic evidence of a severe myopathy initiated two to five weeks post partum (20). Myofiber necrosis and mineralization is typical of that seen in DMD and GRMD but there is usually no evidence of fibrosis. Unlike the situation in DMD and GRMD, regeneration in the mdx mouse appears to be successful. Regeneration may even overcompensate and totally mask the loss of myofibers (114). The cycle of myofiber degeneration and regeneration does continue, however, and serum CK levels remain consistently elevated.

An X-linked, dystrophin deficiency of cats has been described (28) which seems almost intermediate in clinical severity between mdx and GRMD. Despite marked myofiber necrosis and mineralization, overt weakness did not develop in the cats described, but progressive stiffness was seen which resulted in difficulty in walking by two years of age. The most striking feature was the severe muscle hypertrophy affecting most muscles, including the tongue and diaphragm, which was associated with a gross increase in myofiber diameter. Histologic findings included myofiber necrosis and mineralization. These cats showed no evidence of a demonstrable deletion in genomic DNA by Southern blot analysis using the entire human cDNA as a probe. Dystrophin deficiency was confirmed by Western blot and tissue immunohistochemical analyses. Two other cats suffering from a similar disorder, and showing clinical signs of myopathy with respiratory distress and muscle hypertrophy, have also been reported (113). Histopathologic features were again typical of dystrophin deficiency, but analysis for the dystrophin gene and gene product could not be performed.

The disorder affecting Irish terriers was the first X-linked myopathy to be described in any species other than humans (119). Although the status of the dystrophin gene or gene product could not be ascertained in this condition, it bears such striking similarities to GRMD that it very likely represents another spontaneous defect at this locus. Of a litter of eight puppies, five of seven males were affected and the one female was normal. Males from the dams previous two litters had also shown similar signs. Dysphagia was the first sign noticed at eight weeks, followed by gait abnormalities at 13 weeks. Drooling of saliva, trismus, kyphosis, and muscle atrophy were progressive. Serum CK levels were dramatically elevated and tended to decrease with age. Bizarre high frequency discharges on EMG were described as myotonia, but no dimpling on muscle percussion was present as occurs in true myotonia. Post mortem studies revealed general muscle atrophy, but with marked enlargement of the tongue and diaphragm. Light microscopy demonstrated hyaline fibers, myophagocytosis, regeneration, and the presence of mineralized fibers.

In 1988, it was found that dogs with GRMD appeared to lack both dystrophin transcript and protein in their muscles (36). Both Western blot (36) and histochemical analysis (73) of skeletal muscle from affected dogs revealed no dystrophin immunoreactivity. These were perhaps the most important of the many phenotypic similarities reported between GRMD and DMD, and suggested that the disorders shared a true genetic homology. Despite earlier findings of a number of disease associated polymorphisms on Southern blot analysis (13,37), more detailed studies failed to detect any evidence of a rearrangement within the dystrophin gene of GRMD dogs (13). The defect in this model is now known (see Sharp et al, this volume). Analytical comparison of mRNA between normal and GRMD dogs, using polymerase chain reaction (PCR) amplification of first strand cDNA, demonstrated a truncation of the 5' portion of the dystrophin transcript in affected dogs in the region of the seventh exon. Sequence analysis of both the mRNA/PCR products as well as the genomic segment flanking this exon revealed this truncation to be due a transition mutation (A to G) in the consensus splice donor site of intron six. Thus, exon seven was skipped during mRNA processing, altering the open reading frame and resulted in a premature termination of dystrophin translation (see Sharp et al., this volume).

More recently, two other potential X-linked canine myopathies have been discovered in addition to those described in the Irish terrier (119), Alaskan malamute (27) and golden retriever. These have occurred in a family of Samoyed dogs in Norway (Prestus, personal communication) and in a single male Rottweiler (See Cooper, et al., this volume). In DMD the mutation rate is the highest for any genetic disease observed in man (8), with one out of every three patients thought to be a new mutant. It should therefore not be surprising that sporadic cases of mutations affecting the canine dystrophin gene continue to be identified. It is for this reason that we prefer the term golden retriever muscular dystrophy over that of canine X-linked muscular dystrophy (CXMD) used to describe the same condition by the group at Cornell University (109).

The reasons underlying the differing manifestations of dystrophin deficiency across species are not clear. It has been suggested that dystrophin deficiency per se is not the primary cause of disease, as the mdx mouse clearly can function without this protein. Even in young boys with DMD and dogs with GRMD, signs of muscle weakness are delayed for some time, despite the histopathologic features and enzyme leakage associated with dystrophin deficiency that are apparent at or before birth. The primary pathogenesis may be of non-muscle origin, such as the fibrosis that accompanies these two disorders but is much less prominent in mdx mice. Conversely, it may be a function of the inability of muscle to successfully regenerate in DMD and GRMD (60). It is also possible that another protein in the dystrophin family, such as the one located on chromosome six (79), might act as a successful substitute in mdx mice. The basic cause underlying the progressive pathology of dystrophin deficiency in humans, dogs, and to a lesser extent cats, is an important issue. A number of other factors may play a role in pathogenesis including the size of the organism or its myofibers, muscle mass, longevity, and the role of vascular smooth muscle or neurons (60).

Of the available models for dystrophin deficiency, GRMD appears to be the most useful at both a phenotypic and genetic level (12,36,73, and Sharp et al, this volume). Differences do exist between it and DMD including the decreased growth rate in GRMD, and the fact that dogs retain the ability to walk far longer relative to boys with DMD, who require a wheelchair well before maturity. However, the wheelchair becomes necessary not as a result of the patients inability to stand, but more from a difficulty maintaining balance of his upper body. The transition into a wheelchair is associated with the development of severe joint, thoracic and spinal deformities, combined with respiratory insufficiency (3). The inherent stability of a quadruped means that the ability to walk is preserved in affected dogs and the deterioration associated with enforced recumbency is avoided (109). The increased mean myofiber diameter seen in GRMD also differs from the findings in DMD (46), although it has been suggested that a true hypertrophy may also occur in DMD (47). Although many aspects of the cardiac involvement in these two disorders are shared, the reason for cardiac insufficiency being such an important cause of death in GRMD is unknown, unless continued ambulation and increased cardiac work-load are precipitating causes (47).

The importance of an animal model for therapeutic intervention in DMD cannot be overemphasized. The two broad categories of potential treatments for DMD are either myoblast transplantation or genetic therapy. Myoblast therapy has received considerable attention recently. As muscle exists as a multinucleate syncytium, and undergoes regeneration by mononuclear stem cells called myoblasts, it has been proposed that injection of myoblasts from a normal individual might create a functional population of mosaic myofibers. This would be analogous to the situation in a carrier female. The idea of myoblast transplantation therapy has already been shown to be feasible by localized injection of myoblasts into individual muscles of mdx mice (98). Myoblast transplants have also been conducted in DMD boys on a limited basis, but face considerable ethical and legal concerns. However, successful demonstration of dystrophin in the immediate vicinity of an injection site is a very long way from a systemic cure. In addition, myoblast transplants have little chance for correcting the defects of smooth and cardiac muscle, and cardiomyopathy might become more important if improved patient mobility were attained. The problems associated with correcting the defect in all important muscle groups of one individual patient are far beyond the scope of these initial studies. These problems will require the development of new approaches such as intravascular delivery of myoblasts or enhancing the migration of injected cells beyond the few millimeters shown to date, for example by use of chemotactic agents. These hypotheses will be best tested initially in mdx mice. X-irradiation has been used to suppress the successful mdx regenerative response and convert it to a more faithful model of myofiber loss in DMD (114). The irradiated mdx mouse model is still less than ideal for assessing many phenotypic aspects of the disease other than dystrophin deficiency. Evaluation of treatment methods in GRMD, and their refinement for an organism of greater mass, is seen by many as an essential step in the pursuit of myoblast therapy in DMD (99).

Genetic therapy either by direct injection of naked DNA (1,121), by use of a viral vector, by dystrophin minigene (1,48) or full length construct (1,45,77), or by homologous recombination (26), will also require technology that needs to be perfected before being employed in patients. Knowledge of the exact nature of the defect in a given animal model, and of its consequences for the dystrophin gene products, is desirable to allow for accurate interpretation of experimental results.

A proportion of DMD patients with undetermined mutations will almost certainly be found to have point mutations similar to the situation in mdx mice (22). This mechanism does not, however, result in a reading frame error as is found in the majority of patients with DMD. A reading frame error is found in DMD deletion mutants, appears likely in many patients with presumed splicing abnormalities, and is the basis of the defect in GRMD. The mdx mouse will therefore not be as useful a model as GRMD to study the possibility of differential splicing (54,81) and its effect on the resultant disease phenotype (33).

Differential splicing has been proposed (54,81) as one potential mechanism to explain the eight per cent of patients with deletions in their dystrophin gene who do not obey the reading frame hypothesis (66). These patients nearly always have mutations at the 5' end of the dystrophin gene. In a series of 29 patients with deletions in this region, six had frameshifting deletions of exons 3-7 inclusive and were classified as BMD. Seven patients with the same deletion were classified as outliers of intermediate severity, and two patients with DMD also had this defect (81). Twenty out of 258 patients in another series failed to obey the frameshift hypothesis (66). Ten were classified as BMD, of whom seven had deletions of exons 3-7 (five DMD patients in this series also showed this same deletion). The reasons underlying the variable effects of the exon 3-7 deletion are unknown. The intron that follows exon seven is one of the largest introns known, being 110 kb in size (23). The amount and nature of preserved sequence in this intron could cause considerable variation in the effects of exon 3-7 deletions (33,66). This in turn could result in a variety of differential splicing events for subsequent exons. Of 258 patients with characterized dystrophin gene defects, all of the BMD and intermediate cases with out-of-frame deletions would produce in-frame mRNA if there were differential splicing of the first exon beyond the distal breakpoint (66).

Winnard et al (120) have suggested that differential splicing may, in fact, occur in such patients. They have provided tentative evidence for the existence of this mechanism in one patient with an exon 3-7 deletion phenotype. More recently, Chelly et al (33) provided the first clear evidence of differential splicing in BMD patients as a mechanism to overcome frameshift. Three minor alternative transcripts were found at the 5' end of the dystrophin gene by PCR amplification of mRNA from normal muscle. These transcripts resulted from splicing of exons 2 to 10, 1 to 8 and 1 to 10. In two BMD patients with exon 3-7 deletions, the exon 2 to 10 minor transcript was present at ten times the concentration found in normal muscle. This concentration was still only 1-2% of the major out-of-frame species (exon 2 to 8) that results from the deletion in genomic DNA. The protein produced by these two patients corresponded in size to that predicted by the exon 2 to 10 minor transcript. It was proposed that the deletion in genomic DNA juxtaposed these exons, and so facilitated the alternative splicing event (33). This work provides further support for the intron-breakpoint theory of Koenig et al (66).

The other potential explanation for BMD patients with frameshifting deletions is a reinitiation of dystrophin translation downstream of the out-of-frame stop signal in exon eight. One of the three potential in-frame ATG codons in exon eight conforms to Kozak's consensus sequence (73) even better than the start codon in exon one (8)1. A variation of this mechanism is the suggestion that transcription might begin at a postulated promoter in intron seven that could then initiate protein synthesis from the same putative translational start site. Despite the fact that intron seven is one of the largest intron, there is no evidence to support an additional promoter in the DMD/BMD gene in the seventh intron (81). Neither mechanism is sufficient to explain the different manifestations of exon 3-7 deletions in DMD and BMD patients (33).

Study of the various internally deleted dystrophin molecules in BMD patients is a further way to increase understanding of the functional regions of this protein (59). A tentative functional map of dystrophin has been proposed, which suggests that deletions in the N-terminal domains would predict BMD phenotypes, whereas deletions of the cysteine rich or first half of the carboxy-terminal domain predict DMD phenotypes (66). The fate of the protein product in DMD is another gap in our knowledge. It has been suggested that truncated dystrophin molecules are never observed and that there exists a tight post-translational regulation of dystrophin which results in degradation of such products (59). A similar regulatory mechanism seems to operate with regards to spectrin, a closely related protein (76). This putative mechanism may be active in BMD patients who often show dramatic reductions in the levels of their internally deleted dystrophin molecules (59).

More recent evidence contradicts these assertions and suggests that complete degradation of dystrophin gene products does not occur. The 5' portion of the dystrophin transcript is known to be preserved in DMD patients and it might therefore be expected that they would produce protein corresponding at least to this portion of the message (97). This contrasting hypothesis is supported by the findings of Nicholson et al (91), who found minor dystrophin bands on Western analysis of skeletal muscle from six out of nine DMD patients. The size of the dystrophin band was unrelated to the position of the deletion in the patients DNA. Eight of these nine DMD patients also showed occasional positive fibers on immunohistochemical analysis of sections from frozen muscle. The antibody used in these studies was Dy4/6D3, a monoclonal directed to the rod domain of dystrophin. Similar, though less definitive results were also found using amino-terminal antibodies on frozen tissue (123). These studies in DMD and BMD patients suggest that the predicted amino-terminal peptide in GRMD may be translated in addition to the larger species already identified.

From the results of positive dystrophin immunolabelling on Western blots and tissue sections, it can be seen that truncated forms of this protein are found in nearly all patients with DMD and BMD, and that these patients represent the full spectrum of disease phenotypes (91). It would appear that the original frameshift hypothesis, although valid for most patients (66), is an oversimplification (33,91). This is in agreement with the previous findings of Malhotra et al (81). The existence of a putative mechanism to overcome the frameshift error in DMD and BMD (91) has been confirmed by Chelly et al (33). Their conclusion was that besides having a qualitative effect on the reading frame, deletions exert an impact on phenotype through differential quantitative effects on dystrophin mRNA. A similar differential quantitative effect may also be operative in GRMD.

The abnormality of RNA processing in GRMD, which has now been confirmed at the genomic level (See Sharp et al, this Volume), is the first evidence that dystrophin deficiency can be due to a processing error without deletion of portions of the dystrophin coding sequence. This is an important finding for the one third of DMD and BMD patients with undetermined mutations. The use of mRNA/PCR to detect the processing error in the GRMD model, provides evidence for the utility of this technique to detect all frame-shift mutations as altered PCR products. This method has now been demonstrated for the mutation hot-spots in the DMD gene in the segment 2a and segments 7-8 regions of the cDNA (101) for mutant dystrophin protein. The mRNA/PCR will also recognize those BMD patients with in frame processing errors caused by in frame deletions, or alternately processed transcripts (33).

The strong foundation now laid in the study of the GRMD model at the phenotypic and molecular level, as reported at this meeting, confirms that the GRMD mutation is homologous to the vast majority of the defects found in the DMD phenotype. Development of future cell-tranplantation, gene or pharmicological strategies may now use this information to allow for maximum use to be made of the GRMD model in the search for potential therapies for DMD and BMD.

REFERENCES

1. Acsadi, G., Dickson, G., Love, D.R., Jani, A., Walsh, F.S., Gurusinghe, A., Wolff, J.A., Davies, K.E. (1991): Human dystrophin in mdx mice after intramuscular injection of DNA constructs. *Nature,* 352: 8915-8918.
2. Angelini, C., Beggs, A.H., Hoffman, E.P., Fanin, M., Kunkel, L.M. (1990): Enormous dystrophin in a patient with Becker muscular dystrophy. *Neurology,* 40:808-812.
3. Appel, S.H., Roses, A.D. (1978): Muscular dystrophies. Metabolic basis of inherited disease (4th edition). Stanbury, J.B., Wyngaarden, J.B., Fredrickson, S., eds. McGraw-Hill, New York, pp. 1260-1281.
4. Arahata, K., Ishiura, S., Ishiguro, T., Tsukahara, T., Suhara, Y., Eguchi, C., Ishihara, T., Nonaka, I., Ozawa, E., Sugita, H. (1988): Immunostaining of skeletal and cardiac muscle surface membrane with antibody against Duchenne muscular dystrophy peptide. *Nature,* 333: 861-863.
5. Arahata, K., Ishihara, T., Kakamura, K., Tsukahara, T., Ishiura, S., Baba, C., Matsumoto, T., Nonaka, I., Sugita, H. (1989): Mosaic expression of dystrophin in symptomatic carriers of Duchenne's muscular dystrophy. *New Engl. J. Med.,* 320:138-142.
6. Baaker, E. (1989): Duchenne muscular dystrophy: Carrier detection and prenatal diagnosis by DNA analysis. New mutation and mosaicism. Thesis. Leiden. CIP-DATA Koninklijke Bibliotheek, Den Haag.
7. Bar, S. Barnea, E., Levy, Z., Neuman, S., Yaffe, D., Nudel, U. (1990): A novel product of the Duchenne muscular dystrophy gene which greatly differs from known isoforms in its structure and tissue distribution. *Biochem. J.,* 272:557-560.
8. Barnea, E., Zuk, D., Simantov, R., Nudel, U., Yaffe, D. (1990): Specificity of expression of the muscle and brain dystrophin gene promotors in muscle and brain cells. *Neuron,* 5:881-888.
9. Bartlett, R.J., Monaco, A., Kunkel, L., Pericak-Vance, M.A., Lanman, J., Siddique, T., Roses, A.D. (1985): Segregation of Duchenne dystrophy associated with an Xp21.2 deletion detected by probe pert 87-8. *Am. J. Hum. Genet.,* 37(4), Supplement, 422.
10. Bartlett, R.J., Pericak-Vance, M.A., Koh, J., Yamaoka, L.H., Chen, J.C., Hung, W-Y., Speer, M.C., Wapanaar, M.C., Van Ommen, G.J.B., Bakker, E., Pearson, P.L., Kandt, R.S., Siddique, T., Gilbert, J.R., Lee, J.E., Sirotkin-Roses, M.J., Roses, A.D. (1988): Duchenne muscular dystrophy: High frequency of deletions. *Neurology,* 38:1-4.
11. Bartlett, R.J., Walker, A.P., Laing, N.G., Koh, J., Secore, S.L., Speer, M.C., Pericak-Vance, M.A., Hung, W-Y., Yamaoka, L.H., Siddique, T., Kandt, R. Roses, A.D.: (1989) An inherited deletion at the Duchenne

dystrophy locus in a normal male: a second distal deletion of two exons distinguishes the affected sibling. *Lancet*, March 4, 496.

12. Bartlett, R.J., Sharp, N.J.H., Hung, W-Y., Kornegay, J.N., Roses, A.D. (1990): Molecular markers for myoblast transplantation in GRMD. In Advances in Experimental Medicine and Biology, Eastwood, A.B., Griggs, R.C., Karpati, G., eds. (Plenum Publishing Corporation, NY) 280, 273-278.

13. Bartlett, R.J., Sharp, N.J.H., Secore, S.L., Hung, W-Y., Kornegay, J.N., Roses, A.D. (1990): The canine and human DYS genes are highly conserved. *J. Neurol. Sci.* 98, (Suppl) 165.

14. Bartley, J.A., Patil, S., Davenport, S., Goldstein, D., Pickens, J. (1986): Duchenne muscular dystrophy, glycerol kinase deficiency, and adrenal insufficiency associated with Xp21 deletion. *J. Pediatr.*, 108, 189-192.

15. Beggs, A.H., Koenig, M., Boyce, F.M., Kunkel, L.M. (1990): Detection of 98% of DMD/BMD gene deletions by polymerase chain reaction. *J. Human Genetics*, 86: 45-48.

16. Blondon, L.A.J., Grootscolton, P.M., den Dunnen, J.T., Bakker, E., et al (36 other authors) (1991): 242 Breakpoints in the 200-kb deletion prone P20 region of the DMD gene are widely spread. *Genomics*, 10: 631-639.

17. Bonilla, E., Samitt, C.E., Miranda, A.F., Hays, A.P., Salvati, G., DiMauro, S., Kunkel, L.M., Hoffman, E.P., Rowland, L.P. (1988): Duchenne muscular dystrophy: deficiency of dystrophin at the muscle cell surface. *Cell*, 54:447-452.

18. Bonilla, E., Schmidt, B., Samitt, C.E., Miranda, A.F., Hays, A.P., DeOliveira, A.B., Chang, H.W., Servidei, S., Ricci, E., Younger, D.S., DiMauro, S. (1988): Normal and dystrophin-deficient muscle fibers in carriers of the gene for Duchenne muscular dystrophy. *Am.J.Pathol.*, 133:440-445.

19. Botstein, D., White, R.L., Skolnick, M., Davis, R.W. (1980): Construction of a genetic linkage map in man using restriction fragment length polymorphisms. *Am. J. Hum. Genet.*, 32:314-331.

20. Boyd, Y., Buckle, V.J. (1986): Cytogenetic heterogeneity of translocations associated with Duchenne muscular dystrophy. *Clin. Genet.*, 29:108-115.

21. Bulfield, G., Siller, W.G., Wight, P.A.L., Moore, K.J. (1984): X-chromosome-linked muscular dystrophy (mdx) in the mouse. *Proc. Natl. Acad. Sci. USA*, 81:1189-1192.

22. Bulman, D. et al., point mutation. (Personal cummunication.)

23. Burghes, A.H.M., Logan, C., Hu, X., Belfall, B., Worton, R.G., Ray, P.N. (1987): A cDNA clone from the Duchenne/Becker muscular dystrophy gene. *Nature*, 328:434-437.

24. Burghmeister, M., Monaco, A.P., Gillard, E.F., Van Ommen, G-J. B., Affara, N.A., Ferguson-Smith, M.A., Kunkel, L.M., Lehrach, H. (1988): A 10 Megabase physical map of human Xp21, including the Duchenne muscular dystrophy gene. *Genomics*, 2:189-202.

25. Campbell, K.P., Kahl, S.D. (1989): Association of dystrophin and an integral membrane glycoprotein. *Nature*, 338:259-262.

26. Capecchi, M.R. (1989): Altering the genome by homologous recombination. *Science*, 244:1288-1292.

27. Cardinet, G.H., Holliday, T.A. (1979): Neuromuscular diseases of

domestic animals: A summary of muscle biopsies from 159 cases. *Ann. N.Y. Acad. Sci.*, 317, 290-311.

28. Carpenter, J.L., Hoffman, E.P., Romanul F.C.A., Kunkel, L.M., Rosales, R.K., Ma, N.S.F., Dasbach, J.J., Rae, J.F., Moore, F.M., McAfee, M.B., Pearce, L.K. (1989): Feline muscular dystrophy with dytrophin deficiency. *Am. J. Path.*, 135:909-919.

29. Carpenter, S., Karpati, G., Zubrzycka-Gaarn, E.E., Bulman, D.E., Ray, P.N., Worton, R.G. (1990): Dystrophin is localized to the plasma membrane of human skeletal muscle fibers by electron-microscopic cytochemical study. *,Muscle and Nerve,* 13:376-380.

30. Chamberlain J.S., Gibbs, R.A., Ranier, J.E., Nguyen, P.N., Caskey, C.T. (1988): Deletion screening of the Duchenne muscular dystrophy locus via multiplex DNA amplification. *Nucleic Acids Res.*, 16, 11141-11156.

31. Chamberlain, J.S., Pearlman, J.A., Muzny, D.M., Gibbs, R.A., Ranier, J.E., Reeves, A.A., Caskey, C.T. (1989): Expression of the murine Duchenne muscular dystrophy gene in muscle and brain. *Science*, 239, 1416-1418.

32. Cheely, J., Kaplan, J.C., Maira, P.(1988): Transcription of the dystrophin gene in human muscle and non-muscle tissue. *Nature*, 333: 858-860 .

33. Chelly, J., Gilgenkrantze, H., Lambert, M., Hamard, G., Chafey, P., Recan, D., Katz, P., de la Chappelle, A., Koenig, M., Tome, T., Kahn, A., Kaplan, J-C. (1990): Effects of dystrophin gene deletions on mRNA levels and processing in Duchenne and Becker muscular dystrophies. *Cell*, 63:1239-1248.

34. Cooke, A., Lanyon, W.G., Wilcox, D.E., Dornan, E.S., Kataki, A., Gillard, E.F., McWhinnie, A.J.M., Morris, A., Ferguson-Smith, M.A., Connor, J.M. (1990): Analysis of Scottish Duchenne and Becker muscular dystrophy families with dystrophin cDNA probes. *J. Med. Genet.*, 27: 292-297.

35. Cooper, B.J., Valentine, B.A., Wilson, S., Patterson, D.F., Concannon, P.W. (1988): *J. Hered.*, 79: 405-408.

36. Cooper, B.J., Winand, N.J., Stedman, H., Valentine, B.A., Hoffman, E.P., Kunkel, L.M., Oronzi Scott, M., Fischbeck, K.H., Kornegay, J.N., Avery, R.J., Williams, J.R., Schmickel, R.D., Sylvester, J.E.(1988): The homologue of the Duchenne locus is defective in X-linked muscular dystrophy of dogs. *Nature* , 334: 154-156.

37. Cooper, B.J. (1989): Animal models of Duchenne and Becker muscular dystrophy. Molecular genetics of muscle disease - Duchenne and other dystrophies. Buller, A.J., Goodfellow, J., Newsom-Davies, J.M., eds. Churchill Livingstone Inc., New York, pp. 703-718.

38. Cullen, M.J., Walsh, J., Nicholson, L.V.B., Harris, J.B. (1990): Ultrastructural localization of dystrophin in human muscle by using gold immunolabelling. *Proc. R. Soc. Lond.*, B240, 197-210.

39. Darras, B.T., Blattner, P., Harper, J.F., Spiro, A.J., Alter, S., Francke, U. (1988): Intragenic deletions in 21 Duchenne muscular dystrophy (DMD)/ Becker muscular dystrophy (BMD) families studied with the dystrophin cDNA: Location of breakpoints on HindIII and BglII exon-containing fragment maps, meiotic and mitotic origin of the mutations. *Am. J. Hum. Genet.*, 43, 620-629.

40. Davidson, M.D., Critchley, D.R. (1988): Alpha-actinins and the DMD

protein contain spectrin-like repeats. *Cell,* 52, 159-160.

41. Davies, K.E., Pearson, P.L., Harper, P.S., Murray, J.M., O'Brien, T., Sarfarazi, M., Williamson, R. (1983): Linkage analysis of two cloned DNA sequences flanking the Duchenne muscular dystrophy locus on the short arm of the X-chromosome. *Nucleic Acids Res.,* 11, 2303-2312.

42. Davies, K.E., Smith, E., Bundey, S., Read, A.P., Flint, T., Bell, M.,and Speer, A. (1988): Mild and severe muscular dystrophy associated with deletions in Xp21 of the human X-chromosome. *J. Med. Genet.,* 25, 9-13.

43. Den Dunnen, J.T., Baaker, E., Klein Breteler, E.G., Pearson, E.L., Van Ommen, G-J.B. (1987): Direct detection of more than 50% of the Duchenne muscular dystrophy mutations by field inversion gels. *Nature,* 329, 640-642.

44. Dickson, G., Pizzey, J.A., Elsom, V.E., Love, D., Davies, K.E. Walsh, F.S. (1988): Distinct dystrophin mRNA species are expressed in embryonic and adult mouse skeletal muscle. *FEBS Lett.,* 242: 47-52.

45. Dickson, G., Davies, K.E., Love, D. Walsh, F.S (1991): *Journal of Cellular Biochemistry,* (Supplement 15C): 37, 1991.

46. Dubowitz, V., Brooke, M.H. (1973): Muscle biopsy: A modern approach. Vol. 2. Major Problems in Neurology. W.B. Saunders, London pp. 74-102, 168-252.

47. Emery, A.E.H. (1987): Duchenne muscular dystrophy. Oxford University Press Oxford.

48. England, S.B., Nicholson, L.V.B., Johnson, M.A., Forrest, S.M., Love, D.R., Zubrzycka-Gaarn, E.E., Bulman, D.E., Harris, J.B., Davies, K.E. (1990). Very mild muscular dystrophy associated with the deletion of 46% of dystrophin. *Nature,*343, 180-182.

49. Ervasti, J.M., Ohlendieck, K., Kahl, S.D., Gaver, M.G., Campbell, K.P. (1990): Deficiency of a glycoprotein component of the dystrophin complex in dystrophic muscle. *Nature,*345: 315-319.

50. Fardeau, M., Tome, F.M., Collin, H., Augier, N., Pons, F., Leger, J. (1990): Presence of dystrophin-like protein at the neuromuscular junction in Duchenne muscular dystrophy and mutant mice. *Comptes Rendus de l'Academie des Sciences-Serie Iii. Sciences de la Vie,* 311: 197-204.

51. Feener, C.A., Koenig, M., and Kunkel, L.M. (1989): Alternative splicing of human dystrophin mRNA generates isoforms at the carboxy terminus. *Nature,* 338: 509-511.

52. Forrest, S.M., Cross, G.S., Speer, A., Robson, K.J.H., Davies, K.E. (1988): Further studies of gene deletions that cause Duchenne and Becker muscular dystrophies. *Genomics,* 2: 109-114.

53. Francke, U., Ochs, H.D., deMartinville, B., Giacolone, J., Lindgren, V., Disteche, C., Pagon, R.A., Hofker, M.H., van Ommen, G.-J.B., Pearson, P.L., Wedgewood, R.J. (1985): Minor Xp21 chromosome deletion in a male associated with expression of Duchenne muscular dystrophy, chronic granulomatouc disease, retinitis pigmentosa, and McLeod syndrome. *Amer. J Hum. Genet.,* 37: 250-268.

54. Gillard, E.F., Chamberlain J.S., Murphy, E.G., Duff, C.L., Smith, B., Burghes, A.H.M., Thompson, M.W., Sutherland, J., Oss, I., Bodrug, S.E., Klamut, H.J., Ray, P.N., Worton R.G. (1989). Molecular and phenotypic analysis of patients with deletions in the deletion-rich region of the Duchenne muscular dystrophy (DMD) gene. *Am. J. Hum. Genet.,* 45: 507-520.

55. Hoffman, E.P. Monaco, A.P. Feener, C.C., Kunkel, L.M. (1987): Conservation of the Duchenne muscular dystrophy gene in mice and humans. *Science*, 238: 347-350.

56. Hoffman, E.P., Knudson, C.M., Campbell, K.C., and Kunkel, L.M. (1987). Subcellular fractionation of dystrophin to the triads of skeletal muscle. *Nature,* 330: 754-758.

57. Hoffman, E.P., Brown, R.H. Jr., Kunkel, L.M. (1987). Dystrophin: the protein product of the Duchenne muscular dystrophy locus. *Cell,* 51: 919-928.

58. Hoffman, E.P., Hudecki, M.S., Rosenberg, P.A., Pollina, C.M., Kunkel, L.M. (1988). Cell and fiber-type distribution of dystrophin. *Neuron,* 1: 411-420.

59. Hoffman, E.P., Fischbeck, K.H., Brown, R.H., Johnson, M.J., Medori, R., Loike, J.D., Harris, J.B., Waterston, R., Brooke, M., Specht, L., Kupsky, W., Chamberlain, J., Caskey, C.T., Shapiro, F., Kunkel, L.M. (1988): Dystrophin characterization in muscle biopsies from Duchenne and Becker muscular dystrophy patients. *New Engl. J. Med.,* 31: 1363-1368.

60. Hoffman, E.P., Kunkel, L.M. (1989): Dystrophin abnormalities in Duchenne/Becker muscular dystrophy. *Neuron,* 2: 1019-1029.

61. Hu, X., Burghes, A.H.M., Ray, P.N., Thompson, M.W., Murphy, E.G., Worton, R.G. (1988). Partial gene duplication in Duchenne and Becker muscular dystrophy. *J.Med.Genet.,* 25: 369-376.

62. Khurana, T.S., Hoffman, E.P., Kunkel, L.M. (1990): Identification of a chromosome 6-encoded dystrophin-related protein. *Journal of Biological Chemistry,* 265: 16717-16720.

63. Kingston, H.M., Thomas, N.S.T., Pearson, P.L., Sarfarazi, M. Harper, P.S. (1983): Genetic linkage between Becker muscular dystrophy and a polymorphic DNA sequence on the short arm of the X-chromosome. *J. Med. Genet.,* 20: 255-258.

64. Koenig, M., Hoffman, E.P., Bertelson, C.J., Monaco, A.P., Feener, C., Kunkel, L.M. (1987): Complete cloning of the Duchenne muscular dystrophy (DMD) cDNA and preliminary genomic organization of the DMD gene in normal and affected individuals. *Cell ,* 50: 509-517.

65. Koenig, M., Monaco, A.P., Kunkel, L.M. (1988): The complete sequence of dystrophin predicts a rod-shaped cytoskeletal protein. *Cell,* 53: 219-228.

66. Koenig, M., Beggs, A.H., Moyer, M., Scherpf, S., Heindrich, K., Bettecken, T., Meng, G., Muller, C.R., Lindlof, M., Kaarianen, H., de la Chapelle, A., Kiuru, A., Savontaus, M-L., Gilgenkrantz, H., Recan, D., Chelly, J., Kaplan, J-C., Covone, A.E., Archidiancono, N., Romeo, G., Leichti-Gallati, S., Schneider, V., Braga, S., Moser, H., Darras, B.T., Wrogemann, K., Blonden, L.A.J., van Paassen, H.M.B., van Ommen, G.J.B., Kunkel, L.M.. (1989): The molecular basis for Duchenne versus Becker muscular dystrophy: correlation of severity with type of deletion. *Am.J.Hum. Genet.,* 45: 498-506.

67. Koh, J., Bartlett, R.J., Pericak-Vance, M.A., Speer, M.C., Yamaoka, L.H., Phillips, K., Hung, W.Y., Ray, P.N., Worton R.G., Gilbert, J.R., Lee, J.E., Siddique, T., Kandt, R.s., Roses, A.D. (1987): Inherited deletion at Duchenne dystrophy locus in normal male. *Lancet,* 1114-1115.

68. Kornegay, J.N. (1984): Golden retriever muscular dystrophy. In

Scientific Proceedings, 2nd Annual Veterinary Medical Forum. Washington, D.C., American College of Veterinary Internal Medicine pp. 193-196.

69. Kornegay, J.N. (1986): Golden retriever myopathy. In Current Veterinary Therapy IX, Kirk, R.W., ed. W.B. Saunders Co., Philadelphia, pp. 792-794.

70. Kornegay, J.N. (1988): Golden retriever muscular dystrophy: a model of Duchenne muscular dystrophy. Discuss. *Neurosci.*, 5: 118-123.

71. Kornegay, J.N., Tuler, S.M., Miller, D.M., Levesque, D.C. (1988): Muscular dystrophy in a litter of golden retriever dogs. *Muscle and Nerve*, 11: 1056-1064.

72. Kornegay, J.N., Sharp, N.J.H., Bartlett, R.B., Van Camp, S.D., Burt, C.T., Hung, W.Y., Kwock, L., Roses, A.D.(1990): Golden retriever muscular dystrophy: Monitoring for success. In Advances in Experimental Medicine and Biology, Eastwood, A.B., Griggs, R.C., Karpati, G., eds. (Plenum Publishing Corporation, NY) 280: 267-272.

73. Kozak, M. (1987): An analysis of 5' non-coding sequences from 699 vertebrate messanger RNA's. *Nucleic Acids Res.*, 15: 8125-8132.

74. Kunkel, L.M., Monaco, A.P., Middlesworth, W., Ochs, S.D., and Latt, S.A. (1985): Specific cloning of DNA fragments absent from the DNA of a male with an X-chromosome deletion. *Proc. Natl. Acad. Sci. USA.*, 82: 4778-4782.

75. Kunkel, L.M., et al. (1986). Analysis of deletions in DNA from patients with Becker and Duchenne muscular dystrophy. *Nature*, 322: 73-77.

76. Lazarides, E. (1987): From genes to structural proteins: The genesis and epigenesis of a red blood cell. *Cell*, 51:345-356.

77. Lee, C.C., Pearlman, J.A., Chamberlain, J.S., Caskey, C.T. (1991): Expression of recombinant dystrophin and its location to the cell membrane. *Nature*, 349: 334-336.

78. Lidov, H.G.W., Byers, T.J., Watkins, S. and Kunkel, L.M. (1990). Localization of dystrophin to postsnyaptic regions of central nervous system cortical neurons. *Nature*, 348: 725-728.

79. Love, D.R., Hill, D.F., Dickson, G., Spurr, N.K., Byth, B.C., Marsden, R.F., Walsh, F.S., Edwards, Y.H., Davies, K.E. (1989): An autosomal transcript in skeletal muscle with homology to dystrophin. *Nature*, 339: 55-58.

80. Love, D.R., Davies, K.E. (1989): Duchenne muscular dystrophy: The gene and the protein. *Mol. Biol. Med.*, 6, 7-17.

81. Malhotra, S.B., Hart, K.A., Klamut, H.J., Thomas, N.S.T., Bodrug, S.E., Burghes, A.H.M., Bobrow, M., Harper, P.S., Thopmson, M.W., Ray, P.N., Worton, R.G. (1988): Frame-shift deletions in patients with Duchenne and Becker muscular dystrophy. *Science*, 242: 755-758.

82. Menke, A. Jockusch, H. (1991). Decreased osmotic fragility of dystrophin-less muscle cells from *mdx* mice. Nature, 349: 69-71.

83. Mokri, B., Engel, A.G. (1975): Duchenne muscular dystrophy: Electron microscopic findings pointing to a basic or early abnormality in the plasma membrane of the muscle fiber. *Neurology*, 25: 1111-1120.

84. Monaco, A.P., Bertelson, C.J., Middlesworth, W., Colleti, C.-A., Fischbeck, K.H., Bartlett, R.J., Perick-Vance, M.A., Roses, A.D., Kunkel, L.M. (1985): Detection of deletions spanning the Duchenne muscular dystrophy locus using a tightly linked DNA segment. *Nature*, 316: 842-845.

85. Monaco, A.P., Neve, R.L., Colleti-Feener, C., Bertelson, C.J., Kurnit, D.M., Kunkel, L.M. (1986): Isolation of candidate cDNA's for protions of the Duchenne muscular dystrophy gene. *Nature,* 323: 646-650.

86. Monaco, A.P., Bertelson, C.J., Colleti-Feener, C., Kunkel, L.M. (1987): Localization and cloning of Xp21 breakpoints involved in muscular dystrophy. *Hum. Genet.,* 75: 221-227.

87. Monaco, A.P., Kunkel, L.M. (1987): A giant locus for the Duchenne and Becker muscular dystrophy gene. *Trends Genet.,* 3:33-37.

88. Monaco, A.P., Bertelson, C.J., Liechti-Gallati, S., Moser, H., Kunkel, L.M. (1988): An explanation for the phenotypic differences between patients bearing partial deletions of the DMD locus. *Genomics,* 2: 90-95.

89. Murray, J.M., Davies, K.E., Harper, P.S., Meredith, L., Mueller, C.R., and Williamson, R. (1982): Linkage relationship of a cloned DNA sequence on the short arm of the X-chromosome to Duchenne muscular dystrophy. *Nature,* 300: 69-71.

90. Nicholson, L.V.B., Davison, K., Falkous, G., Harwood, C., O'Donnell, E., Slater, C.R., Harris, J.B. (1989): Dystrophin in skeletal muscle. I. Western blot analysis using a monclonal antibody. *J. Neurol. Sci.,* 94: 125-136.

91. Nicholson, L.V.B., Davison, K., Johnson, M.A., Slater, C.R., Young, C., Bhattacharya, S., Gardner-Medwin, D., Harris, J.B. (1989): II. Immunoreactivity in patients with Xp21 muscular dystrophy. *J. Neurol. Sci.,* 94: 137-146.

92. Nicholson, L.V.B., Johnson, M.A., Bhattacharya, S., Gardner-Medwin, D., Harris, J.B. (1990): Heterogeneity of dystrophin expression in patients with Duchenne and Becker muscular dystrophy. *Acta. Neuropath.,* 80: 239-249.

93. Noegel, A., Witke, W., Schleicher, M. (1987): Calcium-sensitive non-muscle alpha-actinin EF-hand structures and highly conserved regions. *FEBS Lett.,* 221: 391-396.

94. Nordenskjold, M., Nicholson, L., Edstrom, L., Anvret, M., Eiserman, M., Slater, C., Stolpe, L. (1990): A normal male with an inherited deletion of one exon within the DMD gene. *Hum. Genet.,* 84: 207-209.

95. Nudel, U., Zuk, D., Einat, P., Zeelon, E., Levy, Z., Neuman, S., Yaffe, D. (1989). Duchenne muscular dystrophy gene product is not identical in muscle and brain. *Nature,* 337: 76-78.

96. Ohlendieck, K., Ervasti, J.M., Snook, J.B., Campbell, K.P. (1991). Dystrophin-glycoprotein complex is highly enriched in isolated skeltal muscle sarcolemma. *J. Cell Biol.,* 112: 135-148.

97. Oronzi-Scott, M., Sylvester, J.E., Heiman-Patterson, T., Shi, Y.-J., Fieles, W., Stedman, H., Burghes, A., Ray, P., Worton, R., Fischbeck, K.H. (1988): Duchenne muscular dystrophy gene expression in normal and diseased human muscle. *Science,* 239, 1418-1420.

98. Partridge, T.A., Morgan, J.E., Coulton, G.R., Hoffman, E.P., Kunkel, L.M. (1989). Conversion of mdx myofibres from dystrophin-negative to -positive by injection of normal myoblasts. *Nature,* 337: 176-179.

99. Partridge, T.A. Myoblast transplantation: (1991): A possible therapy for inherited myopathies? *Muscle and Nerve* , In Press.

100. Ray, P.N., Belfall, B., Duff, C., Logan, C., Kean, V., Thompson, M.W., Sylvester, J.E., Gorski, J.L., Schmickel, R.D., Worton, R.G. (1985): Cloning of the breakpoint of an X:21 translocation associated with Duchenne muscular dystrophy. *Nature,* 318: 672-675.

101. Roberts, R.G., Bentley, D.R., Barby, T.F.M., Manners, E. Bobrow, M. (1990): Direct diagnosis of carriers of Duchenne and Becker muscular dystrophy by amplification of lymphocyte RNA. *Lancet*, 336: 1523-1525.
102. Roses, A.D., Herbstreith, M.H., and Appel, S.H. (1975): Membrane protein kinase alteration in Duchenne muscular dystrophy. *Nature*, 254: 350-351.
103. Rowland, L.P. (1988): A triumph of reverse genetics and the end of the beginning. *New Engl. J Med.*, 318: 1392-1394.
104. Royer-Pokora, B., Kunkel, L.M., Monaco, A.P., Goff, S.C., Newburger, P.E., Baehner, R.L., Cole, F.S., Curnette, J.T., and Orkin, S.H. (1986): Cloning the gene for an inherited human disorder - chronic granulomatous disease - on the basis of its chromosomal location. *Nature,* 322: 32-38.
105. Samitt, C.E., Bonilla, E. (1990): Immunocytochemical study of dystrophin at the myotendinous junction. *Muscle and Nerve* 13: 493-500.
106. Sicinski, P., Geng, Y., Ryder-Cook, A.S., Barnard, E.A., Darlison, M.G., Barnard, P.J. (1991): The molecular basis of muscular dystrophy in the *mdx* mouse is a point mutation. *Science*, 244: 1578-1579.
107. Valentine, B.A.,Cooper, B.J.,Cummings, J.F., deLahunta, A. (1986). Progressive muscular dystrophy in a golden retriever dog: light microscopic and ultrastructural features at 4 and 8 months. *Acta Neuropath (Berl.)* , 71: 301-310.
108. Valentine, B.A., Cooper, B.J., Dietze, A.E. Noden, D.M. (1988): Canine congenital diaphragmatic hernia. *J. Vet. Int. Med.,* 2: 109-112.
109. Valentine, B.A., Cooper, B.J., deLahunta, A., O'Quinn, R., and Blue, J.T. (1988). Canine X-linked muscular dystrophy. An animal model of Duchenne muscular dystrophy: clinical studies. *J. Neurol. Sci.* 88: 69-81.
110. Valentine, B.A., Cooper, B.J., Cummings, J.F., and de Lahunta, A. (1990). Canine X-linked muscular dystrophy: morphologic lesions. *J.Neurol. Sci.*, 97: 1-23.
111. Van Ommen, G-J.B., Verkerk, J.M.H., Hofker, M.H., Monaco, A.P., Kunkel, L.M., Ray, P., Worton, R., Wieringa, B., Bakker, E. Pearson, P.L.(1986) A physical map of 4 million bp around the Duchenne muscular dystrophy gene on the human X-chromosome. *Cell,* 47: 499-504.
112. Verellen-Dumoulin, C., Freund, M., De Meyer, R., Laterre, C., Frederic, J., Thompson, M.W., Markovic, V.D., and Worton, R.G. (1984): Expression of an X-linked muscular dystrophy in a female due to translocation involving Xp21 and non-random inactivation of the normal X-chromosome. *Hum. Genet.*, 67: 115-119.
113. Vos, J.H., van der Linde-Sipman, J.S., Goedegeburre, S.A. Dystrophy-like myopathy in the cat. *J. Comp. Path.*, 96: 335-341.
114. Wakeford, S., Watt, D.J. Partridge, T.A. (1991): X-irradiation improves mdx mouse muscle as a model of myofiber loss in DMD. *Muscle and Nerve,* 14:42-50.
115. Walker, A.P., Bartlett, R.J., Laing, N.G., Hung, W.Y., Yamaoka, L. H., Secore, S.L., Holsti, M., Speer, M.C., Mechler, F., Denton, M., Siddique, T., Pericak-Vance, M.A., Roses, A.D. (1989): A partial Taq I map of the Duchenne muscular dystrophy gene: use of small cDNA fragments in deletion and RFLP analysis. *Am.J.Human Genet.* 45: A166.
116. Walker, A P., Laing, N.G., Yamada, T., Chandler, D C., Kakulas, B.A., Bartlett, R J. A TaqI map the dystrophin gene useful for deletion

and carrier status analysis. *Jour. Med. Genetics*, in press.
117. Watkins, S.C., Hoffman, E.P., Slayter, H.S., Kunkel, L.M. (1988): Immunoelectron microscopic localization of dystrophin in myofibers. *Nature*, 333: 863-866.
118. Webster, C., Silberstein, L., Hays, A.P., et al. (1988): Fast muscle fibers are preferentially affected in Duchenne muscular dystrophy. *Cell.*, 52: 503-513.
119. Wentink, G.H., van der Linde-Sipman, J.S., Meier, H., Hendriks, H.J. (1972). Myopathy with a possible X-linked mode of inheritance in a litter of Irish terriers. *Vet. Path.*, 9: 328-349.
120. Winnard, A. , Mendell, J.R., Florence, J., Brooke, M., Burghes, A.H.M. (1990): Detection of point mutations and examination of translational frameshift exceptions in Duchenne and Becker dystrophy. *Am. J. Hum. Genet.*, 47: A242.
121. Wolff, J.A., Malone, R.W., Williams, P. Chong, W., Ascadi, G., Jani, A., Felgner, P.L. (1990): Direct gene transfer into mouse muscle in vivo. *Science*, 247: 1465-1468.
122. Worton, R.G., Duff, C., Sylvester, J.E., Schmickel, R.D., and Willard, H.F. (1984): Duchenne muscular dystrophy involving translocation of the dmd gene next to ribosomal RNA genes. *Science*, 224: 1447-1449.
123. Zubrzycka-Gaarn, E.E., Bulman, D.E., Karpati, G., Burghes, A.H.M., Belfall, B., Klamut, H.J., Talbot, J., Hodges, R.S., Ray, P.N., and Worton, R.G. (1988): The Duchenne muscular dystrophy gene product is localized in sarcolemma of human skeletal muscle. *Nature*, 333: 466-470.

DISCUSSION

Dr. Manfred W. Beilharz:

I just want to get your speculations on the lattice model, in view of what you are saying about the differences between the DMD and the Becker patients. You are saying the N and C terminals are always there with the Beckers at least, and you are basically losing a lot of the molecule in the DMD cases. When you look at the antibody staining of the Beckers one has that sporadic pattern on the outside of the membrane. Have you ever speculated using the lattice model that you were showing us. What we are physically seeing with the immunostain may be a result of alterations in the ability to form a lattice?

Assistant Professor Richard J. Bartlett:

Many of the Becker patients have mutations which are located in the first 10 exons (amino terminal end) and, therefore, may not be expressing these sequences. This would be the case if any have initiation of translation occurring from the AUG codon in exon 8. The main point to note here is that the Becker patients, regardless of their mutation, will maintain a reading frame which will permit expression of the carboxy-terminus. Thus, this end of the molecule is the suggestive attachment point for the membrane bound glyco-protein complex. Should an interaction with the amino terminal portion of the protein be discovered in the future, then these defective proteins from patients with deletions in the exon 1-10 region may lack that association, but still maintain the carboxy-terminal capacity. As to which is the more important, one can only speculate.

Dr. Miranda D.Grounds
I realise that it would be a very difficult thing to do, but I wonder if anyone has attempted to look at the surface of the muscle fibre to see what the actual organization of the dystrophin molecules was from that point of view. Perhaps I should address this question to John Harris.

Professor John B. Harris:
We have not yet made such experiments, but we are planning to isolate sheets of plasma membrane so that we can study the organisation of the dystrophin lattice after various degrees of stretch.

Dr. Miranda D. Grounds:
I presume that you remove the external lamina.

Professor John B. Harris:
Yes

Dr. Miranda D. Grounds:
So that itself might affect the distribution ofthe molecules.

Professor John B. Harris:
Yes.

Dr. Terence A. Partridge:
On the matter of the relationship between dystrophin abnormalities and lattice formation, another area to look at would be the carriers. In particular a comparison of the lattices of Duchenne and Becker carriers should be interesting because Becker carriers should be making both normal and abnormal sized dystrophin molecules which should disturb lattice structure while Duchenne carriers should make only normalized dystrophin of a type which would associate with the muscle plasmalemma and so should form a normal lattice.

Assistant Professor Richard J. Bartlett:
One would presume that a carrier would produce two different sized products which would have the potential to form heterodimers. These would be predicted to form an asymmetrical lattice which may be weaker than the symmetrical counterpart. These weakened structures may gradually be replaced by homodimers through some potential repair process in the muscle fibre. This might explain some of the patchy staining seen in manifesting carriers and young carriers.

Dr. Terence A. Partridge:
There might be a few Duchenne carriers making membrane-associated dystrophin whereas all Becker carriers would be making abnormal and normal dystrophin and both would become membrane associated.

Professor Allen D. Roses:
It may or may not be true because the x-chromosome doesn't express itself like we presume autosomes do because of lyonization. In fact one of the things neuropathologists have been pointing out for a long time from biopsies which have been taken from carriers, is that they are seeing single normal fibres in a sea of otherwise abnormal fibres.

Dr. Terence A. Partridge:
George Karpati and ourselves have looked at mdx carriers and Barry Cooper has looked at the hearts of dystrophic carrier dogs. In both species you find mosaicism which suggests a roughly 50/50 expression of normal and abnormal X-chromosomes so you might expect the same in skeletal muscle. In skeletal muscle of carriers there is some evidence for a patchy expression of dystrophin in the early stages, suggesting that the normal and defective genes of the two types of "lyonized" myonuclei are expressed equally.

Dr Barry J. Cooper:
I think the point that Terry is making is that the skeletal muscle fibres are multinuclear, therefore both genes should be expressed. What we don't know is whether an abnormal dystrophin molecule is being expressed along side a normal one and whether an abnormal one would be competed out by the normal. I guess it is a difficult question to answer.

Dr. Terence A Partridge:
This could be resolved by immunoblotting. You should find both normal and abnormal dystrophin from skeletal muscles of Becker carriers.

Professor George Karpati:
Another interesting type of mutation that was recently reported from Lou Kunkel's lab is a patient in whom there was no deletion in the genomic DNA but in the dystrophin messenger RNA an exon was missing. I think they postulate that here there is likely a point mutation in an intron that introduced an abnormal splice site which takes out the transcript of an exon in the message and, as a result, abnormal messages can be formed. It is likely that this probably will be responsible for at least some of the non-deleted cases, because a point mutation in an exon that was recently found in Toronto probably is going to be very rare.

Professor Byron A. Kakulas:
That is a nice herald for Nick's talk this afternoon.

Professor Allen D. Roses:
An exon skipping mutation was exactly what they found in the dog.

Professor John B Harris:
I wish to comment on the supposition that the organisation of the lattice should vary according to the length of the dystrophin molecule. That view presupposes that the lattice depends on the length of the protein. If however, the protein is considered highly flexible, a short form of dystrophin may stretch so that it can attach itself to normally spaced anchoring points at the periphery of the muscle fibre. Our quantitative measurements on the distribution of gold labelling in the muscle of the patient with a 50% deletion in the gene (see fig 8, Harris and Cullen this volume) suggests that this is, in fact the case. The implication would be that if the anchoring points are distributed as in normal muscle and the integrity of the N- and C-termini is preserved in the abnormal dystrophin, the lattice will not be disrupted.

Professor George Karpati:
Excuse me, how about the hinges? A lattice implies bending points and if the hinges are missing the molecule will not bend to form the presumptive hexagonal lattices.

Professor John B Harris:
We have one patient with an in-frame deletion affecting a putative hinge region. He has a severe Duchenne phenotype despite being in-frame.

Professor Byron A. Kakulas:
No one has mentioned the name Don Shotland in this discussion. His many freeze fracture studies have shown abnormalities in the membrane in DMD. I wonder if there has been any attempt to correlate his early findings with what you have shown today?

Dr. Terence A. Partridge:
He did try. He looked at the mdx mouse before it was known to be a Duchenne homologue and found no abnormalities in the distribution of caveoli of the type described in other animal models of dystrophin.

DUCHENNE MUSCULAR DYSTROPHY: Animal Models
and Genetic Manipulation, edited by Byron A. Kakulas,
John McC. Howell, and Allen D. Roses.
Raven Press, Ltd., New York © 1992.

5

Expression of C-Terminal Domain of Dystrophin in Duchenne Muscular Dystrophy and *mdx* Mouse

Hideo Sugita, Kiichi Arahata, Masakazu Takemitsu,
Ritsuko Koga, Shoichi Ishiura, and Ikuya Nonaka

National Institute of Neuroscience,
National Center of Neurology and Psychiatry
4-1-1 Ogawahigashi, Kodaira, Tokyo, 187 Japan.

INTRODUCTION

Dystrophin is the protein product of Duchenne muscular dystrophy (DMD) gene, which is now thought to be a membrane associated cytoskeletal component of muscle fiber (5). Amino acid sequence analysis predicts a 427 kDa dystrophin protein composed of 3,685 amino acids arranged in 4 distinct domains (10).

The fourth, 420 amino acids carboxy(C)-terminal domain was supposed to have no relation to any previously characterized proteins, until the discovery of a new sequence, B3 which has high homology to this region (9). In addition, the strong evolutionary conservation of the C-terminal coding and 3'untranslated regions between human and chicken emphasizes the functional and structural importance of the C-terminus of dystrophin molecule (8).

The work reported here was conducted to clarify the expression of the C-terminal domain in Duchenne/Becker muscular dystrophy and *mdx* mouse by using mono- and polyclonal antibodies against 50 amino acids sequence of the C-terminal domain of dystrophin.

MATERIALS AND METHODS

The limb-muscle specimens from Duchenne/Becker muscular dystrophy (BMD) and other neuromuscular diseases (OND) were obtained for diagnostic purposes, with informed consent and kept at -85 °C.

The hindlimb muscles were obtained from *mdx* mice at various developmental stages and after denervation. B10 mice were used as control.

The 50 residues (peptide IV, 3495-3544: LISLESEERGELERILA DLEEENRNLQAEYDRLKQQHEHKGLSPLPSPPE) of the carboxy terminal domain of human skeletal muscle dystrophin were synthesized as described previously (15). This amino acid sequence has 70% homology to the corresponding region in B3 (9).

The antiserum was raised by repeated injection of peptide IV mixed with Freund's complete adjuvant into New Zealand white rabbit. The monoclonal antibody against peptide IV (the antibody is designated as 4C5), which is specific for dystrophin, was used in this experiment (3).   Immunoblotting and immunofluorescence were conducted by the procedures described in our previous papers (1,7).

RESULTS AND DISCUSSION

(1) Expression of C-terminal Domain of Dystrophin in DMD/BMD and OND

The abundance and molecular weight of dystrophin were examined using 4C5 (3) as well as anti-peptide IV antiserum. OND showed a 400 kDa band as observed in Fig. 1.

Dystrophin was undetectable in all cases of DMD, but patients with BMD showed a dystrophin of altered size and/or abundance (Fig.1).

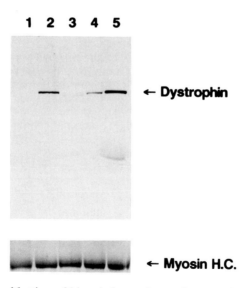

FIG. 1.   Immunoblotting of biopsied muscle specimens using anti-peptide IV antiserum. Lane 1, DMD; Lanes 2 and 5, OND; Lanes 3 and 4, BMD.

In immunohistochemistry with 4C5, all 24 OND patients showed clear immunostaining at the surface membrane as shown in our previous papers using anti-peptide II antiserum (1,15). In contrast, none of 21 DMD patients had detectable staining of the surface membrane (3).

In all 30 BMD patients, the immunostaining with 4C5 was fainter than normal and the pattern was "patchy" (3), which is essentially the same as reported by using anti-peptide II antiserum (2).

It was confirmed that all BMD have dystrophin gene products which include the C-terminal domain using a monoclonal antibody directed specifically against the C-terminal portion of dystrophin molecule. While in DMD, the C-terminus is absent in all cases studied.

These observations strongly suggest that the C-terminal domain is crucial for generation of the proper function and stability of dystrophin molecule.

Bulman and his co-workers (4) have also revealed that the truncated immunoreactive dystrophin band was demonstrated in 11 out of 25 DMD patients when immunoblotting was performed with antiserum directed against the N-terminus but not C-terminus of dystrophin.

These results mentioned above, however, do not coincide with those of Vainzof et al. (17) who observed partially stained fibers with antibodies against both N-terminal and C-terminal regions of the protein in 13 and with only N-terminus in 7 out of 22 cases of DMD.

(2) Expression of C-terminal Domain of Dystrophin in Relation to Dystrophin Related Protein in *mdx* Mouse

Adult *mdx* Mouse

As already reported with the anti-peptide II antiserum (1), a single 400 kDa band was observed in B10 mouse with anti-peptide IV antiserum (Fig.2) (7).

In mdx mouse, a very faint, but a single immunoreactive band of 400 kDa was also observed. (Fig. 2).

Immunohistochemically, the anti-peptide IV antiserum stained the surface membrane and also neuromuscular junctions (NMJ) of B10 mouse skeletal muscle as observed with anti-peptide II antiserum (Fig. 3a).

In adult *mdx* mouse, the antibody did not stain the surface membrane, but clear immunoreactivity was observed at the NMJ as shown in Fig. 3b.

Embryonic and Denervated *mdx* Mouse

A single band of 400 kDa was observed in the 14th and 20th embryonic day mdx mouse skeletal muscles which is stronger than that observed in adults (Fig. 2.) Limb muscles obtained 8 days after denervation showed an immunoreactive band of the same molecular weight as shown in Fig. 2.

In immunohistochemistry, the anti-peptide IV antiserum stained the surface membrane of 20 day embryonic *mdx* mouse muscle faintly (Fig. 4a) (16). Several studies have reported that in mammalian muscles, dystrophin is particularly concentrated at the NMJ (12,14).

Pons and his co-workers (13) have reported that polyclonal antibodies against N-terminal, central region and C-terminal domain of dystrophin molecule immunostained the NMJ of DMD patients and NMJ and sarcolemma of normal controls. They showed that those 3 polyclonal antibodies bind to a protein of 400 kDa which is present in extracts of *mdx* muscle including NMJ and is absent from extracts without NMJ. However, this NMJ-associated homologue has 2 epitopes, which are different to the usual Xp21 coded dystrophin expressed along the sarcolemma of normal muscles. This protein was also expressed in NMJ of DMD who lacks the first 52 exons of dystrophin gene.

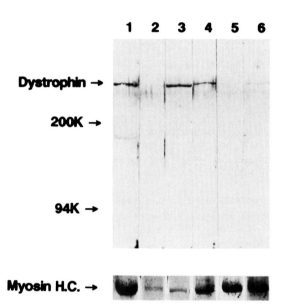

FIG. 2. Immunoblotting of *mdx* mouse muscle using anti-peptide IV antiserum. Lane 1, B10 mouse; Lanes 2 to 6, *mdx* mouse. Lane 2, 14-day embryo; Lane 3, 20-day embryo; Lane 4, 1-week neonate; Lane 5, 1-year old adult; Lane 6, 8-day denervated muscle.

Since the sarcolemma was not stained in *mdx* mouse, the crossreactive NMJ-associated homologous protein must be a distinct but dystrophin-like protein. The plausible candidate might be chromosome 6-encoded dystrophin related protein (DRP) (11).

According to Khurana and his coworkers (11), the molecular weight of DRP is 400 kDa which is the same as that of dystrophin.

As the peptide IV has 70% homology to the corresponding sequence in B3 reported by Love et al. (9), it is highly possible that the antiserum against peptide IV crossreacts with both dystrophin and DRP.

Therefore, the location of the positive immunofluorescence shown in various stages of *mdx* mouse suggests the developmental expression of DRP in mouse skeletal muscle.

DRP is expressed along the surface membrane in 14 and 20 day embryonic *mdx* muscles and localized at NMJ when the muscle is matured.

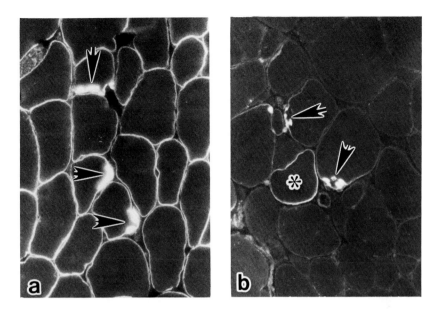

FIG. 3. Immunohistochemistry of adult B10 and *mdx* mouse skeletal muscle with anti-peptide IV antiserum; 3a. B10 mouse (x150); 3b. *mdx* mouse (x150). Arrows indicate neuromuscular junctions. Asterisk indicates a revertant muscle fiber stained with the antiserum.

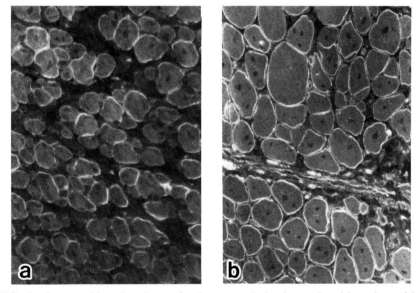

FIG. 4. Immunohistochemistry of *mdx* mouse skeletal muscle with anti-peptide IV antiserum; 4a. 20-day embryo (x200); 4b. 8-day denervated muscle (x150).

Our result on immunoblotting is in accord with the result of Khurana et al. who reported a higher expression of DRP in fetal than in adult mouse skeletal muscle (11).

The reappearance of DRP in the surface membrane of *mdx* mouse 8 days after denervation closely resembles the formation of extra-junctional acetylcholine receptor (AchR) areas along the surface membrane after denervation (6). A similar expression of DRP and AchR during embryonic development and after denervation suggests that DRP could serve a role in molecular organization of AchR.

CONCLUSIONS

Immunoblotting and immunostaining experiments were conducted by using mono- and polyclonal antibodies against a 50 amino acid sequence of C-terminal domain of dystrophin molecule.

It was clarified by monoclonal antibody that the C-terminus is preserved in BMD, but not in DMD.

The result strongly emphasizes the importance of the C-terminal domain for differential diagnosis and confirms the validity of the reading frame hypothesis for DMD/BMD.

In *mdx* mouse, the polyclonal antibodies against the middle of the C-terminal domain of the dystrophin molecule which has high homology with B3 protein was used. This antiserum is supposed to crossreact with both dystrophin and B3 protein.

It was suggested that the chromosome 6-encoded B3 protein, dystrophin related protein is expressed at the surface membrane in the embryonic stage, localized at the neuromuscular junction when muscle matured, and reappeared at the surface membrane of the skeletal muscle after denervation.

ACKNOWLEDGEMENTS

This work was supported by a Research Grant for Nervous and Mental Disorders of the Ministry of Health and Welfare, Japan.

REFERENCES

1.   Arahata, K., Ishiura, S., Ishiguro, T., Tsukahara, T., Suhara, Y., Eguchi, C., Ishihara, T., Nonaka, I., Ozawa, E., and Sugita, H. (1988): Immunostaining of skeletal and cardiac muscle surface membrane with antibody against Duchenne muscular dystrophy peptide. *Nature,* 333:861-863.
2.   Arahata, K., Hoffman, E.P., Kunkel, L.M., Ishiura, T., Tsukahara, T., Ishihara, T., Sunohara, N., Nonaka, I., Ozawa, E., Sugita, H. (1989): Dystrophin diagnosis: comparison of dystrophin abnormalities by immunofluorescence and immunoblot analyses. *Proc. Natl. Acad. Sci. U.S.A.,* 86:7154-7158.
3.   Arahata, K., Beggs, A.H., Honda, H., Ito, S., Ishiura, S., Tsukahara, T., Ishiguro, T., Eguchi, C., Orimo, S., Arikawa, E., Kaido, M., Nonaka, I., Sugita, H., Kunkel, L.M. (1991): Preservation of the C-terminus of dystrophin molecule in the skeletal muscle from Becker muscular dystrophy. *J. Neurol. Sci.,* 101:148-156.

4. Bulman, D.E., Gordon Murphy E., Zubrzycka-Gaarn, E.E., Worton, R.G., Ray, P.N. (1991): Differentiation of Duchenne and Becker muscular dystrophy phenotypes with amino-and carboxy-terminal antisera specific for dystrophin. *Am. J. Hum. Genet.,* 48:295-304.
5. Hoffman, E.P., Kunkel, L.M. (1989): Dystrophin abnormalities in Duchenne/Becker muscular dystrophy. *Neuron,* 2:1019-1029.
6. Howe, P.R.C., Telfer, J.A., Austin, L. (1976): *Exp. Neurol.,* 52:272-284.
7. Ishiura, S., Arahata, K., Tsukahara, T., Koga, R., Anraku, H., Yamaguchi, M., Kikuchi, T., Nonaka, I., Sugita, H. (1990): Antibody against the C-terminal portion of dystrophin crossreacts with the 400 kDa protein in the pia mater of dystrophin-deficient mdx mouse brain. *J. Biochem.,* 107:510-513.
8. Lemaire, C., Heilig, R., Mandel, J.L. (1988): The chicken dystrophin cDNA: striking conservation of the C-terminal coding and 3' untranslated regions between human and chicken. *EMBO J.,* 7:4157-4162.
9. Love, D.R., Hill, D.F., Dickson, G., Spurr, N.K., Byth, B.C., Marsden, R.F., Walsh, F.S., Edwards, Y.H., Davies, K.E. (1989): An autosomal transcript in skeletal muscle with homolgy to dystrophin. *Nature,* 339:55-58.
10. Koenig, M., Monaco, A.P., Kunkel, L.M. (1988): The complete sequence of dystrophin predicts a rod-shaped cytoskeletal protein. *Cell,* 53:219-228.
11. Khurana, T.S., Hoffman, E.P., Kunkel, L.M. (1990): Identification of a chromosome 6-encoded dystrophin-related protein. *J. Biol. Chem.,* 265:16717-16720.
12. Miyatake, M., Miike, T., Zhao, Ji-en, Yoshioka, K., Uchino, M., Usuku, G. (1991): Dystrophin localization and presumed function. *Muscle and Nerve,* 14:113-119.
13. Pons, F., Augier, N., Léger.J.O.C., Robert, A., Tomé, F.M.S., Fardeau, M., Voit, T., Nicholson, L.V.B., Mornet, D., and Léger, J.J. (1991): A homologue of dystrophin is expressed at the neuromuscular junctions of normal individuals and DMD patients, and of normal and mdx mice. *FEBS. Lett.,* 282:161-165.
14. Shimizu, T., Matsumura, K., Sunada, Y., Mannen, T. (1989): Dense immunostainings on both neuromuscular and myotendon junctions with an anti-dystrophin monoclonal antibody. *Biomed. Res .,* 10:405-409.
15. Sugita, H., Arahata, K., Ishiguro, T., Suhara, Y., Tsukahara, T., Ishiura. S., Eguchi, C., Nonaka, I., Ozawa, E., (1988): Negative immunostaining of Duchenne muscular dystrophy (DMD) and mdx mouse muscle surface memberane with antibody against synthetic peptide fragment predicted from DMD cDNA. *Proc Japan Acad.,* 64:210- 212.
16. Takemitsu, M., Ishiura, S., Koga, R., Arahata, K., Nonaka, I., Sugita, H.: A dystrophin homologue on the surface membrane of embryonic and denervated mdx mouse muscle fibres. *Proc. Japan Acad.,* in press.
17. Vainzof, M., Zubrzycka-Gaarn, E.E., Rapaport, D., Passos-Bueno, M.R., Pavanello, R.C.M., Pavanello-Filho, I., Zatz, M. (1991): Immuno-fluorescence dystrophin study in Duchenne dystrophy through the concomitant use of two antibodies directed against the carboxy-terminal and the amino-terminal region of the protein. *J Neurol. Sci.,* 101:141-147.

DISCUSSION

Professor George Karpati:
I think Dr. Sugita deserves congratulations and our appreciation for generating this very important antibody which is monospecific for this dystrophin-related protein (DRP). It is presumably the one that is coded on chromosome 6, although we cannot be absolutely sure. Until this time, the antibodies that people have used to display DRP have cross-reacted with dystrophin and you never knew whether you saw dystrophin or DRP, except if you used mdx or DMD muscle in which Xp21 dystrophin cannot be present. But, with those antibodies, the data were extremely confusing. I feel that you have clarified the situation beautifully, in that DRP is only expressed at the neuromuscular junction in the normal adult muscle. However, in embryonic and denervated muscle it is also expressed over the entire surface membrane just like dystrophin. My question is: what about the myotendinous junctions in normal muscle?

Professor Hideo Sugita:
We are planning to study the localization of dystrophin related protein in the myotendinous junctions, but so far we have no data.

Prof. George Karpati
This point is very important because people had hoped that a molecule which is a dystrophin analogue could compensate for dystrophin deficiency in DMD and mdx but what we have heard here seems to cast doubt upon such a supposition.

Professor Allen D. Roses:
There are a number of patients with myasthenia gravis that do not have circulating antibodies of the acetylcholine receptor site. Have you worked on this possibility?

Professor Hideo Sugita
We also have the same idea as you have mentioned, but we have no data.

Professor Allen D. Roses:
This is of interest because many of these myasthenia patients have had "antimuscle antibodies" that are not the acetylcholine receptor.

GENERAL DISCUSSION

Morning Session

Leaders: Allen D. Roses and John B. Harris

Professor Allen D. Roses:
I am going to play tag with John and let the discussion start with some of the questions regarding your paper. George?

Professor George Karpati:
John Harris was good enough to lend me this slide in which the details of our own experimental concentric versus eccentric contraction results are summarized in mdx versus normal mice by a novel technique.

It is well known that in normal muscle the vulnerability of muscle fibres to necrosis after lengthening contraction is significantly greater than after concentric contraction. What should be emphasized however, is that in the mdx muscle the prevalence of necrosis after lengthening contraction is approximately 5-6 times greater after concentric than eccentric contraction. Nevertheless, what is more to the point is that in normals the prevalence of necrosis after eccentric contraction is 0.7% while in the mdx it is 3.28%, which represents an approximate 5-fold increase. So the message here is, that eccentric or lengthening contractions in mdx muscle produce a much higher frequency of muscle fibre necrosis than in non-dystrophic control muscle.

Professor Allen D. Roses:
George, can you just add one thing as clarification for some of us, what is the definition of eccentric and concentric contractions?

Professor George Karpati:
Very simply, when a muscle shortens during contraction it is then called a concentric contraction. If, during contraction the muscle is stretched by a load, it is then called an eccentric or lengthening contraction. During our daily activities many of our muscles undergo lengthening contractions, in particular, the antigravity muscles of the lower extremities, especially during such activities as walking downstairs. We have suggested that perhaps this might be one of the factors which makes these particular muscles vulnerable to earlier and more profound damage in DMD than other muscles.

Professor Byron A. Kakulas:
Allen, if you permit me I wish to refer to the work of Richard Edwards, a clinical physiologist, who earlier drew attention to the damage that can be caused by eccentric contractions. George, I wonder if you agree, that rather than using the term "contractions" which in itself implies shortening we should refer to "force generation while lengthening" to describe this type of muscle function.

75

Professor George Karpati:

Yes, it would do away with a term that is really an oxymoron. Allen, could I also make a couple of additional comments here in relation to John Harris' talk. I think that his calculations were made on the basis of dystrophin being a monomer not a dimer, and a square lattice instead of a hexagonal lattice. Probably the difference between square and hexagonal would not affect his calculations but being a monomer versus a dimer would make a difference in the marking density. So this would mean either that the marking efficiency is about half what he says it is, if it is a dimer, or it is not a dimer.

Professor John B Harris:

The only evidence I am aware of suggesting that dystrophin is organized as a dimer is based on the evidence that the molecule polymerizes when it has been extracted from muscle.

Professor George Karpati:

There is also the analogy with spectrin.

Professor John B Harris:

The analogy of spectrin is neat, but it is not evidence in favour of the view that dystrophin is organized as a dimer in vivo. I prefer to consider dystrophin organized as a monomer in vivo, because it makes the quantitative analysis of our gold labelling easier to handle.

Professor George Karpati:

I would like to make one other comment, which is that the tightness with which dystrophin is linked to the plasma membrane is remarkable and that reference has been made to the fact that it probably occurs by attachment of the C-terminus to the plasma membrane though linkage proteins which were described by Kevin Campbell. The best evidence of this tight linkage comes from studies we performed with the late Dr Zubrycke-Gaarn of Toronto and Dr Hunter of Glasgow in which we vesiculated plasma membrane of muscle fibres by a well-known technique and the plasma membrane blebs that formed contained dystrophin on the correct side (inside) of it, instead of dystrophin remaining behind the surface of the fibre. The last point I wish to make concerns John Harris' observation about the appearance of dystrophin in regenerating fibres after notexin-induced necrosis, where he wonders why it is a late phenomenon with other specific molecules appearing much earlier. I would suggest, therefore, you consider the fact that in myoblasts, dystrophin is not yet inserted into the surface membrane, so a steady-state equilibrium has to be obtained in regenerating cells before the surface membrane is fully saturated, which takes time. To put it simply, 7 days may not be enough for that.

Dr. Manfred W. Beilharz:

I have a question growing out of an observation that Richard Bartlett made on the complexity of the expression of the dystrophin gene product. His observation on the hot spots where deletions frequently occur made me think that perhaps there must be some recombinase proteins or something like that, that normally maintain the system. This made me think of the family studies that have been done, of deletions which have occurred and been traced from generation to generation. Has anyone ever looked to see whether the frequency with which a new mutation occurs is in fact higher in these families or groups of families than in the general population?

Professor Allen D. Roses:

I will start and then I will pass it over to others. The answer to some is yes and some is no. I have been very interested from the mid-70's in the rate of new mutations and I would like to bring you back in time to tell you what the situation was in 1975. It is clear that the way disease stays in the population is because of a high rate of new mutations. It is almost generally assumed that one-third of cases would be due to new mutation, and that is true. What was not true and what was proven not to be true, was the way that it was applied clinically. The way that it has been applied clinically was that if you were the first child born in a family that had Duchenne dystrophy and your mother did not have an elevated CK, the probability was that there was a new mutation and a lot of these people were counselled that they were "safe". Now since the disease would only occur in one out of every four births, if they were genetic carriers, doctors were right 75% of the time. If they were wrong, the patients never went back to see the same doctors. So if you did this study to look at those people who had a second born, with no prior family history, which we did at that time, we found that they switched clinics, but then they would be defined as genetic carriers. So our interest in this was a clinical interest, where do the new mutations occur and do the new mutations lead? Is it in fact, most of the time, occurring so that a carrier is born and sneaks into the population, having another daughter, perhaps as a carrier, and 3 generations later being the first time that the family is ascertained, and therefore detection of carriers has become a major focus of the laboratories. For years we collected the DNA from every female in the family and all of their children. One of the outcomes of this study, is the finding of multiple mutations. In the study of single families, for instance in one of the families we were using XJ1.1 and we were following it through, but in fact another boy, or another person, in that family had a second mutation we were seeing these things in the context of generations of people spinning out new mutations within the families that we were studying. I do not think the answer to the question is about where these new mutations occur, whether certain families have a propensity of doing it, because those families turn up as families with boys with disease and those families are the only ones we can study. But in fact in families where these new mutations have been documented, in some cases a second mutation has also been documented in these very same families in a later generation.

Dr. Manfred W. Beilharz:

If I can just follow that up, I can appreciate your first point, but the other point that I am not clear on is that there is just no data which would allow you to pin point the rate of spontaneous mutation in the normal population as opposed to the families studied?

Professor Allen D. Roses:

I know, but epidemiologically you can estimate what the rate of that is. There is some data in the literature that you just have to deal with. If you assume that a carrier is going to have in every two pregnancies a male, she is going to have one that is going to be affected on the average, and one that is unaffected. Then we can use standard genetic epidemiology techniques and come down to one third of the cases needing to be by new mutation. A different fact has happened in the last 5 years which is not well publicised. If you do prenatal diagnosis on carriers, what you happen to find is that there are more "normal" male pregnancies than there are "abnormal" male pregnancies.

Professor John B Harris:
We have found that the routine introduction of genetic analysis at gene-level and the examination of protein expression in patients with neuromuscular disorders has resulted in a major revision of our estimates of the incidence and prevalence of Xp21 muscular dystrophy. This in turn has a significant effect on our counselling services, because several of the affected men have families who have never been counselled. I am sure our experience is common to other large centres.

Assist. Professor Richard J. Bartlett:
I wish to amplify part of what Allen has described. We initially had a family with an intronic deletion in both normal and DMD affected male siblings. This deletion was inherited from the mother who had a haploid complement of this segment. When the cDNA became available for testing, the affected male was found to have a new, second mutation in the high frequency deletion region in segment 7/8. One wonders if genetic counselling may be required of the daughters of the unaffected sibling with the intronic deletion. They may in fact repeat the process that occurred with their grandmother to produce their affected uncle. The second case to examine is the family which appears to have a deletion segregating from a mother who is a new mutation, but lacks any evidence of a deletion in her peripheral blood. It is presumed that this is a case of ovarian mosaicism, but that may be only one cause. The second possible cause would be an instability created by the meiotic pairing of two X-chromosomes in repeated events in the ovary which produce the same or very similar deletion events. With the available probes, we can now begin to test this sort of possiblity.

Dr. Nigel G. Laing:
We have investigated a pedigree (3) where two family members were diagnosed as having Becker muscular dystrophy, but in whom we could not identify a mutation in the dystrophin gene. However, in a foetus from the family, terminated on the basis of sex and which had been stored in liquid nitrogen, we did identify a deletion of the gene. So here is one family with multiple people affected and with 2 distinct mutations in the Duchenne gene. The deletion is an out of frame deletion, suggesting that if the foetus, had been born it would have had Duchenne muscular dystrophy. So some families where you see different phenotypes may well have multiple mutations and again with the molecular techniques available, this can be looked at. I know of one other family where this has been seen but I notice that you John were nodding your head and Richard was talking about everybody seeing such families. We have looked for mutations in 11 families from Western Australia with more than one affected family member and we found one with multiple mutations. Perhaps suggesting to me, in response to your question Manfred, that in families segregating Duchenne or Becker dystrophy the mutation rate in the gene may be higher than in the "normal population".

Dr. Manfred W. Beilharz:
So you agree with what I have suggested in that there may be some controlling protein which is governing the successful maintenance of this very complex gene and its expression?

Dr. Nigel G. Laing:
I have no idea, I do not want to speculate. All that I am saying is that in Duchenne and Becker families the mutation rate may be higher than in the general population. But a proper study of this question, to prove it one way or the other, would require a multi-centre, multinational collaboration to obtain sufficient numbers to perform the statistical analysis.

Professor Allen D. Roses:
It is sort of interesting to go back. We use to have great difficulty in making the distinction between Becker muscular dystrophy and Duchenne muscular dystrophy and arguments would rage at meetings because there would be both in the same family. Of course everyone knew that Becker muscular dystrophy was at a different locus, near colour blindness at the other end of the chromosome and it was very hard to make sense of this. Going back to those families, we had a very interesting family where the older boy is 29 now and is still walking, the younger boy was in a wheelchair at 11 years old and again this now turns out most probably to be a difference in a mutation in a degree of what has happened to a gene in this family. I think that the data should be looked at from that angle, in that there seems to be an increased incidence of new mutations in families that probably already carry something. Whether this is a controlling protein because it does not line up right, meiosis or whatever, it is unclear.

Assist. Professor Richard J. Bartlett:
The paper that appeared in "Cell" (1) had two patients who had exon 50 deleted. In one, the mRNA processing created an in frame mutation corresponding with a Becker phenotype whereas the other had an alternative splicing which created an out of frame mutation leading to a Duchenne phenotype.

Dr. Nigel G. Laing:
In relation to that, we are studying one West Australian family which does have the exon 3-7 deletion which may produce either a Becker or Duchenne phenotype (2). This family historically has shown variable phenotype with some members severely affected and others not. To look at the alternate splicing in family members with variable phenotype would be interesting, but the severely affected family members are dead and we do not have any stored tissue.

Professor Allen D. Roses:
One of the things I guess we are probably not as concerned with in this conference is that there are other dystrophinopathies that really do not look like what we call "standard" Duchenne and "standard" muscular dystrophy and there are some that have looked like spinal muscular atrophy patients. Implications of that for therapy, I think are very important because what we may do for Duchenne dystrophy may have implications for all dystrophinopathies and will include a wider range of disease spectra and their models than what we are basically concerned with. I think that within the next day or so we will be working into the models themselves and I think some interesting questions may be anticipated,such as why the mdx mouse is a healthy little mouse, as compared to what we see in the dog and what are the implications for therapeutic consequences of what we find.

REFERENCES

1. Chelly, J., Gilgenkrantz, H., et al (1990): Effect of dystrophin gene deletions on mRNA levels and processing in Duchenne and Becker muscular dystrophies. *Cell,* 63:1239-1248.
2. Koenig, M., Beggs, A.H., et al (1989): The molecular basis of Duchenne versus Becker muscular dystrophy: correlation of severity with type of deletion. *Am. J. Hum. Genet.,* 45:498-506.
3. Laing, N.G., Layton, M.G., Johnsen R.D., Chandler, D.C., Mears, M.E., Goldblatt, J., Kakulas, B.A. (1991): Two distinct mutations in a dystrophin gene: chance occurrence or pre-mutation? *Am. J. Med. Genet.,* (In Press).

DUCHENNE MUSCULAR DYSTROPHY: Animal Models
and Genetic Manipulation, edited by Byron A. Kakulas,
John McC. Howell, and Allen D. Roses.
Raven Press, Ltd., New York © 1992.

6

Immunocytochemical Analysis of Dystrophin in Muscular Dystrophy

Eri Arikawa, Kiichi Arahata, Nobuhiko Sunohara,
Shoichi Ishiura, Ikuya Nonaka, Hideo Sugita

*Division of Neuromuscular Research,
National Institute of Neuroscience, NCNP,
4-1-1 Ogawahigashi, Kodaira, Tokyo 187, Japan.*

INTRODUCTION

Recent advances in molecular genetics have revolutionized the diagnostic approach to patients with muscular dystrophy.
Complete cloning of the coding sequence for the DMD gene(13,14) and discovery of the gene product, dystrophin(10,11), are great successes in muscular dystrophy research. Dystrophin testing(12) with both protein and DNA-based analyses is quite useful in distinguishing DMD, BMD and patients with other neuromuscular disorders. Furthermore these tests are also very useful for detecting DMD/BMD carriers.
We have established region specific anti-dystrophin antibodies. We synthesized four oligopeptides deduced from the DMD cDNA corresponding to different regions of the dystrophin molecule, peptide I corresponding to the amino acid sequence 215-264, peptide II to 440-489, peptide III to 2359-2408, and IV to 3459-3544(1,4,13). Using these oligopeptides, several polyclonal and monoclonal antibodies specific to dystrophin were raised. This battery of antisera allows us to detect the presence or absence of several different regions of dystrophin.

DYSTROPHIN DIAGNOSIS OF
DUCHENNE/BECKER MUSCULAR DYSTROPHY

Although in normal individuals, dystrophin is detected immuno-cytochemically as a homogeneous ring around the periphery of all muscle fibers(1,15), muscle from DMD patients has little or no detectable staining(1,8,15), while muscle from BMD patients shows variable staining and occasionaly patchy and/or faintly stained fibers. By immunoblot analysis, dystrophin is generally undetectable in muscle samples from DMD patients. But, muscle biopsies from BMD patients show abnormal dystrophin protein of either altered molecular weight, or amount, or both(3). For DMD carriers, immunocytochemistry is a most useful method for detecting patches of negative fibers among positive ones(2). However, it should be noted that even if there are no negative fibers we can not rule out the diagnosis of a DMD carrier. DNA-based deletion analysis and linkage analysis are currently performed for clinical diagnosis. Using 18 pairs of multiplex primers designed by Chamberlain(9) and Beggs(7), up to 98% of gene deletions can be identified by PCR analysis(7). Thus PCR analysis is becoming useful because it is capable of rapid deletion detection on small quantities of DNA. However, duplications are harder to detect by the PCR, so patients with no detectable mutations should be analized further by the Southern blot test.

Table. 1   **Differential diagnosis of DMD/BMD**

	DMD	**BMD**	**Manifesting carrier of DMD**	**Normal muscle**
Immuno-staining pattern	negative	faint &/or patchy	mosaic	normal (continuous)
Amount of dystrophin	<3%	normal or decrease	normal or decrease	normal
Molecular weight of dystrophin	undetect-able	larger or smaller	normal	normal (427kd)
Gene abnormality	yes	yes	heterozygote	no

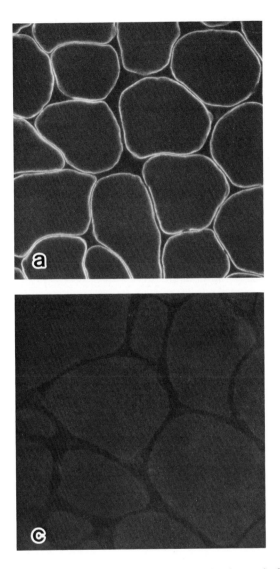

FIG. 1. (a and c):   Frozen sections of biopsied skeletal muscle from control (1-a) and DMD(1-c) immunostained with monoclonal anti-dystrophin antibody raised against peptide IV. Note the complete absence of immunostaining in DMD muscle compared with clear immunostaining of all the surface membrane in control muscle.

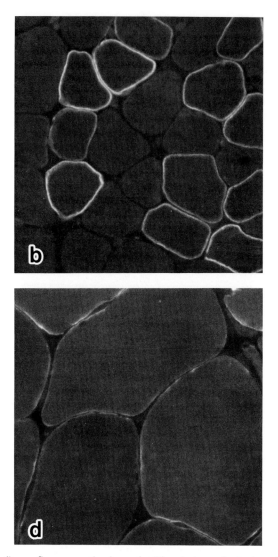

FIG. 1. (b and d): Some methods as in Fig. 1 (a and c) showing immuno-staining of manifesting carrier (1-b) and BMD patient (1-d). The BMD patient shows faint and patchy immunostaining. The manifesting carrier of DMD shows mosaic of positive and negative immunostaining.

QUADRICEPS MYOPATHY (QM)
FORME FRUSTE OF BECKER MUSCULAR DYSTROPHY

Patients with mild and slowly progressive muscle wasting and weakness limited to the quadriceps femoris muscle have been diagnosed as QM, which has been regarded as a disease entity including a heterogeneous group of disorders such as limb-girdle muscular dystrophy(LGD), spinal muscular atrophy, and polymyositis . We examined dystrophin in muscle biopsy specimens from 4 male patients with QM(16). All 4 patients had clear abnormalities of dystrophin, and were considered as having BMD by both immunofluorescence and immunoblot tests. Dystrophin of an abnormal molecular mass was visualized in cryosections of muscle as patchy immunostaining at the surface membrane of the muscle fibers. From these results we concluded that the syndrome called QM includes a group of form fruste of BMD.

DYSTROPHIN ANALYSIS IN FUKUYAMA
CONGENITAL MUSCULAR DYSTROPHY (FCMD).

FCMD, an autosomal recessive disorder endemic to Japan but rarely observed in other countries, is a congenital muscular dystrophy with associated central nervous system involvement. Although a gene abnormality has not been detected, histopathological changes of skeletal muscle in FCMD are similar to those seen in DMD or even more severe when compared with age-matched DMD. We examined dystrophin expression patterns of skeletal muscles in 36 FCMD patients by immunocytochemical methods(6). Basically, 34 out of 36 FCMD patients showed positive immunoreaction. However, occasional fibers (mean=28%) were negative or reacted abnormality (partially deficient, fluffy, or intense) for dystrophin immunostaining. In contrast, muscle fibers in age-matched non FCMD patients showed a significantly lower percentage (mean=4%) of negative and abnormal staining for dystrophin. Interestingly, immunoreaction for spectrin, a membrane associated cytoskeletal protein related to dystrophin, was preserved in DMD muscle (9%) much better than in FCMD muscle (mean=25%). Most of the abnormally immunoreacting fibers for dystrophin and spectrin were acridine orange positive early regenerating fibers or C9 positive necrotic fibers. However, some of these fibers were normal-looking fibers without C9 immunostaining. Immunocytochemical abnormalities of dystrophin and spectrin in FCMD muscle may represent secondary events, but the presence of some primary factor(s) associated with membrane damage can not be excluded. Dystrophin was undetectable in 2 out of 36 patients by both immunocytochemical and immunoblot analyses the dystrophin test is useful to differentiate some DMD patients from FCMD patients.

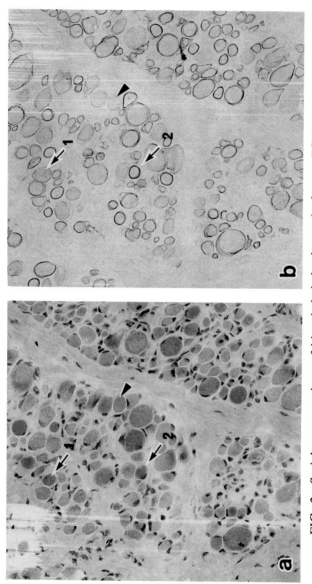

FIG. 2. Serial cross sections of biopsied skeletal muscle from a FCMD patient stained with haematoxylin and eosin(2-a), and immunostained for dystrophin (2-b). Note the heterogeneous pattern of immunostaining for dystrophin, i.e. negative (arrowhead), partially deficient (arrow 1), intense (arrow 2), and normal fibers in the section.

DYSTROPHIN ABNORMALITIES IN PATIENTS WITH A CLINICAL DIAGNOSIS OF LIMB-GIRDLE MUSCULAR DYSTROPHY (LGD)

LGD is a descriptive diagnosis which may represent a genetically heterogeneous group of disorders. We have analyzed over 40 cases for dystrophin in muscle by both immunofluorescence and immunoblot(5). We identified 5 male patients with an abnormal dystrophin pattern diagnostic of BMD, and 2 female patients with a dystrophin pattern consistent with manifesting carriers of DMD. Thus, approximately 20% of patients with the clinical diagnosis of LGD showed abnormalities of dystrophin. Using PCR analysis, we found dystrophin gene deletions in all 5 male patients.

ACKNOWLEDGEMENTS

We would like to thank Mmes. Kanako Goto, Ritsuko Koga, and Ms. Harumi Anraku. for their expert technical assistance.
This work was supported by a Research Grant for Nervous and Mental Disorders of the Ministry of Health and Welfare, Japan.

REFERENCES

1. Arahata, K., Ishiura, S., Ishiguro, T., Tsukahara, T., Suhara, Y., Eguchi., C., Ishihara, T., Nonaka, I., Ozawa, E., Sugita, H. (1988): Immunostaining of skeletal and cardiac muscle surface membrane with antibody against Duchenne muscular dystrophy peptide. *Nature*, 333:861-863.
2. Arahata, K., Ishihara, T., Kamakura, K., Tsukahara, T., Ishiura, S., Baba, C., Matsumoto, T., Nonaka, I., Sugita, H. (1989): Mosaic expression of dystrophin in symptomatic carriers of Duchenne muscular dystrophy. *N. Eng. J. Med.,* 320:138-142.
3. Arahata, K., Hoffman, EP., Kunkel, LM., Ishiura, S., Tsukahara T., Ishihara T., Sunohara, N., Nonaka, I., Ozawa, E., Sugita H. (1989): Dystrophin diagnosis: comparison of dystrophin abnormalities by immunofluorescent and immunoblot analysis. *Proc. Natl. Soc. Acad. Sci. USA.,* 86:7154-7158.
4. Arahata, K., Beggs, A.H., Honda, H,. Ito, S., Ishiura, S., Tsukahara, T., Ishiguro, T., Eguchi, C., Orimo, S., Arikawa, E., Kaido, M., Nonaka, I., Sugita, H., Kunkel, L.M. (1991): Preservation of C-terminus of dystrophin molecule in the skeletal muscle from Becker muscular dystrophy. *J. Neurol. Sci.,* 101:148-156.
5. Arikawa, E., Ishihara, T., Nonaka, I., Sugita, H., Arahata, K. (1991): Immunocytochemical analysis of dystrophin in congenital muscular dystrophy. *J Neurol. Sci.,* (in press).
6. Arikawa, E., Hoffman, E.P., Kaido, M., Nonaka, I., Sugita, H. Arahata, K. (1991): The frequency of patients having dystrophin abnormalities in a limb-girdle patient population. *Neurology,* (in press).

7. Beggs, A.H., Koenig, M,. Boyce, M., Kunkel, L.M. (1991): Detection of 98% of DMD/BMD gene deletions by polymerase chain reaction. *Hum. Genet.*, 86:45-48.
8. Bonilla, E., Samitt, C.E., Miranda, A.F., Hays, A.P., Salvatore, G., DiMauro, S., Kunkel, L.M., Hoffman, E.P., Rowland, L.P.(1988): Duchenne muscular dystrophy:deficiency of dystrophin at the muscle cell surface. *Cell*, 54:447-452.
9. Chamberlain, J.S., Gibbs, R.A., Ranier, J.E., Nguyen P.N., Caskey, C.T. (1988): Deletion screening of Duchenne muscular dystrophy locus via multiplex DNA amplification. *Nucl . Acids Res.*, 23:11141-11156.
10. Hoffman, E.P., Brown, R.H. Jr, Kunkel, L.M. (1987): Dystrophin: the protein product of the Duchenne muscular dystrophy locus. *Cell*, 51:919-928.
11. Hoffman, E.P., Kunkel, L.M. (1989): Dystrophin abnormalities in Duchenne/Becker muscular dystrophy. *Neuron.*, 2:1019-1029.
12. Hoffman, E.P., Kunkel, L.M., Angelini, C., Clarke, A., Johnson M., Harris, J.B. (1989): Improved Diagnosis of Becker muscular dystrophy via dystrophin testing. *Neurology*, 39:1011-1017.
13. Koenig. M., Hoffman, E.P., Bertelson, C.J., Monaco, A.P., Feener, C., Kunkel, L.M. (1987): Complete cloning of the Duchenne muscular dystrophy (DMD)cDNA and preliminary genomic organization of DMD gene in normal and affected individuals. *Cell*, 50:509-517.
14. Koenig, M., Monaco, A.P., Kunkel, L.M. (1988): The complete sequence of dystrophin predicts a rod-shaped cytoskeletal protein. *Cell*, 53:219-228.
15. Sugita, H., Arahata, K., Ishiguro, T., Suhara, Y., Tsukahara, T., Ishiura, S., Eguchi, C., Nonaka, I., Ozawa, E. (1988): Negative immunostaining of Duchenne muscular dystrophy (DMD) and mdx mouse muscle surface membrane with antibody against synthetic peptide from DMD cDNA. *Proc. Japan Acad.*, 64:210-212.
16. Sunohara,N,. Arahata, K., Hoffman, E.P., Yamada, H., Nishimiya, J., Arikawa, E., Kaido, M., Nonaka, I., Sugita, H. (1990): Quadriceps myopathy: form fruste of Becker muscular dystrophy. *Ann. Neurol.*, 28:634-639.

DISCUSSION

Professor Allen D. Roses:
Has anybody looked genetically at the Fukuyama disease with probes for spectrin?

Dr. Eri Arikawa:
As far as I know, no molecular genetical study has been performed on FCMD, but I do not think FCMD is caused by an abnormality of the spectrin gene, because change of spectrin seems to me a secondary phenomenon, not primary.

Professor Byron A. Kakulas:
You have not told us whether you thought the changes were primary or secondary. Do you believe that there is a deletion or an abnormality of the Duchenne gene in these patients?

DUCHENNE MUSCULAR DYSTROPHY: Animal Models
and Genetic Manipulation, edited by Byron A. Kakulas,
John McC. Howell, and Allen D. Roses.
Raven Press, Ltd., New York © 1992.

7

Relevance of Animal Models for Human Disease

J. McC. Howell

School of Veterinary Studies,
Murdoch University,
Murdoch, Western Australia

Duchenne Muscular Dystrophy was first described in, and is of great importance in, boys. It was then described in a number of other mammals, in which it is of importance, because the disease in animals other than man can serve as a model for the disease in boys. The second mammal in which the disease was discovered was the mouse (4), then several years later the condition was found in dogs (13), and more recently in cats (5). Colonies of affected mice and dogs have been established and work on these models is reported elsewhere in this book (2,6,12,17,18,19).

This paper will indicate in general terms the value of animal models of human disease, how they might best be used for the benefit of people and other animals, comment about their use in the evaluation of therapies and preventive regimes, and give some examples of valuable positive and negative results which have been obtained in therapy trials.

A large number of animal models for human disease have been described. Reports of many of them have been published in the American Journal of Pathology and the Comparative Pathology Bulletin. They have been brought together in the fascicles of the Handbook: Animal Models of Human Disease published by the Registry of Comparative Pathology of the Armed Forces Institute of Pathology in Washington D.C. In 1989 the US National Institutes of Health held a conference which they called "Modelling in Biomedical Research" (1). The purpose of the conference was to assess the status and potential of models to studies in cardiovascular/pulmonary function and diabetes. The motivating hypothesis was that "continued innovation and development in model systems is important to progress in improving the health of the nation". The conference considered mathematical, computer, physical, tissue culture, mammalian and non-mammalian models. The conclusion was that biomedical research would be most effectively advanced by the continued application of a combination of models used in a complimentary and interactive manner.

Many animal models have been of diseases with a significant genetic component. This might involve a mutation of the homologous gene or an interference with the message or function of the gene product. The phenotypic characteristics of a genetic disease which occurs in several species will be modified by differences within those species. When the disease occurs in humans and in animals the various expressions of the disease may act as multiple models, and if we are clever we can use the similarities and differences found within the species to extend our knowledge of pathogenesis and treatment of the disease.

The disease state cannot be fully comprehended until there is an understanding of the animal in normality. Animal models have been of immense value in helping to develop an understanding of the normal structure and function of tissues and of physiological and biochemical processes in health and in disease. I will give three examples. The giant axon of the squid was the key experimental system at the birth of modern neuroscience. Much of our knowledge of microvascular physiology and of the fundamental importance of microvascular changes in acute inflammation came from studies made on the mesentery of the frog. The basic work on the role of insulin in glucose metabolism and its importance in the disorder diabetes melitus was carried out in the dog.

Studies on diabetes mellitus revealed that it was not a single disease and it has been divided into two major types. Type 1 diabetes mellitus is insulin dependent and has many characteristics of an autoimmune disease. Type 11 diabetes mellitus is non-insulin dependant and usually has a late onset. There is a genetic component to both diseases. Animal models of both genetic forms of the disease occur in rodents, there are naturally occurring models in domesticated animals and models can be produced experimentally by surgical removal of the pancreas, the administration of streptozocin or alloxan, or by overfeeding. Morphological and functional changes may develop in the kidneys, eyes and nerves of the laboratory animal models, and although the changes may not be identical to those found in these tissues in man, they may be used to investigate pathogenetic mechanisms and to evaluate treatments. Studies using animal models have shown that transplanted islet tissue has reversed experimentally induced diabetes mellitus in rat, mouse, pig and dog (9). However, immune rejection is a major problem. Advances have been made in developing techniques utilising pancreatic transplants without immunosuppression by the use of foetal islet tissue cultured in an atmosphere of 95% oxygen and 5% carbon dioxide (3). Work is continuing on this aspect of the problem and has been greatly aided by the use of animal models.

A study of animal models of diseases found in humans may have the following advantages :

• Humans are mammals, and as a group, mammals contain similar anatomical and functional systems which may respond in a similar manner to metabolic upsets, pathogens and therapies.

• Mammalian models can be found in which diseases develop and respond to therapy in a similar way to people. Therefore they can be used to investigate new treatments and new ways of delivering treatments.

Mammalian models offer the only reliable means of testing the collective response of the whole system. A response in which not only does the target organ react but in which the complex array of detoxification, metabolism, immunity and inflammation can come into play.

Animal models are properly subject to concerns for their welfare, and are subject to legal and moral constraints. However they are more amenable to investigative procedures than are human patients.

The time of onset, or even the presence or absence of clinical, biochemical and morphological changes can be predicted more accurately.

In most instances the desired number of animals can be fitted into each experimental and positive or negative control group.

With suitable constraints and precautions invasive techniques can be more readily carried out. Samples of tissues for morphological and biochemical examination can be readily obtained.

Postmortem examinations can be carried out in all cases.

Mammalian models are accepted by Federal Governments for mandated testing of new drugs.

The limitations are:-

Different species may respond in different ways because of a difference in anatomy. A drug will not inflame the gall bladder of a horse because it does not have one.

All animal models may not respond in the same way because of differences in their physiology. If a safe dose for the toxin fluroacetate had been determined in Western Australian marsupials the amount would have been lethal for almost every other animal, for Western Australian marsupials have evolved an efficient detoxifying pathway for fluroacetate, a compound which exists in some native plants (15).

Some mammalian models are difficult and/or costly to acquire and maintain.

The use of animal models will undoubtedly facilitate the quest for treatments for Duchenne Muscular Dystrophy. It has already done so in the area of myoblast transfer. Myoblast supply the genetic material that is absent in the muscles. Bone marrow cells have also been used to supply missing genetic material. Positive results have been reported in bone marrow transplantation therapy trials involving a number of animal models of lysosomal storage diseases (10). These have included fucosidosis (alpha-fucosidase deficiency) mucopoly-saccharidosis 1 (alpha-L-iduronidase deficiency) and mucopoly-saccharidosis V11 (beta-glucuronidase deficiency) in dogs; the twitcher - globoid cell leucodystrophy - (galactosylceramidase deficiency) and mucopolysaccharidosis V11 (beta-glucuronidase deficiency) in mice; and mucopolysaccharidosis 1 (alpha-L-iduronidase deficiency) mucopoly-saccharidosis V1 (arylsulphatase deficiency) GM1 gangliosidosis (beta-galactosidase deficiency) Gm2 gangliosidosis (hexosaminidase deficiency) and alpha-mannosidosis (alpha-mannosidase deficiency) in cats.

There are a number of problems associated with replacement therapies. These include: 1) targeting the replacement gene or protein to the appropriate site and 2) the development of immune rejection. Targeting to the central nervous system is a major problem but a number of successes have been claimed in animal studies including the recently reported bone marrow transplantation in fucosidosis, globoid cell leucodystrophy and mucopolysaccharidosis 1 (10).

Immune rejection can be a severe complication in transplantation therapy trials. The use of an animal model may overcome this difficulty and allow a clearer evaluation of the uncomplicated effect of replacement. Di Marco *et al* (8) reported that adding acid alpha glucosidase to cultures of muscle from cattle with Pompe's Disease resulted in the uptake of the enzyme and a reduction of glycogen to normal concentrations. Thus demonstrating a positive result for enzyme replacement therapy *in vitro* and indicating that such replacement may be feasible *in vivo* in this disease. Bone marrow transplantation had been tried unsuccessfully in children (20) and it was possible that immune rejection could have played a significant part in this.

In twin calves the placentae join, and the calves receive bone marrow precursor cells from one another *in utero* before the immune system develops. They become lymphoreticular chimeras and the bone marrow transplants are not subject to immune rejection. Using embryo transfer techniques twin calves were produced, one of which had Pompe's Disease and the other was normal. Because of the chimeric state, circulating leucocytes in both the normal and affected calves produced active acid alpha glucosidase. In the affected twins the activity of the enzyme in leucocytes was always significantly greater than in affected single calves and in one affected twin there was no significant difference in activity to that found in normal single calves. The activity of the enzyme was higher than that found in affected single animals in a number of other tissues, but this was only statistically significant in biopsies of semitendinosus muscle and in spleen, lymph node and diaphragm removed at the time of death. The concentration of glycogen was significantly lowered in liver, spleen and lymph node of the affected twins but was not lowered in any of the muscles examined and the progress and degree of muscle damage and the development of clinical signs were not affected (11). This negative result indicates that bone marrow transplantation will not be effective as a treatment for Pompe's Disease.

Bone marrow transplantation and myoblast transfer are a means of supplying a normal gene to an animal that is deficient in that particular gene and therefore in that particular gene product. Recent work has shown that Duchenne Muscular Dystrophy is associated with the absence of a normally functioning dystrophin gene (16). The supply of the normal functioning gene - gene therapy - must be considered in the treatment of this group of muscular dystrophies. There are a number of problems associated with gene therapy and they again include targeting and the possibility that the gene product may evoke an immune response.

There are also specific problems related to the supply of genes which include failure of expression of the introduced gene and the problem of location of the introduced gene.

The gene may be placed into the cell but it is not possible to put it into its normal position in the chromosome. If the DNA which is added integrates into the middle of a functioning gene the function of that gene is likely to be disrupted. This may not be important in somatic cells but could be of great importance in germ cells.

Work on animal models has been of great help in progressing the use of genes towards therapy. Much experimental work has been done on adding normally functioning genes to somatic cells and to germ cells. Bone marrow stem cells have commonly been used and DNA has been inserted by calcium phosphate precipitation or by the use of retroviruses. The treated bone marrow cells have then been returned to the host where they have lodged in the bone marrow and multiplied. However only a small proportion of the bone marrow cells have expressed the gene. Following insertion of the gene into a fertilised ovum, the gene is distributed to all cells. It usually functions well in the cells in which it normally expresses and does not function in those cells in which it is not normally expressed (7).

Positive results with gene therapy have been obtained in animal models. Wolff *et al* (21) used an animal model - the mouse - to demonstrate the expression of beta-galactosidase and luciferase activity in muscle following the direct injection of the appropriate genes without the use of special delivery systems. Kyle *et al* (14) demonstrated the correction of mucopolysaccharidosis V11 in the mouse model by using a human beta-glucuronidase gene. The DNA fragment was injected into male pronuclei of F1 and F2 zygotes. Homozygous mucopolysaccharidosis V11 mice produce virtually no murine beta-glucuronidase. However, the transgenic mice homozygous for the mucopolysaccharidase V11 mutation expressed high levels of human beta-glucuronidase activity in all tissues examined and were phenotypically normal. This experiment using transgenic animals illustrates the values and the problems of gene therapy, for in the animals in which it was successful it worked well. But expression was only produced in 4 out of the 29 animals born from the injected zygotes.

Germ cell treatments may tell us many things about the action of the gene and its product in the whole body, but will germ cell gene therapy ever be used for the treatment of genetic disease? Insertion of the gene into a fertilised egg would involve the use of *in vitro* fertilisation. There would be no point in inserting a gene into a normal fertilised egg. Indeed harm might be done by this procedure. Therefore one would have to distinguish a normal from an abnormal fertilised egg. Having done so it would be much more sensible to implant the normal fertilised egg and to discard the abnormal one rather than to treat and implant it. Germ cell gene therapy will be a useful experimental tool but is unlikely to make an impact as a means of clinical treatment (7).

I believe that the use of animal models is an integral component of the work that is being undertaken to increase understanding of the pathogenesis of disease and that such models are essential in the development of therapies.

ACKNOWLEDGEMENTS

I wish to thank my colleagues Drs. P.R. Dorling and C.R. Huxtable for useful discussions.

REFERENCES

1.   Anon (1989): An NIH Conference Modelling in biomedical research: An assessment of current and potential approaches. U.S. Department of Health and Human Services, Bethesda.
2.   Bartlett, R.J. (1991): Potential strategies for gene therapy in GRMD. In: Animal Models for Duchenne Muscular Dystrophy and Genetic Manipulation Workshop.
3.   Bowen, K.M., Lafferty, K.J. (1980): Reversal of diabetes by allogeneic islet transplantation without immunosuppression. *Aust. J. Exp. Bio. Med. Sci* . 58:441.
4.   Bulfield, G., Siller, W.G., Wright, P.A.L., Moore, K.Y. (1984): X-chromosome-linked muscular dystrophy (mdx) in the mouse. *Proc. Natl. Acad. Sci.* USA. 81:1189.
5.   Carpenter, J.L., Hoffman, R.P., Romanul, R.C., Kunkel, L.M., Rosales,

R.K., Ma, N.S., Dasbach, J.J., Rae, J.F., Moore, F.M., McAfee, M.B. Pearce, L.K. (1989): Feline muscular dystrophy with dystrophin deficiency. *Am. J. Pathol* . 135:909.

6. Cooper, B.J. (1991): In: Animal Models for Duchenne Muscular Dystrophy and genetic Manipulation Workshop.

7. Danks, D.M. (1988): DNA and clinical medicine. *Aust. NZ. Med.* 18:339.

8. Di Marco, P.N., Howell, J. McC., Dorling, P.R. (1985): Bovine glycogenosis type II. Uptake of lysosomal alpha-glucosidase by cultured skeletal muscule and reversal of glycogen accumulation. *FEBS Letters* 190:301.

9. Eloy, R., Doillon, C., Dubois, P. (1980): Fetal pancreatic transplantation - Review of experimental data. *Trans. Proc.* 12: Suppl. 2.

10. Haskins, M., Baker, H.J., Burkenmeier, E., Hoogerbrugge, P.M., Poorthuis, B.J.H.M., Sakiyama, T., Shull, R.M., Taylor, R.M., Thrall, M.A., Walkley, S.U. (1991): Transplantation in Animal Model Systems. In: Proceedings of the 5th International Congress on inborn Errors of Metabolism (In the press).

11. Howell, J.McC., Dorling, P.R., Shelton, J.N., Taylor, E.G., Palmer, D.G., DiMarco, P.N. (1992): Natural bone marrow transplantation in cattle with Pompe's disease. *Neuromus. Disorders* (in press).

12. Kornegay, J.N. (1991): Golden Retriever muscular dystrophy: the model and relevance to developmental therapeutics. In: Animal Model for Duchenne Muscular Dystrophy and Genetic Manipulation Workshop.

13. Kornegay, J.N., Luler, S.M., Miller, D.M., Levesque, D.C. (1988): Muscular dystrophy in a litter of Golden Retriever dogs. *Muscle and Nerve* 11:1056.

14. Kyle, J.W., Birkenmeier, E.H., Gwynn, B., Vogler, C., Hoppe, P.C., Hoffman, J.W., Sly, W.S. (1990): Correction of murine mycopolysaccharidosis VII by a human -glucuronidase transgene. *Proc. Natl. Acad. Sci* . USA 87:3914.

15. Mead, R.J., Oliver, A.J., King, D.R., Hubach, P.H. (1985): The co-evolutionary role of fluoroacetate in plant - animal interactions in Australia. *OIKOS* 44:55.

16. Monaco, A.P., Neve, R.L., Colletti-Feener, C., Bertelson, C.J., Kirnit, D.M., Kunkel, L.N. (1986): Isolation of candidate cDNAs for portions of the Duchenne muscular dystrophy gene. *Nature* 323:646.

17. Partridge, T.A. (1991): Mdx mouse : A model of Duchenne Muscular Dystrophy. In: Animal Models for Duchenne Muscular Dystrophy and genetic Manipulation Workshop.

18. Partridge, T.A. (1991): Results of myoblast transplantation in the mdx mouse. In: Animal Models for Duchenne Muscular Dystrophy and genetic Manipulation Workshop.

19. Sugita, H. (1991): Expression of C-terminal domain of dystrophin in Duchenne/Becker Muscular Dystrophy and mdx mouse. In: Animal Models for Duchenne Muscular Dystrophy and genetic Manipulation Workshop.

20. Watson, J.G., Gardner-Medwin, D., Goldfinch, M.E., Pearson, A.D.J. (1986). Bone marrow transplantation for glycogen storage disease type II (Pompe's disease). *N. Eng. J. Med.* 314: 385.

21. Wolff, J.A., Balone, R.W., Williams, P., Chong, W., Ascadi, G., Jani, A., Felgner, P.L. (1990): Direct gene transfer into mouse muscle *in vivo*. *Science*. 247:1465.

DUCHENNE MUSCULAR DYSTROPHY: Animal Models and Genetic Manipulation, edited by Byron A. Kakulas, John McC. Howell, and Allen D. Roses. Raven Press, Ltd., New York © 1992.

8

The *mdx* Mouse: A Model of Duchenne Muscular Dystrophy

T. A. Partridge, J.E. Morgan, G.R. Coulton*

*Departments of Histopathology and *Biochemistry, Charing Cross & Westminster Medical School, Fulham Palace Road, London W6 8RF, U.K.*

DISCOVERY AND EARLY DESCRIPTIONS

Prior to the discovery of the *mdx* mouse in the early 1980's (4), all animal genetic models of muscular dystrophy were autosomally inherited. By virtue of the well established principle of conservation of X-chromosome linkage of genes within placental mammals (24), this disqualified them from homology with the commonest and most severe human muscular dystrophies, namely the X-linked Duchenne (DMD) and Becker (BMD) dystrophies. The only possible exception was the chicken muscular dystrophy model. Thus, the finding of a mouse (*mdx*) which leaked muscle enzymes into its serum and which exhibited extensive muscle fibre necrosis, as X-chromosome-linked traits, excited some interest (4).

Unfortunately, the myopathy did not live up to expectation as a model of DMD, or indeed of any other human dystrophy, and the *mdx* mouse fell into disuse until interest was rekindled by the discovery that it suffered from the same biochemical defect as Duchenne children, i.e. it lacked the protein dystrophin (14). Much debate has since been directed at the paradox - for it is commonly seen as such - of how two species with a common biochemical lesion can exhibit such different clinico-pathological phenotypes. This article will examine some of the suggested resolutions of this paradox and will discuss the uses and limitations of the *mdx* mouse in the investigation of muscular dystrophy and in the search for therapeutic strategies.

THE *mdx* MUTATION

One of the earliest directions to be explored in search of an explanation of the clinical eccentricity of the *mdx* mouse was the idea that it was not truely a genetic homologue of DMD and that some property of the particular lesion of the dystrophin gene in this animal might account for its mild phenotype. Analysis of the dystrophin gene in the *mdx* mouse revealed that the genetic defect was a point mutation involving a single base change within an exon which should produce a full-length mRNA with a 'stop' signal about 27% along its length whereas the majority of DMD cases arise from detectable deletions(27). This, on translation, would be predicted to generate a truncated protein lacking the C-terminus. Perhaps because a large section of the message is never occupied by ribosomes, it is rapidly degraded and, although found at the expected full length, is present at only 10% of the normal concentration (7).

Since the original discovery of the spontaneous *mdx* mutant, 3 further mdx mutations have been generated deliberately by treatment of male mice with ethyl-nitroso-urea, a point mutagen (8). It is likely that all of these will be point mutations, each differing from the original. PCR analysis supports the second of these expectations (Chamberlain, personal communication). Superficially at least, these new *mdx* mice are indistinguishable from the original mutation, arguing that the mild nature of the myopathy is attributable to the murine background rather than to a particular mutation.

This rationale can be applied more generally, for example, between 0.1% and 0.01% of muscle fibres in the *mdx* mouse stain positively for dystrophin(16). The fact that these 'revertant' fibres are also seen at similar frequencies in the 3 new *mdx* mutants as well as in a large proportion of DMD muscle biopsies, argues for some generalized mechanism for circumventing arrest of translation arising from errors in the dystrophin gene (and probably in other genes as well), rather than a specific mechanism applicable to a precise mutation, e.g. a high rate of new point mutation in the affected codon. At the same time, knowledge of the precise defect in the original *mdx* mutant, gives the opportunity to test specific hypotheses as to the mechanism of sporadic expression of dystrophin in these animals.

All of the *mdx* mice differ from the majority of human DMD mutations, which are detectable deletions or duplications. At the biochemical level, however, the *mdx* mouse is as devoid of dystrophin as the majority of DMD patients (14) and the argument that this animal survives by somehow making a product from its dystrophin gene is no longer widely held.

HISTOPATHOLOGICAL FEATURES

In several of the earliest pathological studies of the *mdx* mouse, it was recognized (4,5,10,29) that some of the histopathological features resembled quite closely those seen in DMD while others did not fit at all well. Certainly, the early pathological changes, with scattered hyaline fibres, focal groups of necrotic myofibre segments and associated grouped regenerating myotubes, are reminiscent of the picture seen in early DMD biopsies. But the distinct attenuation of these pathological changes in older mice, together with the retention of muscle fibre mass and lack of fibrous and fatty infiltration, lead to an overall picture quite distinct from DMD. More disconcerting still, is the increase in muscle mass (2) and proportionately supernormal absolute muscle strength (11), which put this disease outside any normal definition of a 'dystrophy'.

Gradually, it has become accepted that this dual picture represents interspecific pathogenetic divergence; the early myonecrotic changes are clearly a feature common to dystrophin deficiency in man and mouse, the later phases - fibro-fatty proliferation and loss of muscle bulk in man - muscle fibre hypertrophy in the mouse - are determined by the individual responses of the two species to this initial degenerative process.

That interspecies differences play a major part in determining the pathogenetic outcome of dystophin deficiency, is supported by the observations on two other animal models of this condition, the X-linked dystrophic dog (9,20,31) and the cat (6). The X-linked canine dystrophy resembles DMD in that the muscles become progressively fibrotic and weak while the cat displays a true muscle hypertrophy even more spectacular than that of the mouse. Together, these four examples defy any attempt to construct single parameter explanations of disease severity, e.g. by correlation with size, growth span or longevity. The precise nature of these interspecific differences is a matter of some interest, for we must infer that quite minor variations can make the difference between a devastating disease in man and a mildly debilitating condition in the mouse.

DYSTROPHIN-LIKE PROTEINS

One of the more popular speculations as to the mildness of the *mdx* myopathy is that the mouse is able to substitute for dystrophin another protein of similar function. This idea was boosted by the finding of an autosomal homologue of dystrophin (21). Such explanations cannot be tested critically at present, first because we do not yet have sufficiently well-characterized antibodies to determine absolutely which protein we are looking at and, second, because the two genes are insufficiently well-characterized in terms of their total content of exons and alternative-splicing options. Thus, most polyclonal and many monoclonal antibodies cross-react between the X-chromosome encoded and autosomally encoded proteins. And, even when a particular antibody is known to be specific for one or other protein, this is so with certainty only for the particular splicing isoform containing the exon for which that antibody is specific. Although these essentially technical problems will be resolved with time, specific immunolocalization of these two proteins remains uncertain for the present.

In the meantime, evidence has arisen suggesting that there may be other explanations for the failure of *mdx* muscle to progress to a DMD-like pathology. In very old mice, fibrotic changes have been noted in some muscles (15), and, more recently, it has been reported that the diaphragm and to a lesser extent the intercostal muscles of mdx mice become progressively replaced by fibrotic and fatty tissue (28). It is suggested, on the basis of these studies, that the pattern of work plays an important part in directing the progression of pathological changes in muscle degenerating and regenerating as a result of a lack of dystrophin.

A second factor which looks likely to have a bearing on the mildness of the *mdx* myopathy is the phasic nature of the myonecrosis. In most *mdx* muscle studied, there are no abnormalities at birth and only minor pathological features up to about 20 days of age, whereupon there occurs a sudden bout of severe multifocal necrosis, each focus involving up to several hundred contiguous fibre profiles. Beyond the age of 80-100 days, these lesions become less frequent (and possibly less extensive, although these two qualities are difficult to separate). Over this period, muscle fibre segments undergo a limited number of rounds of degeneration/regeneration, probably ranging from zero to <10 and, in consequence, intense inflammatory processes, with their fibrogenic aftermath, operate only for a short period in mdx muscle.

Attention turns, then, to the reason for the phasic manifestation of the disease process in the *mdx* mouse. The absence of myonecrosis in young mice has been attributed to the small fibre cross sectional area, invoking the size-related increase in stress on the muscle cell surface during contraction as the source of lesions (18). This explanation does not, however, account for the great diminution in incidence of myofibre necrosis in older *mdx* mice, where most muscle fibres are considerably larger than those undergoing necrosis in younger mice. It is interesting to note that leakage of muscle enzymes into the serum remains high throughout the growth period of the *mdx* mouse and falls to lower - but still abnormally high - levels as growth ceases at 100-120 days (10), raising the possiblity that myofibre necrosis may stem from processes associated with growth *per se* rather than from absolute size of muscle fibres. Whether this relationship between growth phase and disease extends to other species is also worth consideration. Certainly, reports on the X-linked dystrophic dog indicate (20,31) a rapid decline over the first year followed by a stabilization extending over some years. In man too, it is reported that levels of muscle enzyme in the serum decline in older DMD and BMD patients and in carrier females. This too is interpretable as a lessening of disease activity as opposed to the conventional explanation that it represents a loss of susceptible muscle mass.

Such comparative pathological studies deserve attention for the insight they give into the relationship between dystrophin-deficiency and overt myopathology. Understanding at this basic level will aid our attempts to determine the function of dystrophin and, quite separately, may suggest ways of minimizing the pathological consequences of the lack of this protein.

USES OF THE *mdx* MOUSE

As discussed above, the discrepancy between the *mdx* mouse myopathy and that in man, is one of the most valuable assets of the mouse, both as a source of basic information and as a source of ideas for therapy. In addition, the mdx mouse possesses a number of specific qualities which make it the best model currently available for studying the primary pathological link between the lack of dystrophin and the sporadic death of muscle fibres.

At a purely utilitarian level, the *mdx* mouse provides the cheapest and most readily accessible source of pathological material around which to construct experiments. Just the murine background, with the opportunity it offers to study the defective gene in a variety of reproducible genetic backgrounds and to use transgenes and genes modified by homologous recombination as accessory experimental tools, is sufficient to assure the place of the *mdx* mouse as an experimental animal model.

These are largely the reasons for the relative ease with which it has been possible to perform well-controlled grafting experiments with a high level of success in the mdx mouse. It is a relatively simple matter to choose breeds or to cross-breed and select so as to make use of strain-specific markers and to avoid immune rejection. By these means it was shown that the spontaneous myonecrosis of mdx muscle was retained when the muscle was placed in a normal host and that normal muscle remained normal in an *mdx* host, thus ruling out the neurogenic hypothesis of muscle disease in dystrophin-deficiency (23). Similar strategies have made it possible to perform detailed and controlled studies of myoblast transplantation (24, 26). With the advent of newly available genetic and transgenic markers of nuclei, it will be possible to make more detailed and rigorous studies of the cell biology of *mdx* muscle than will be possible in the foreseeable future with any other species.

Speed of breeding and cheapness have been invaluable in the study of dystrophin distribution in mosaic fibres of female *mdx*/+ heterozygotes (19,32) and the changes which occur with time.

Availability is also the basis of attempts to probe, from a variety of aspects, the function of dystrophin. In this regard, the lack of secondary fibrofatty change is a most useful feature, for it is likely that this secondary pathology and more remote consequences, will themselves give rise to distortions of muscle fibre metabolism with associated pathological changes. There is, indeed, a considerable literature dedicated to observations on DMD muscle of what can be seen, in retrospect, to be secondary, tertiary etc. effects of the lack of dystrophin. The relative lack of such distractions in mdx muscle means that observed difference are likely to be closely associated with the primary pathology and therefore with the functional deficit arising directly from the lack of dystrophin. Even so, no comprehensive hypothesis, backed by critical evidence, has yet appeared to explain why dystrophinless skeletal muscle fibres are susceptible to necrosis at particular stages of the life of the mdx mouse.

Over the past few years, reports have appeared describing defects in Ca^{++} handling within *mdx* muscle fibres (13,30). It should be noted however that a breakdown of Ca^{++} homeostasis is almost inevitable at some stage in the pathogenetic process and there is no experimental evidence to place this event at the crucial point of irreversible induction of myonecrosis. More recently, it has been shown that mdx muscle fibres are more susceptible to osmotic stress than normal muscle fibres (22). This excessive fragility of mdx fibres persists at all ages and so cannot, alone, explain the 'recovery' of mdx mouse muscle in later life. At a biochemical level, dystrophin deficiency has been shown to be associated with a lack of certain plasmalemmal proteins and glycoproteins which, in normal muscle, are strongly bound to dystrophin (12).

Opponents of animal experimentation often justify their cause by pointing, quite correctly, at the fact that man differs significantly from each of the animals used to model human disease and that results of studies on these animals cannot, therefore, be applied directly to man. Although it has been available for only a short time, the *mdx* mouse epitomizes the value of animal models. First and foremost, it provides reliable material for characterizing the primary pathological processes linking the absence of dystrophin to necrosis in muscle fibres. In the diaphragm(28), the more severe DMD-like effects may extend the usefulness of this animal model to cover some of the secondary and tertiary changes which characterize DMD. In addition, tests of the feasibility of therapeutic strategies, such as myoblast transfer (2, 4, 17, 26) and direct gene transfection (1), made on the *mdx* mouse, have laid the path without which it would be very difficult to justify subsequent experiments with these same techniques on human volunteers.

ACKNOWLEDGEMENTS

Our work in this field, over a number of years, has been supported by the Muscular Dystrophy Group of Great Britain and Northern Ireland.

REFERENCES

1. Acsadi, G., Dickson, G., Love, D.R., Jani, A., Walsh, F.S., Gurusinghe, A., Wolff, J.A., Davies, K.E. (1991): Human dystrophin expression in *mdx* muscle after injection of DNA constructs. *Nature*, 352:815-818.
2. Anderson J.E., Bressler B.H. Ovalle W.K. (1988): Functional regeneration in the hindlimb skeletal muscle of the mdx mouse. *J. Muscle Res. Cell Motil.*, 9:499-415.
3. Bridges L.R. (1986): The association of cardiac muscle necrosis and inflammation with the degenerative and persistent myopathy of *mdx* mice. *J. Neurol. Sci.* 72:147-157.
4. Bulfield, G., Siller, W.G., Wight, P.A.L. Moore, K.J. (1984): X chromosome-linked muscular dystrophy (*mdx*) in the mouse. *Proc. Natn. Acad. Sci. U.S.A.*, 81:1189-1192.
5. Carnwath, J.W. Shotton, D.M. (1987): Muscular dystrophy in the *mdx* mouse: histopathology of the soleus and extensor digitorum longus muscles. *J. Neurol. Sci.* , 80:39-54.
6. Carpenter, J.L., Hoffman, E.P., Romanul, F.C.A., Kunkel, L.M., Rosales, R.K., Ma, N.S.F., Dasbach, J.J., Rae, J.F., Moore, F.M., McAfee, M.B. Pearce, L.K. (1989): Feline muscular dystrophy with dystrophin deficiency. *Am. J. Path.*, 135:909-919.
7. Chamberlain, J.S., Pearlman, J.A., Muzny, D.M., Gibbs, R.A., Ranier, J.E., Reeves, A.A. Caskey, C.T. (1988): Expression of the murine Duchenne muscular dystrophy gene in muscle and brain. *Science,* 239:1416-1418.
8. Chapman, V.M., Miller, D.R., Armstrong, D. Caskey, C.T. (1989): Recovery of induced mutations for X chromosome-linked muscular dystrophy in mice. *Proc. Natn. Acad. Sci. U.S.A.*, 86:1292-1296.
9. Cooper, B.J., Winand, N.J., Stedman, H., Valentine, B.A., Hoffman, E.P., Kunkel, L.M., Scott, M-O., Fishbeck, K.H., Kornegay, J.N., Avery, R.J., Williams, J.R., Schmickel, R.D. Sylvester, J.E. (1988): The homologue of the Duchenne locus is defective in X-linked muscular dystrophy of dogs. *Nature,* 334:154-156.
10. Coulton, G.R., Morgan, J.E., Partridge, T.A. Sloper, J.C. (1988): The *mdx* mouse skeletal muscle myopathy: I, a histological, morphometric and biochemical investigation. *Neuropath. Appl. Neurobiol.*, 14:53-70.
11. Coulton, G.R, Curtin, N.A., Morgan, J. Partridge, T.A. (1988): The *mdx* mouse skeletal muscle myopathy: II, contractile properties. *Neuropath. Appl. Neurobiol.* 14:299-314.
12. Ervasti, J.M., Ohlendieck, K., Kahl, S.D., Gaver, M.G. Campbell, K.P. (1990): Deficiency of a glycoprotein component of the dystrophin complex in dystrophic muscle. *Nature,* 345:315-319
13. Franco, A. Lansman, J.B. (1990): Calcium entry through stretch-inactivated ion channels in *mdx* myotubes. *Nature*, 344:670-673.

14. Hoffman, E.P., Brown, R.H. Kunkel, L.M. (1987): Dystrophin: the protein product of the Duchenne Muscular Dystrophy locus. *Cell,* 51:919-928.
15. Hoffman, E.P. Gorospe, J.R. (1991): The animal models of Duchenne muscular dystrophy: windows on the pathophysiological consequences of dystrophin deficiency. In; *Topics in Membranes,* edited by J. Morrow & M. Mooseker, Academic Press, New York, in press.
16. Hoffman, E.P., Morgan, J.E., Watkins, S.C., Slayter, H.S. Partridge T.A. (1990): Somatic reversion/suppression of the mouse *mdx* phenotype in vivo. *J. Neurol. Sci.,* 99:9-25.
17. Karpati, G., Pouilot, Y., Zubrzycka-Gaarn, E., Carpenter, S., Ray, P.N., Worton, R.G. Holland, P. (1989): Dystrophin is expressed in *mdx* skeletal muscle fibers after normal myoblast implantation. *Am. J. Pathol.,* 135: 27-32.
18. Karpati, G., Carpenter, S. Prescott, S. (1988). Small-caliber skeletal muscle fibers do not suffer necrosis in mdx mouse dystrophy. *Muscle and Nerve,* 11:795-803.
19. Karpati, G., Zubrzycka-Gaarn, E.E., Carpenter, S., Bulman, D.E., Ray, P.N. Worton, R.G. (1990): Age-related conversion of dystrophin-negative to -positive fibre segments of skeletal muscle but not cardiac muscle fibres in heterozygote *mdx* mice. *J. Neuropath. Exp. Neurol.,* 49: 96-105.
20. Kornegay, J.N., Tuler, S.M., Miller, D.M. Levesque D.C. (1988): Muscular dystrophy in a litter of golden retriever dogs. *Muscle and Nerve,* 11:1056-1064.
21. Love, D.R., Hill, D.F., Dickson, G., Spurr, N.K., Byth, B.C., Marsden, R.F., Walsh, F.S., Edwards, Y.H. & Davies, K.E. (1989): An autosomal transcript in skeletal muscle with homology to dystrophin. *Nature,* 339:55-58.
22. Menke, A. and Jockusch, H. (1991): Decreased osmotic stability of dystrophin-less muscle cells from the mdx mouse. *Nature,* 349:69-71.
23. Morgan, J.E., Coulton, G.R. Partridge,T.A. (1989): *Mdx* muscle grafts retain the *mdx* phenotype in normal hosts. *Muscle and Nerve,* 12:401-409.
24. Morgan, J.E., Hoffman, E.P. Partridge, T.A. (1990): Normal myogenic cells from newborn mice restore normal histology to degenerating muscles of the *mdx* mouse. *J. Cell Biol.,* 111; 2437-2449.
25. Ohno, S., Becak, W. Becak, M.L. (1964): X-autosome ratio and the behaviour pattern of individual X-chromosomes in placental mammals. *Chromosoma,* 15:14-30.
26. Partridge, T.A., Morgan, J.E., Coulton, G.R., Hoffman, E.P., Kunkel, L.M. (1989): Conversion of *mdx* myofibres from dystrophin-negative to positive by injection of normal myoblasts. *Nature,* 337:176-179.
27. Sicinski, P., Geng, Y., Ryder-Cook, A.S., Barnard. E.A., Darlison, M.G. Barnard, P.J. (1989): The molecular basis of muscular dystrophy in the *mdx* mouse: a point mutation. *Science,* 244:1578-1580.
28. Stedman, H.H., Sweeney, H.L., Shrager, J.B., Maguire, H.C., Pannettieri, R.A., Petrof, B., Narusawa, M., Leferovich, J.M., Sladky, J.T. Kelly, A.M. (1991): The *mdx* mouse diaphragm reproduces the degenerative changes of Duchenne muscular dystrophy. *Nature,* 352:536-539
29. Torres, L.B.F. & Duchen, L.W. (1987): The mutant *mdx*: inherited myopathy in the mouse. Morphological studies of nerves, muscles and endplates. *Brain,* 110:269-299.

30. Turner. P.R., Westwood. T., Regen. C.M., Steinhardt, R.A. (1998):
    Increased protein degradation results from elevated free calcium levels
    found in muscle from *mdx* mice. *Nature,* 335:735-738.
31. Valentine, B.A., Cooper, B.J., Cummings, J.F. de Lahunta, A. (1990):
    Canine X-linked muscular dystrophy: morphologic lesions. *J. Neurol.
    Sci.,* 97:1-23.
32. Watkins, S.C., Hoffman, E.P., Slayter, H.S. Kunkel L.M. (1989):
    Dystrophin distribution in heterozygote *mdx* mice. *Muscle and Nerve,*
    12:861-868.

DISCUSSION

Professor George Karpati:
This was a very nice expose`. I should like to comment on a couple of the more
tantalizing aspects of your presentation. One is the appearance of large clusters
of necrotic muscle fibres instead of single ones. As you have suggested, it is
probably not a direct consequence of the dystrophin deficiency but it is due to
some secondary and tertiary effects. One of the possibilities which has been
suggested is that a single necrotic fibre invites a lot of macrophages and while
they are in the neighbourhood they invade not only the single fibre, which was
destined to die, but many other ones around it.
To test this hypothesis we have treated *mdx* mice starting at age 10 days (when
there is not yet any necrosis) with a variety of agents which suppress the activity
of macrophages. Different groups of *mdx* mice were given either prednisone or
azathioprine or cyclophosphamide or cyclosporin-A. We were looking for the
prevalence of necrosis in these groups as compared to untreated *mdx* muscles. I
would say that these interventions did not change the pattern of the natural
history. So we must look for other mysterious factors to explain the large group
necrosis. This is also interesting because as you know, prednisone has a
beneficial effect on the natural history of Duchenne dystrophy. This is not the
case in *mdx* mice, which points out the difference between humans and mice.
Another point that I wanted to make is the prevalence of necrosis of *mdx* mice
as a function of age. As you show, necrosis continues to occur throughout the
lifespan of the animals, but in our colonies, the prevalence of necrosis declines
enormously after age 100 days. We have never actually quantitated this but did
a short-cut. We gamma irradiated (20 Gray) leg muscles of *mdx* mice at 100
days to see if, after radiation, the older animals continue to lose muscle fibres
which would indicate significant continued necrosis. However, the rate of
muscle fibre loss after 100 days in mdx animals up to one year is much less than
if you radiate them at 10 days. There is no question that regenerated *mdx*
muscle fibres, though they are still dystrophin-deficient and some of them are,
as you say, bigger than normal, somehow develop a relative resistance to
necrosis. This fact underscores your comment that mdx offer a reliable chance
to figure out why the *mdx* muscle fibre can develop compensation for dystrophin
deficiency, which the dog model does not.
I think that the other point that you were making is that if you gamma irradiate
muscles of *mdx* mice at the early age of 10 days or so, in a year the muscle will
disappear except about 5% of the fibres. I feel that this 5% of fibres represents
those satellite cells which have escaped "reproductive death" by irradiation.

Dr. Terence A. Partridge:
I think that fibrotic scar tissue becomes the limiting factor in regeneration in DMD, not the necrosis. It is a fact that muscle fibres do disappear and that degeneration does figure conspicuously, particularly over the first few weeks.

Professor John B Harris:
I think one of the worst decisions I have ever made in Newcastle was to advise my colleagues to stop working on the *mdx* mouse. I was convinced that the pattern of focal degeneration seen in affected muscles implied that the origin of the problem was ischaemia.

Dr. Terence A. Partridge:
I feel that the ischaemia had been ignored as a part of the disease process but I am not sure how it is implicated.

Professor John B Harris:
I was going to ask you that. If that is the case and you get the ischaemia in the transplanted muscles then it suggests that there is something inherent within the muscle which prevents the formation of a normal microcirculation.

Dr. Terence A. Partridge:
We have two contrary sets of observations about the vascularization of the lesions. The invasion of inflammatory cells and the wave of regeneration both move from outside to inside suggesting a micro-infarct and a gradual re-vascularization of the lesion from the outside. However Gary Coulton in our department perfused some *mdx* muscles with colloidal carbon and found apparently normal vascularization even in early lesions.

Assoc. Professor John K McGeachie:
Terry, I just wanted to ask about the diaphragm of the mouse with DMD you showed on the slide. Do you have any comments to make? Why is the diaphragm the single muscle in the model which looks like a DMD situation.

Dr. Terence A. Partridge:
The idea of the authors of this paper on *mdx* diaphragm[1] is that the pattern and type of work undertaken by this muscle is such as to push the pathological process along a similar pathway to that in human muscles that are severely affected by DMD.

Professor George Karpati:
In response to this if you denervate an *mdx* muscle before the necrotic phase sets in, not a single necrotic fibre will be seen in that muscle as long as it remains denervated. After reinnervation, the necrotic cycle continues. We have suggested that this is due to 2 factors; firstly, there was no contraction in the denervated muscle and secondly, the small calibre of the denervated muscle and secondly, the small calibre of the denervated fibres are also protected against necrosis on the basis of Laplace's law.

Professor Allen D. Roses:
Concerning those which did not have dystrophin but still function, what do we know about the differences or any other characteristics of those fibres compared to the fibres which have dystrophin in the normal mouse?

Dr. Terence A. Partridge:
We have looked at the physiology of *mdx* mouse muscles and the differences from normal muscle are very minor. Pierre Moens and Georges Marechal in Brussels, have made detailed studies of the length/tension characteristics of soleus and extensor digitorum longus muscles of *mdx* mice and have found that they are slightly physiologically slower than the equivalent muscles of normal mice. We have collaborated in this study by making orthotopic isografts of these two muscles; when transplanted they both become slightly physiologically faster. Therefore we cannot attribute the slowness of *mdx* muscles to the fact that they have degenerated and regenerated and feel that this might reflect some intrinsic feature of dystrophinless muscle.

DUCHENNE MUSCULAR DYSTROPHY: Animal Models
and Genetic Manipulation, edited by Byron A. Kakulas,
John McC. Howell, and Allen D. Roses.
Raven Press, Ltd., New York © 1992.

9

Golden Retriever Muscular Dystrophy: The Model and Relevance to Developmental Therapeutics

Joe N. Kornegay

College of Veterinary Medicine,
North Carolina State University,
Raleigh, NC, 27606, USA.

The recent discovery of the defective gene in Duchenne muscular dystrophy (DMD) (1) and the protein for which it codes (dystrophin) (2) has allowed for a critical assessment of potential models of this X-linked condition. Until the description of the mdx mouse in 1984 (2,3), no X-linked forms of muscular dystrophy had been well characterized in animals. However, athough mdx mice have pathologic lesions similar to those seen in DMD and lack dystrophin, they do not develop progressive clinical dysfunction. In fact, affected mice have a normal life expectancy. The absence of clinical dysfunction in this model will cause difficulty in evaluating future experimental therapeutic modalities. In contrast, golden retriever dogs with a recently characterized form of muscular dystrophy (GRMD) have progressive clinical dysfunction.

Seven golden retriever dogs with similar clinical features of a presumed inherited myopathy were described between 1958 and 1986 (4). These characteristic features mirrored those of DMD, suggesting that the conditions might be homologous. A colony of dogs with GRMD was established at the College of Veterinary Medicine at Cornell University using one of the dogs originally studied by the author. Studies conducted by the Cornell group have been instrumental in defining the clinicopathologic features of GRMD and its validity as a model of DMD. Among other things, their results, as well as our own (see paper by Sharp et al elsewhere in these proceedings) have indicated that dogs with GRMD lack the DMD gene transcript and dystrophin, thus confirming genetic homology between the two conditions (5). An additional colony of affected dogs has been developed at the College of Veterinary Medicine at North Carolina State University (NCSU-CVM) using dogs provided by the Cornell group. In turn, we have provided dogs to the Association Francaise Contre les Myopathies for development of a colony in France and frozen GRMD semen to investigators in Western Australia. A British colony, sponsored by the Muscular Dystrophy Group of Britain and developed through a collaboration with Cornell, is planned.

Animal models are of course frequently used to define underlying mechanisms of disease. In order for the model to be maximally utilized, however, results from such studies must ultimately have value in defining therapeutic modalities. Thus, to be of maximal benefit, the GRMD model must be used in trials of investigative drugs and other therapies that are of potential value to DMD patients. In fact, as discussed above, considering the lack of distinct clinical involvement in the mdx mouse, studies detailing investigative therapeutics are perhaps the greatest application of the GRMD model. As an example, considerable attention has been focused recently on the value of myoblast transplantation in DMD. In fact, based on promising results achieved in the mdx mouse (6) and a condition termed the dy mouse (7), several groups have initiated preliminary trials in affected boys (8). However, a number of potential problems jeopardize the ultimate value of myoblast transplantation (9). For localized therapy to be successful, multiple muscles will have to be injected. Furthermore, dysfunction related to dystrophin-deficiency in cardiac (10) and smooth (11) muscle will not be reversed. Clearly, a systemic mode of therapy, potentially utilizing progenitor cells that would home to target tissues, is desirable. Studies necessary to address these points, as well as others such as the potential for immunorejection in myoblast transplantation, cannot be ethically performed in DMD patients, and must, therefore, be conducted in appropriate models (9).

Objective criteria of improvement, including multiple pathologic and clinical factors, must be evaluated in defining the value of any therapy. Clinical function tests are clearly the ultimate criterion by which improvement must be judged. Volitional tests of muscle contraction force used in humans will not be readily applicable in dogs. However, tests that provide an objective measurement of strength have been defined in dogs and will potentially be valuable in studies of GRMD. One example is ground reaction force measured by force plate analysis. Methods for determining these forces have been described in dogs and they have been shown to be a reliable indicator of function (13). We have conducted preliminary studies of force plate analysis on normal and GRMD dogs and are unsure whether this method will be sensitive enough to detect changes in strength occurring subsequent to treatment, or for that matter, differences between GRMD-affected and normal dogs. In one force plate analysis study, variably-aged DMD patients did not differ from normal, age-matched boys (14). Alternatively, contraction force generated by electrically stimulated muscles can be measured. We have initiated studies in dogs with a modification of a method originally used in rabbits (15).

Electrodiagnostic studies offer an objective indication of neuromuscular function, often showing deterioration or improvement in advance of clinical signs. Accordingly, electrodiagnostic techniques, especially quantitative forms of electromyography, will have a critical role in assessing improvement of DMD or GRMD patients. Single fiber electromyography should be of particular value in evaluating muscle regeneration occurring secondary to a therapy such as myoblast transplantation. This method allows determination of fiber density and the sequence of myofiber reinnervation (16), both of which will obviously be of critical importance to assessing transplant success. Methods for single fiber electromyography have been developed in dogs (17). The mean consecutive difference (MCD) in latency of single fiber potentials for the peroneus longus muscle was 17.2 μsec, which is similar to the value reported for the extensor digitorum communis muscle in humans. Methodology for certain other quantitative forms of electromyography must be developed in dogs.

The GRMD model is also particularly suited for studies detailing the risks of immunorejection of transplanted myoblasts. There is already considerable information on canine transplantation immunology. The dog was, in fact, the first random-bred animal in which the relevance of in vitro histocompatibility testing for the outcome of bone marrow transplantation was shown (18). Several international workshops have defined the canine major histocompatibility complex, which has been termed dog lymphocyte antigen (DLA) (19,20). Antisera to serologically-defined antigens are available, and assay methodology has been standardized through international symposia (20). More recently, restriction length polymorphisms (RFLP) have been used to show allelic polymorphism within the DLA complex (21) and will be valuable, together with mixed lymphocyte reactions, in determining MHC compatibility of donor/recipient pairs used in myoblast transplantation. Monoclonal antibodies to canine equivalent CT4+ and CT8+ lymphocytes are also available, thus allowing critical assessment of lymphocyte subsets that may be involved in immunorejection.

The GRMD model is now established as perhaps the most appropriate animal model of DMD. Colonies have been, or are being, established on several continents. Studies conducted in GRMD dogs should be invaluable in answering questions pertinent to developmental therapeutics. In order to maximize the value of the GRMD model, however, investigators must take advantage of existing methods of evaluation and strive to develop other more critical means of assessment.

ACKNOWLEDGEMENTS

Supported by the Muscular Dystrophy Association of America, March of Dimes Birth Defects Foundation, Association Francaise Contre les Myopathies, and the State of North Carolina.

REFERENCES

1. Koenig, M., Hoffman, E.P., Bertelson, C.J., et al (1987): Complete cloning of the Duchenne muscular dystrophy (DMD) cDNA and preliminary genomic organization of the DMD gene in normal and affected individuals. *Cell*, 50:509-517.
2. Hoffman, E.P., Brown, R.H., Kunkel, L.M. (1987): Dystrophin: the protein product of the Duchenne muscular dystrophy locus. *Cell*, 51:919-928.
3. Tanabe, Y., Esaki, K., Nomura, T. (1986): Skeletal muscle pathology in X chromosome-linked muscular dystrophy (mdx) mouse. *Acta. Neuropathol.*, (Berl) 69:91-95
4. Kornegay, J.N., Tuler, S.M.,. Miller, D.M., et al (1988): Muscular dystrophy in a litter of golden retriever dogs. *Muscle and Nerve*, 11:1056-

1064.
5. Cooper, B.J., Winand, N.J., Stedman, H., et al (1988): The homologue of the Duchenne locus is defective in X-linked muscular dystrophy of dogs. *Nature*, 334:154-156.
6. Partridge, T.A., Morgan, J.E., Coulton, G.R. et al (1989): Conversion of mdx myofibres from dystrophin-negative to -positive by injection of normal myoblasts. *Nature*, 337:176-179.
7. Law, P.K., Goodwin, T.G., Wang, M.G. (1988): Normal myoblast injections provide genetic treatment for murine dystrophy. *Muscle and Nerve*, 11:525-533.
8. Law, P.K., Bertorini, T.E., Goodwin, T.G. et al (1990): Dystrophin production induced by myoblast transfer therapy in Duchenne muscular dystrophy. *Lancet*, 336:114-115.
9. Partridge, T.A. (1991): Invited review: Myoblast transfer: A possible therapy for inherited myopathies. *Muscle and Nerve,* 14:197-212.
10. Banilowicz D, Rutkowski M, Mgung D: Echocardiography in Duchenne muscular dystrophy. *Muscle and Nerve*, 3:298-303, 1980.
11. Barohn, R.J., Levine, E.J., Olsen, J.O. et al (1987): Gastric hypomotility in Duchenne's muscular dystrophy. *New Engl. J. Med.*, 319:15-18.
12. Budsberg, S.C., Verstraete, M.C., Soutas-Little, R.W. (1987): Force plate analysis of the walking gait in healthy dogs. *Am. J. Vet. Res.*, 48:915-918.
13. Budsburg, S.C., Verstraete. M.C., Soutas-Little, R.W. et al (1988): Force plate analyses before and after stabilization of canine stifles for cruciate injury. *Am. J. Vet. Res.*, 49:1522-1524.
14. Khodadadeh, S., McClelland, M., Patrick, J.H. (1987): Force plate studies of Duchenne muscular dystrophy. *Engineer Med.* 16:177-178.
15. Bolesta, M.J., Garrett, W.E., Ribbeck, B.M. et al (1988): Immediate and delayed neurorrhaphy in a rabbit model: A functional, histologic, and biochemical comparison. *J. Hand. Surg.*, 13A:352-357.
16. Stalberg, E. (1991): Invited review: Electrodiagnostic assessment and monitoring of motor unit changes in disease. *Muscle and Nerve*, 14:293-303.
17. Hopkins, A.L., Howard, J.F., Stewart, C.R. et al (1991): Stimulated single fiber electromyography in normal dogs. *J. Vet. Int. Med.*, 5:136.
18. Epstein, R.B., Storb, R., Ragde, H. et al (1968): Cytotoxic typing antisera for marrow grafting in littermate dogs. *Transplantation*, 6:45.
19. Deeg, H.J., Raff, R.F., Grosse-Wilde, H. et al (1986): Joint report of the third international workshop on canine immunogenetics. I. Analysis of homozygous typing cells. *Transplantation*, 41:111-117.
20. Bull, R.W., Vriensendorp, H.M., Cech, R. et al (1987): Joint report of the third international workshop on canine immunogenetics. II. Analysis of the serological typing of cells. *Transplantation*, 43:154-161.
21. Sarmiento, U.M., Sarmiento, J.I., Storb, R. (1990): Allelic variation in the DR subregion of the canine major histocompatibility complex. *Immunogenetics*, 32:13-19.

DUCHENNE MUSCULAR DYSTROPHY: Animal Models
and Genetic Manipulation, edited by Byron A. Kakulas,
John McC. Howell, and Allen D. Roses.
Raven Press, Ltd., New York © 1992.

10

The *xmd* Dog: Molecular and Phenotypic Characteristics

Barry J. Cooper

Department of Pathology,
New York State College of Veterinary Medicine,
Cornell University, Ithaca, NY 14853, USA.

The recognition of defects in the dystrophin gene as the basis for Duchenne muscular dystrophy has also allowed the identification of the homologous disease in animal models. Canine mutants have been identified and referred to as the *xmd* dog, that closely resemble Duchenne muscular dystrophy in humans. In this report the molecular and phenotypic relationship of the canine disease to DMD are reviewed.

PHENOTYPIC CHARACTERISTICS

Two canine strains with dystrophin defects have been identified, one in the Golden Retriever breed and one in the Rottweiler. In the best characterized of these, the Golden Retriever, overt clinical signs first become apparent at approximately 8 weeks of age (1). Affected pups initially show weakness, stiffness of gait, and difficulty in fully opening the mouth. Clinical signs are progressive, with loss of muscle mass, further stiffness, and contractures becoming apparent. Serum creatine kinase (CK) levels are greatly elevated, and can be used to identify affected dogs within the first few days of life. CK levels are further elevated by exercise (2). Morphologically, the disease is characterized by the presence of numerous swollen, hyalinized fibers, followed by fiber necrosis and infiltration and phagocytosis by macrophages. There is abundant regeneration and muscle fibrosis eventually results. Clinical signs and morphologic lesions are similar in the Rottweiler strain, except that the disease is more severe. The phenotypic expression of canine X-linked muscular dystrophy therefore closely resembles that of Duchenne muscular dystrophy in man.

Dystrophic dogs may also succumb to a fulminant neonatal form of the disease, in which certain muscles, including the tongue, the deltoideus, the trapezius, the diaphragm, and the sartorius, are affected early and severely (3). Studies of such early lesions in our laboratory have revealed that severely affected muscles have larger fibers than those that are affected later. However, comparison of the size of fibers in littermate controls did not reveal significant differences between such muscle groups. We could not, therefore, attribute differences in susceptibility of lesions to inherent differences in fiber size. Rather, we believe that such differences in fiber size in dystrophic animals are due to early and consistent fiber hypertrophy. We also hypothesize that selective involvement of muscles early in the course of the disease may be exercise related.

Dogs with X-linked muscular dystrophy also develop cardiomyopathy (4,5). Lesions first become apparent at about 6 months of age and include myocardial necrosis, and eventual fibrosis. Fibrotic lesions are most prominent within the subepicardial myocardium of the left ventricular free wall, the right ventricular aspect of the septum, and the papillary muscles. Again, these lesions closely resemble those observed in DMD patients.

MOLECULAR RELATIONSHIP TO DMD

Studies in our laboratories have shown the *xmd* dog to be a genetic homologue of DMD. The disease is inherited as an X-linked trait (6) and affected dogs have drastically reduced levels or absence of dystrophin and its message (7). Recent results using highly sensitive Western blotting techniques demonstrate trace amounts of dystrophin of apparently normal size in muscle of dystrophic Golden Retrievers. However, we have been unable to demonstrate any dystrophin in the Rottweiler strain. Linkage analysis using RFLPs confirms that the defect in the Golden Retriever is in or close to the dystrophin locus. Immunohistochemistry confirms that the normal sarcolemmal staining pattern for dystrophin is absent in both skeletal (8) and cardiac muscle.(5)

MOSAICISM IN CARRIERS

Studies of young obligate *xmd* carriers have shown that dystrophin is expressed in a mosaic pattern in skeletal muscle (8). Carriers show variable elevations of serum creatine kinase and occasional necrotic muscle fibers (unpublished observations). Individual muscle fibers show variable expression of dystrophin along their length, indicating that there is a nuclear domain effect for the expression of the protein. However, this effect is transient and mosaicism in skeletal muscle resolves as animals mature (8). We hypothesize that this resolution of mosaicism is due to mobilization of dystrophin within mosaic muscle fibers.

In the heart mosaicism is striking, with about 50% of cardiac myocytes lacking dystrophin completely, the rest expressing apparently normal levels. This mosaicism does not alter with age, and apparently persists for the lifetime of the animal. Recent studies in our laboratory have shown that this persistent mosaicism in the heart of carriers results in cardiac dysfunction (4) and lesions that are qualitatively identical to those of affected animals (unpublished observations).

CONCLUSIONS

Both strains of *xmd* dog represent excellent models of Duchenne muscular dystrophy. The disease results from a mutation in the DMD locus, resulting in the absence, or near absence, of dystrophin in muscle tissues. Lesions show a remarkable resemblance to those of man, and affected animals demonstrate a similar clinical phenotype. These models should therefore be suitable for studies of the pathogenetic factors involved in Duchenne muscular dystrophy as well as for assessing potential therapeutic approaches, including myoblast transfer and gene therapy.

REFERENCES

1. Valentine, B.A., Cooper, B.J., de Lahunta, A., et al. (1989): Canine X-linked muscular dystrophy. An animal model of Duchenne muscular dystrophy: clinical studies. *J. Neurol. Sci..*, 88:69-81.
2. Valentine, B.A., Blue, J.T., Cooper, B.J. (1989): The effect of exercise on canine dystrophic muscle. *Ann. Neurol..*, 26:588.
3. Valentine, B.A., Cooper, B.J. (1991): Canine X-linked muscular dystrophy: Selective involvement of muscles in neonatal dogs. *Neuromusc. Disorders*,1:31-38.
4. Moise, N.S., Valentine, B.A., Brown, C.A., et al. (1990) Duchenne cardiomyopathy in a canine model: electro-cardiographic and echocardiographic studies. *J. Am. Coll. Cardiol.*, 17:812-820.
5. Valentine, B.A., Cummings, J.F., Cooper, B.J. (1989): Development of Duchenne-type cardiomyopathy: Morphologic studies in a canine model. *Am. J. Pathol.*, 135:671-678.
6. Cooper, B.J., Valentine, B.A., Wilson, S., et al. Canine muscular dystrophy: Confirmation of X-linked inheritance. *J. Hered.*, 79:405-408.
7. Cooper, B.J., Winand, N.J., Stedman, H., et al. (1988) The homologue of the Duchenne locus is defective in X-linked muscular dystrophy of dogs. *Nature*, 334:154-156.
8. Cooper, B.J., Gallagher, E.A., Smith, C.A., et al. (1990): Mosaic expression of dystrophin in carriers of canine X-linked muscular dystrophy. *Lab. Invest.*, 62:171-178.

DUCHENNE MUSCULAR DYSTROPHY: Animal Models
and Genetic Manipulation, edited by Byron A. Kakulas,
John McC. Howell, and Allen D. Roses.
Raven Press, Ltd., New York © 1992.

11

Exon Skipping During Dystrophin mRNA Processing in the Canine Homologue of Duchenne Muscular Dystrophy

N.J.H. Sharp*#, J.N. Kornegay#, S.D.Van Camp°,
M.H. Herbstreith*, S.L. Secore*, S. Kettle*, M.J. Dykstra+,
C.D. Constantinou*, A.D. Roses*, R.J. Bartlett*#

*Department of Medicine, Division of Neurology,
Duke University Medical Center, Durham, North Carolina 27710.

#Department of Companion Animal and Special Species Medicine.
+Department of Microbiology, Pathology and Parasitology.
°Department of Food Animal and Equine Medicine.
College of Veterinary Medicine, North Carolina State University,
Raleigh, NC 27606.

Golden retriever muscular dystrophy (GRMD) is a spontaneous, X-linked, progressively fatal disease of dogs. It is also a homologue of Duchenne muscular dystrophy (DMD), a fatal, X-linked, recessive disease of humans that afflicts 1 in 3500 live-born males(15). Approximately two thirds of DMD patients carry detectable deletions in their dystrophin gene (5,9,11,14,16,23,34,35). The defect underlying the remaining one third of DMD patients is undetermined (1). Patients with DMD are severely deficient in both dystrophin protein (12) and its transcript (25).

Dogs with GRMD also lack both dystrophin transcript and protein (8,17). Analysis of the canine dystrophin gene in normal and GRMD dogs fails to demonstrate any detectable loss of exons (2). We have identified a truncated dystrophin transcript in affected dogs using the polymerase chain reaction (PCR) (28). This truncation is caused by a precise deletion of the seventh exon from the dystrophin transcript, despite the fact that this exon is present in the genomic

DNA. Skipping of exon seven is the result of an A to G transition in the 3' splice site of intron six. This is the first example of dystrophin deficiency due to an RNA processing error that is caused by a mutation other than an intragenic deletion.

In order to identify the molecular basis for dystrophin deficiency in GRMD, we have amplified single-stranded dystrophin cDNA prepared from skeletal muscle of normal and affected dogs. All primers for the reverse transcriptase and PCR reactions (Figure 1) were based on the human dystrophin cDNA sequence (15). Products amplified by PCR were visualized after Southern blotting and subsequent hybridization with human skeletal muscle dystrophin cDNA (15).

Primer pair F1/R2 (exons 1-8), amplified a product of expected size (1 kb) from the muscle of three normal dogs (Figure 2A, lanes 1,2,8). The same primer pair amplified a slightly smaller product (approximately 0.88 kb) from each of five different dogs with GRMD (Figure 2A, lanes 3-7). Primer pair F1/R3 (exons 1-11), also amplified a product that was approximately 120 nucleotides smaller in GRMD dogs compared to normal dogs (data not shown). Similar results were obtained using primer pair F1/R4 (exons 1-20, data not shown). In contrast, primer pair F1/R1 (exons 1-5) amplified products of equal size from the first 0.5 kb of normal and GRMD dystrophin cDNA (data not shown). These four experiments suggested that there was a deletion in the GRMD transcript between exons 5-8 (corresponding to nucleotides 565 and 969 of the human dystrophin cDNA) (15).

Complimentary DNA generated by the first three experiments (primer pairs F1/R2, F1/R3, F1/R4) was used as template in a second, asymmetric PCR amplification. Primer pair F2/R2 (exons 5-8) was used to generate single stranded cDNA which was then sequenced to determine the basis for the truncated product from GRMD muscle (Figure 3A). The dystrophin sequence from normal canine muscle corresponded very closely to that of human dystrophin (2,15). The sequence of the truncated dystrophin cDNA from GRMD dogs was equivalent up to and including the last nucleotide of exon six. The next nucleotide in the GRMD sequence corresponded to the first nucleotide of exon eight from the normal dog. Exon seven had been precisely deleted and there was no apparent inclusion of sequence that might correspond to that from the intervening sequences between exons six and eight (Figure 3B). This finding was confirmed in three normal and three affected dogs. The size of the deleted exon corresponded very closely to the difference in PCR products generated in normal and GRMD dogs. Assuming intron-exon junctions in dogs and humans are identical, skipping of exon seven would change the reading frame of exon eight. This would predict a premature termination codon in the eighth codon of the new reading frame (Figure 3B).

In order to demonstrate that the truncated PCR product of GRMD muscle was indeed caused by skipping of exon seven, oligo-nucleotide (F7) was end-labelled (29) and hybridized to the PCR products amplified in the first three experiments. In each case, only products amplified from normal canine muscle produced a signal (Figure 2B).

Screening of genomic blots from normal and GRMD dogs using the entire human dystrophin cDNA as probe has previously detected no major rearrangements (2). A labelled PCR product (30) specific for exon seven (primer pair F7/R7) also revealed identical restriction fragments when hybridized to Southern blots of genomic DNA from normal and GRMD dogs (Figure 4). This confirms that exon seven is present in the genome of GRMD dogs and that there is no obvious deletion or insertion in introns six or seven.

Human Dystrophin cDNA Primers

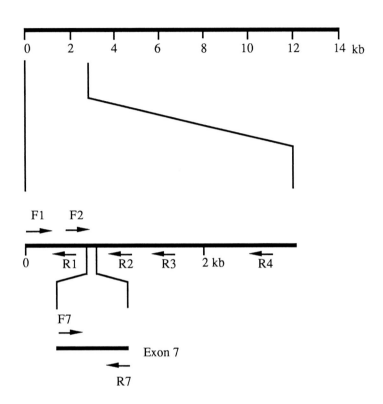

Primer Positions and Sequence

		5'	3'	
F1	(1-24)	GGGATTCCCTCACTTTCCCCCTAC		EXON 1
F2	(529-565)	CTTGGTTTGATTTGGAATATAATCCTCCACTGGCAG		EXON 5
F7	(738-766)	GCCAGACCTGCTTGACTGGAATAGTGTG		EXON 7
R1	(500-479)	CAGTACTTCCAATATTCACTAG		EXON 5
R2	(990-969)	GTCACTTTAGGTGGCCTTGGC		EXON 8
R3	(1518-1476)	GCTACCCTGAGGCATTCCCATCTTGAATTTAGGAGATTCATC		EXON 11
R4	(2709-2679)	GCGATGATGTTGTTCTGATACTCCAGCCAG		EXON 20
R7	(857-829)	CTTCAGGATCGAGTAGTTTCTCTATGCC		EXON 7

FIG. 1. **Oligonucleotide primers used for reverse transcription and cDNA PCR.**
The primers are shown relative to their position in the dystrophin cDNA.15 Forward (F) and reverse (R) primers are depicted by arrows, scale on the dystrophin cDNA is in kilobases. Oligo-nucleotide primers were prepared using DuPont DNA synthesizers (Coder 300 and Generator).

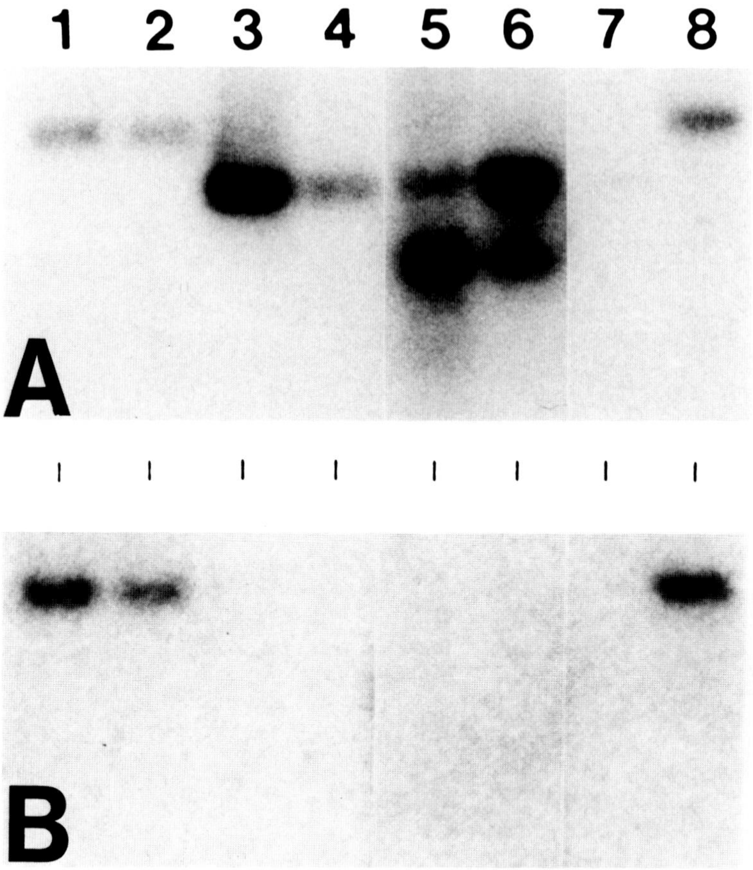

FIG. 2.   **PCR amplification of normal and GRMD transcripts.**
Amplified products of normal(N) and GRMD mRNA were separated
on agarose gels, blotted and hybridized (10).

FIG. 2A.   Probed with 9-7 cloned fragment of human dystrophin cDNA
(nucleotides 1-1500, relative to published cDNA sequence) (15).
Lanes 1,2,8 are samples from normal dogs; lanes 3-7 are samples
from GRMD dogs.

FIG. 2B.   Probed with end-labelled (29) oligo-nucleotide F7 located within exon
seven of the human cDNA.   Lanes are as per Figure 2A.   Size
standards are indicated in base pairs.   Total RNA (4 ug per sample)
from skeletal muscle (limb) was prepared with guanidinium
hydrochloride (6) and reverse transcribed into first strand cDNA with
an oligo-nucleotide primer R2, and Superscript reverse transcriptase
(LTI).   Primer pair F1/R2 was used to amplify first strand cDNA
using 20 cycles, standard buffers and 2.5 units of Taq polymerase
(Cetus).   Annealing was at 37oC for 10 minutes for the first 5 cycles,
then at 55oC for the next 15 cycles. Extension was at 72oC for 2 to 3
minutes, and denaturation was at 94oC for 1 minute.

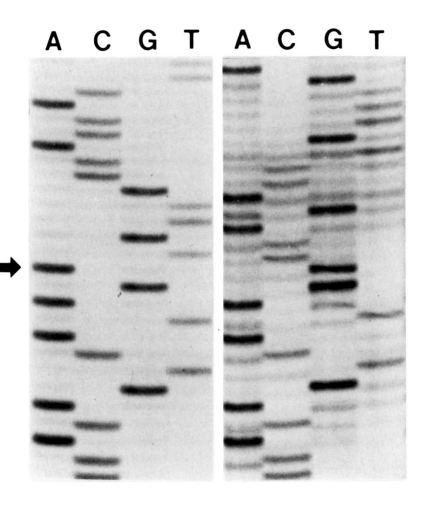

FIG. 3.   **Sequence of the dystrophin cDNA in the region of the mutation.**

FIG. 3A.   Canine dystrophin sequences from normal (4 lanes on right) and GRMD (4 lanes on left) dogs in the region of the mutation. The sequence representing exon seven is deleted from the GRMD dog (arrow) when compared to the normal dog. This change has been observed in three normal and three GRMD dogs, and in different amplification products from the same GRMD mRNA.

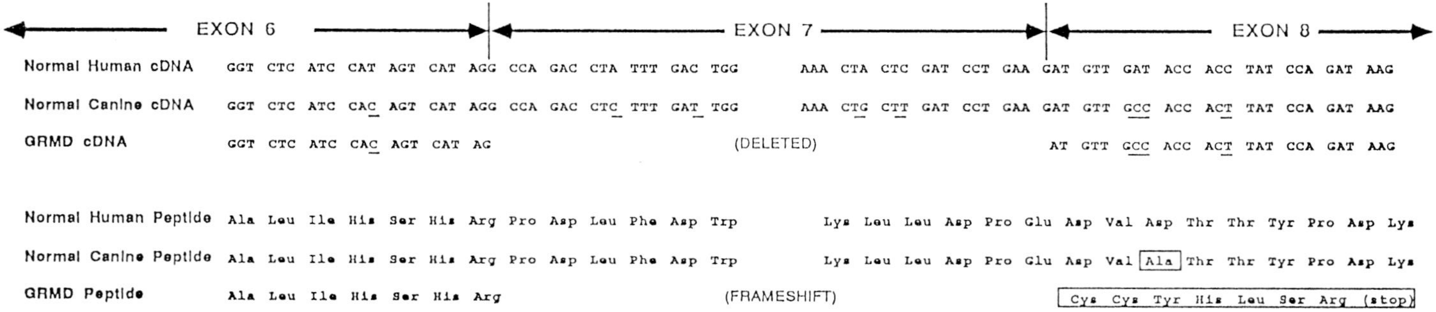

| | ← | EXON 6 | | | | | | | | | | ← | EXON 7 | → | | | | | | | | | | | | | | EXON 8 → |

Normal Human cDNA GGT CTC ATC CAT AGT CAT AGG CCA GAC CTA TTT GAC TGG   AAA CTA CTC GAT CCT GAA GAT GTT GAT ACC ACC TAT CCA GAT AAG

Normal Canine cDNA GGT CTC ATC CAC AGT CAT AGG CCA GAC CTC TTT GAT TGG   AAA CTG CTT GAT CCT GAA GAT GTT GCC ACT TAT CCA GAT AAG

GRMD cDNA GGT CTC ATC CAC AGT CAT AG   (DELETED)   AT GTT GCC ACT TAT CCA GAT AAG

Normal Human Peptide Ala Leu Ile His Ser His Arg Pro Asp Leu Phe Asp Trp   Lys Leu Leu Asp Pro Glu Asp Val Asp Thr Thr Tyr Pro Asp Lys

Normal Canine Peptide Ala Leu Ile His Ser His Arg Pro Asp Leu Phe Asp Trp   Lys Leu Leu Asp Pro Glu Asp Val Ala Thr Thr Tyr Pro Asp Lys

GRMD Peptide Ala Leu Ile His Ser His Arg   (FRAMESHIFT)   Cys Cys Tyr His Leu Ser Arg (stop)

FIG. 3B. The DNA sequences and predicted amino acid sequences from normal and GRMD dogs, and from normal human beings (15) in the region of the mutation. Changes in sequence are underlined (nucleotides) or boxed (amino acids). Primer pair F2/R2 was used to generate single and double stranded cDNA. Single stranded cDNA amplification products were separated by electrophoresis through an agarose gel, purified and sequenced both manually (20) with the Sequenase kit (USB) and by an automated sequence analysis system (DuPont Genesis 2000 DNA sequencer). Double stranded DNA was sequenced manually (4).

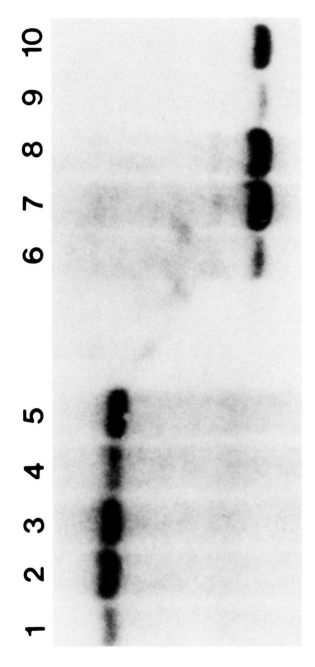

FIG. 4. Southern blot analysis of genomic DNA from normal and GRMD dogs. DNA samples in lanes are as follows: 1,6, GRMD male; 2,3,7 and 8, carrier females; 4,9, normal male; 5,10, normal female. Lanes 1-5 are Eco R1 digested DNA and lanes 6-10 are HindIII digested DNA. Intensity differences reflect X-chromosome dosage effects. Samples were isolated (21), separated by electrophoresis through a 1% agarose gel, transferred to GeneScreenPlus membranes (Dupont) and hybridized to a PCR generated probe (29) representing exon seven made using primer pair F7/R7.

The results observed in GRMD suggested that there was a mutation in one of the consensus splice sites flanking exon seven. To obtain intronic sequence adjacent to exon seven, a normal canine genomic library in bacteriophage was probed with the same PCR product (30) specific for exon seven (primer pair F7/R7). A single positive plaque was isolated and then purified through three cycles (29) The insert from this clone was sequenced for 100-150 bases on either side of the intron-exon junctions using sequencing primers GF1 and GR1 (Figure 5A). Primers GF2 and GR2 were then designed to allow amplification of the intronic sequences flanking and including exon seven (Figure 5A). Identical products of 340 base pairs were amplified from three affected and one normal dog studied previously. Sequencing of these products revealed that the 5' splice site in intron seven was the same in both normal and affected dogs. The 3' splice site in intron six from all three GRMD dogs had an A to G transition mutation in the highly conserved -2 position (Figure 5B). This changes the canonical sequence CAG/G to CGG/G (24), thereby inactivating it as a functional splice acceptor site and causing exon seven to be processed out along with introns six and seven.

Seven mutations affecting the universal consensus sequence for the 3' splice site of mammalian genes have been reported to date (Table 1). Two mutants have been described in the dihydrofolate reductase gene, one in the -1 position (G to A), and one affecting the first nucleotide of the downstream exon (G to T) (22). Five diseases result from an -AG to -GG mutation in the 3' splice site which then causes aberrant pre-mRNA processing (7,13,26,27,33). In human osteogenesis imperfecta, (33) hereditary analbuminemia, (27) and retinoblastoma, (13) as in GRMD, the exon downstream of the mutation was skipped during processing of the major species of transcript. In familial ApoE deficiency (7) and Beta-Thalassemia (26,33) cryptic splice sites were activated and intronic material was included in the transcript.

Table 1:   Other mutations affecting the 3' splice site of mammalian genes.

Species	Gene/Disease	3' Splice Site	Outcome
Hampster (22)	Dihydrofolate reductase	CAA:G	Exon skipped
Hampster (22)	Dihydrofolate reductase	CAG:T	Exon skipped
Human (33)	Osteogenesis imperfecta	CGG:T	Exon skipped
Human (27)	Hereditary Analbuminemia	CGG:T	Exon skipped
Human (13)	Retinoblastoma	CGG:T	Exon skipped
Human (7)	Familial ApoE deficiency	CGG:T	Cryptic splice site activated

Universal consensus: 3' splice site signal:- CAG:T

CANINE GENOMIC SEQUENCING PRIMERS

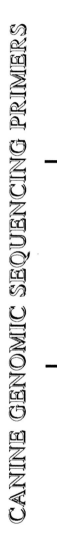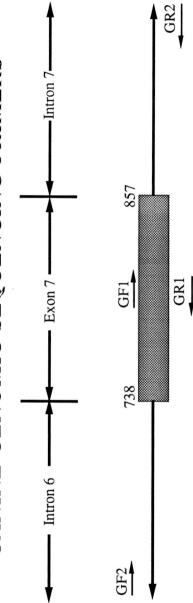

5'   3'

GF1	(817 to 794)	CTGGAACATGCATTCAACATCGCC	EXON 7
GF2	(-134 to -114)	GGGAATCATGGGCATGGG	INTRON 6
GR1	(802 to 782)	TGCATGTTCCAGTCGTTGTGTGGC	EXON 7
GR2	(-103 to -82)	ATGCATAGTTTCTCTTTCATGC	INTRON 7

FIG 5.   **Sequence of the dystrophin gene in the region of the mutation.**

FIG. 5A.   Primers used for amplification and sequencing of the 5' and 3' splice sites flanking exon seven. Genomic DNA template was from the same three affected dogs and one normal dog studied by mRNA PCR. Sequencing of the insert from phage DNA was performed using a kit (double strand DNA cycle sequencing kit, LTI).

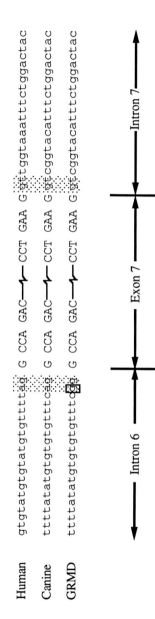

Human	gtgtatgtgtatgtgtttag G CCA GAC—CCT GAA Ggtggtaaatttctggactac
Canine	tttatatgtgtgtgttcag G CCA GAC—CCT GAA Ggtcggtacatttctggactac
GRMD	tttatatgtgtgtgttcgg G CCA GAC—CCT GAA Ggtcggtacatttctggactac

Intron 6 ⟷ Exon 7 ⟷ Intron 7

FIG. 5B. The DNA sequences from normal and GRMD dogs, and from normal human beings (33), in the region of the mutation. The stippled areas represent nucleotides that should be 100% conserved. Single stranded (20) and double stranded DNA (4) was amplified using primers GF2 and GR2 and then sequenced manually using primers GF1, GF2 or GR1.

In DMD, up to 65% of mutations are due to intragenic deletions, the majority of which cause frame-shifts of protein translation and result in severely truncated dystrophin molecules (14,16,23,34,35). Intragenic duplications occur much less commonly (1,9). Mutations responsible for the remainder of patients with DMD are largely unknown (1). A G to T point mutation at position 3714 of the dystrophin cDNA has recently been described which changes a glutamic acid codon to an Amber stop codon (3). A similar point mutation at position 3185 is the molecular basis for the defect in the mdx mouse (32). Additional nonsense mutations will undoubtedly be identified, but it has been predicted that many of the as yet undetermined defects in DMD, are splice site mutations that prevent or alter RNA processing (23).

A processing error has been described in one DMD patient which results from a deletion within exon 19 and does not involve a consensus splice site (19). It was proposed, however, that this deletion prevented correct recognition of the 5' splice site in intron 20. The truncated exon 19 was then skipped entirely during processing to generate a translation termination signal in exon 20. Exon skipping that alters the translational reading frame appears to predict the disease phenotype in a way analogous to that of a genomic deletion causing loss of a single exon. Both genomic deletion of exon 7 alone, (18) and skipping of exon seven as reported here, cause the severe (DMD) phenotype.

The consensus splice site mutation and subsequent exon skipping in GRMD is the first example of dystrophin deficiency due to an error in RNA processing that is caused by a mutation other than an intragenic deletion. This finding supports the suggestion that similar mutations may be found in some DMD patients who lack genomic deletions (2,23,31,34).

ACKNOWLEDGEMENTS

The authors wish to thank L.M. Kunkel for human dystrophin cDNA clones, L. Leinward for human adult myosin heavy chain probe. Support for this research was from the Association Francaise contre les Myopathies (RJB and JNK); Muscular Dystrophy Association (JNK); March of Dimes (JNK); National Institutes of Neurological Disease and Stoke, NS (RJB); LEAD Award AG (ADR); and the Joseph and Kathleen Bryan Alzheimer's Disease Research Center, (ADR).

REFERENCES

1. Angelini, C., Beggs, A.H., Hoffman, E.P., Fanin, M., Kunkel, L.M. (1990): Enormous dystrophin in a patient with Becker muscular dystrophy. *Neurology*, 40: 808-812.
2. Bartlett, R.J., Sharp, N.J.H., Secore, S.L., Hung, W.Y., Kornegay, J.N., Roses, A.D. (1990): The canine and human DYS genes are highly conserved. *J. Neurol. Sci.*, 98: (Suppl), 165.
3. Bulman, D.E., Gangopadhyay, S.B., Bebchuk, K.G., Worton, R.G., Ray, P.N. (1991): Point mutation in the human dystrophin gene: Identification through western blot analysis. *Genomics* 10:457-460.
4. Casanova, J.L., Pannetier, C., Jaulin, C., Kourilsky, P. (1990): Optimal conditions for directly sequencing double-stranded PCR products with Sequenase. *Nucleic Acids Res.*, 18:4028.
5. Chamberlain, J.S., Gibbs, R.A., Ranier, J.E., Nguyen, P.N., Caskey, C.T. (1988): Deletion screening of the Duchenne muscular dystrophy locus

via multiplex DNA amplification. *Nucleic Acids Res.,* 16:11141-11156.

6. Chirgwin, J.M., Przybyla, A.E., MacDonald, R.J., Rutter, W.J. (1979): Isolation of biologically active ribonucleic acid from sources enriched in ribonuclease. *Biochemistry,* 18:5294-5299.

7. Cladaras, C., Hadzopoulou-Cladaras, M., Felber, B.K., Paklakis, G., Zannis, V.I. (1987): The molecular basis of familial Apo E deficiency: An acceptor splice-site mutation in the third intron of the deficient Apo E gene. *J. Biol. Chem.,* 262:2310-2315.

8. Cooper, B.J., Winand, N.J., Stedman, H., Valentine, B.A., Hoffman, E.P., Kunkel, L.M., Oronzi Scott, M., Fischbeck, K.H., Kornegay, J.N., Avery, R.J., Williams, J.R., Schmickel, R.D., Sylvester, J.E.(1988): The homologue of the Duchenne locus is defective in X-linked muscular dystrophy of dogs. *Nature,* 334: 154-156.

9. den Dunnen, J.T., Bakker, A.A., Klein-Breteler, E.G., Pearson, P.L., van Ommen, G.J.-B. (1987): Direct detection of more than 50% of the Duchenne muscular dystrophy mutations by field inversion gels. *Nature,* 329:640-642.

10. Feener, C.A., Koenig M., Kunkel, L.M. (1989): Alternative splicing of human dystrophin mRNA generates isoforms at the carboxy terminus. *Nature,* 338:509-511.

11. Forrest, S.M., Cross, G.S., Speer, A., Gardner-Medwin, D., Burn, J., Davies, K. (1987): Preferential deletion of exons in Duchenne and Becker muscular dystrophies. *Nature,* 329:638-640.

12. Hoffman, E.P., Fischbeck, K.H., Brown, R.H., Johnson, M.J., Medori, R., Loike, J.D., Harris, J.B., Waterston, R., Brooke, M., Specht, L., Kupsky, W., Chamberlain, J., Caskey, C.T., Shapiro, F., Kunkel, L.M. (1988): Dystrophin characterization in muscle biopsies from Duchenne and Becker muscular dystrophy patients. *New Engl. J. Med.,* 31:1363-1368.

13. Horowitz, J.M., Yandell, D.W., Park, S.-H., Canning, S., Whyte, P., Buchkovich, K., Harlow, E., Weinberg, R.A., Dryja, T.P. (1989): Point mutational inactivation of the retinoblastoma antioncogene. *Science,* 243:937-940.

14. Koenig, M., Hoffman, E.P., Bertelson, C.J., Monaco, A.P., Feener, C., Kunkel, L.M. (1987): Complete cloning of the Duchenne muscular dystrophy (DMD) cDNA and preliminary genomic organization of the DMD gene in normal and affected individuals. *Cell,* 50:509-517.

15. Koenig, M., Monaco, A.P., Kunkel, L.M. (1988): The complete sequences of dystrophin predicts a rod-shaped cytoskeletal protein. *Cell,* 53: 219-228.

16. Koenig, M., Beggs, A.H., Moyer, M., Scherpf, S., Heindrich, K., Bettecken, T., Meng, G., Muller, C.R., Lindlof, M., Kaarianen, H., de la Chapelle, A., Kiuru, A., Savontaus, M.-L., Gilgenkrantz, H., Recan, D., Chelly, J., Kaplan, J.-C., Covone, A.E., Archidiancono, N., Romeo, G., Leichti-Gallati, S., Schneider, V., Braga, S., Moser, H., Darras, B.T., Wrogemann, K., Blonden, L.A.J., van Paassen, H.M.B., van Ommen, G.J.B., Kunkel, L.M.. (1989): The molecular basis for Duchenne versus Becker muscular dystrophy: correlation of severity with type of deletion. *Am.J.Hum. Genet.,* 45:498-506.

17. Kornegay, J.N., Sharp, N.J.H., Bartlett, R.B., Van Camp, S.D., Burt, C.T., Hung, W.Y., Kwock, L., Roses, A.D.(1990): Golden retriever muscular dystrophy: Monitoring for success. In: *Advances in Experimental Medicine and Biology.* edited by A.B. Eastwood, R.C. Griggs, G. Karpati. 280: pp.267-272. Plenum Publishing Corporation, New York.

18. Malhotra, S.B., Hart, K.A., Klamut, H.J., Thomas, N.S.T., Bodrug, S.E., Burghes, A.H.M., Bobrow, M., Harper, P.S., Thopmson, M.W., Ray, P.N., Worton, R.G. (1988): Frame-shift deletions in patients with Duchenne and Becker muscular dystrophy. *Science*, 242:755-758.

19. Matsuo, M., Masamura, T., Nishio, H., Nakajima, T., Kitoh, Y., Takumi, T., Koga, J., Nakamura, H. (1991): Exon skipping during splicing of dystrophin mRNA precursors due to an intragenic deletion in the dystrophin gene of Duchenne muscular dystrophy Kobe. *J. Clin. Invest.*, 87: 2127-2131.

20. Mihilovilovic, M., Lee, J.E. (1989): An efficient method for sequencing PCR amplified DNA. *Biotechniques*, 7:14-16.

21. Miller, S.A., Dykes, D.D., Patesky, H.F. (1988): A simple salting out procedure for extracting DNA from human nucleated cells. *Nucleic. Acids Res.*, 16: 1215.

22. Mitchell, P.J., Urlaub, G., Chasin, L. (1986): Spontaneous splicing mutations at the dihydrofolate reductase locus in Chinese hamster ovary cells. *Molec. and Cell Biol.*, 6:1926-1935.

23. Monaco, A.P., Bertelson, C.J., Liechti-Gallati, S., Moser, H., Kunkel, L.M. (1988): An explanation for the phenotypic differences between patients bearing partial deletions of the DMD locus. *Genomics*, 2: 90-95.

24. Mount, S.M. (1982): A catalogue of splice junction sequences. *Nucleic Acids Research*, 10:459-472.

25. Oronzi Scott, M., Sylvester, J.E., Heiman-Patterson, T., Shi, Y.-J., Fieles, W., Stedman, H., Burghes, A., Ray, P., Worton, R., and Fischbeck, K.H. (1988): Duchenne muscular dystrophy gene expression in normal and diseased human muscle. *Science*, 239:1418-1420.

26. Padgett, R.A., Grabowski, P.J., Konarska, M.M., Seiler, S., Sharp, P.A. (1986): Splicing of messenger RNA precursors. *Annu. Rev. Biochem.*, 55:1119-1150.

27. Ruffner, D.E., Dugaiczyk, A. (1988): Splicing mutation in human hereditary analbuminemia. *Proc. Natl. Acad. Sci.*, 85:2125-2129.

28. Saiki, R.K., Gelfand, D.H., Stoffel, S., Scharf, S.J., Higuchi, R., Horn, G.T., Mullis, K.B., Ehrlich, H.A. (1988): Primer-directed enzymatic amplification of DNA with a thermostable DNA polymerase. *Science*, 239:487-491.

29. Sambrook, J., Fritsch, E.F., Maniatis, T. (1989): *Molecular Cloning: A Laboratory Manual.* 2nd edition. Cold Springs Harbour Laboratory, Cold Springs Harbour, New York.

30. Schowalter, D.B., Sommer, S.S. (1989): The generation of radiolabelled DNA and RNA probes with polymerase chain reaction. *Anal. Biochem.*, 177: 90-4.

31. Sharp, N.J.H., Kornegay, J.N., Van Camp, S.D., Herbstreith, M.H., Secore, S.L., Kettle, S., Dykstra, M.J., Constantinou, C.D., Roses, A.D., Bartlett, R.B. A consesus splice-site mutation causes golden retriever muscular dystrophy. *Nature*, (Submitted).

32. Sicinski, P., Geng, Y., Ryder-Cook, A.S., Barnard, E.A., Darlison, M.G., and Barnard, P.J. (1989). The molecular basis of muscular dystrophy in the mdx mouse: a point mutation. *Science*, 244:1578-1580.

33. Tromp, G., Prockop, D.J. (1988): Single base mutation in the pro alpha2 (I) collagen gene that causes efficient splicing of RNA from exon 27 to exon 29 and synthesis of a shortened but in-frame pro alpha2 (I) chain. *Proc. Natl. Acad. Sci.*, 85:5254-5258.

34. Walker, A.P., Bartlett, R.J., Laing, N.G., Hung, W.Y., Yamaoka, L. H.,
     Secore, S.L., Holsti, M., Speer, M.C., Mechler, F., Denton, M.,
     Siddique, T., Pericak-Vance, M.A., Roses, A.D. (1989): A partial Taq I
     map of the Duchenne muscular dystrophy gene: use of small cDNA
     fragments in deletion and RFLP analysis. *Am.J.Human Genet.,* 45:A166.
35. Walker, A.P., Laing, N.G., Yamada, T., Chandler, D.C., Kakulas, B.,
     Bartlett, R.B. (1991): A Taq I map of the dystrophin gene useful for
     detection and carrier status analysis. *J. Med. Genet.,* In Press.

DISCUSSION

Dr. Barry J. Cooper:
This is a technical question for Nick. You stated at one stage that the dystrophin messenger RNA was considerably higher in puppies then in the older dogs. Based on PCR, it is difficult to quantitate. Do you have any backup, western blots, etc?

Dr. Nicholas J.H. Sharp:
No, the quantitative western blot has not been attempted.

Dr. Henry J. Klamut:
The intron sequences that you've shown surrounding exon 7 are highly conserved. Does this sequence conservation extend further into either intron?

Dr. Nicholas J.H. Sharp:
One of the introns was highly conserved initially but the other one started to diverge quickly.

GENERAL DISCUSSION

Afternoon Session

Leaders: Frank L. Mastaglia and Joe N. Kornegay

Professor Frank L. Mastaglia:
Perhaps I could highlight some of the major messages that have come across in today's papers, from my point of view, and someone might like to follow this up. One of the main messages has been that of variability in the phenotypic expression of dystrophin deficiency. Not only variability in expression in different species but also considerable variability in the human dystrophin deficiency states, leading to the emergence of the concept of dystrophinopathies, which I feel is a very important concept that needs to be taken further and has important implications diagnostically and also for the classification of patients with neuromuscular disorders.

It was perhaps not too surprising to hear that patients who, as neurologists we have previously regarded as having myopathies - eg. in conditions such as Becker dystrophy, limb girdle dystrophy or quadriceps myopathy, turn out to be partial forms of expression of dystrophin deficiency, and have been drawn together under this label of **dystrophinopathy**. What is more surprising and more radical is to hear about cases such as those that Byron spoke to us about this morning where on clinical, electromyographic and histological grounds these patients would have been confidently classified as having a neurogenic disorder, with the assumption that the primary derangement was in the motor neuron and not in the muscle, in which similar deletions of the dystrophin gene have been found and this obviously raises the question - how broad is the spectrum of **dystrophinopathy**? Do we yet know its full extent?

I would like to start by asking Dr. Sugita or Byron whether either of them have studied other patients with neurogenic disorders, for example, sporadic cases of spinal muscular atrophy. Dr. Sugita would you like to comment?

Professor Hideo Sugita:
I think Dr. Arikawa is the best person to answer this question.

Dr. Eri Arikawa:
I have not seen any cases of neurogenic diseases with dystrophinopathies in my laboratory.

Professor Byron A. Kakulas:
A number of cases of Kugelberg-Welander that we have looked at have shown a DMD deletion. We still have some, for example, limb girdles that we are still working through.

Dr. Nigel G. Laing:
We have examined cases clinically diagnosed as disorders other than DMD or BMD including 8 with a diagnosis of limb girdle muscular dystrophy (LGMD), 9 with a diagnosis of spinal muscular atrophy (SMA) and 6 with facioscapulohumeral muscular dystrophy. Out of the 17 diagnosed as "SMA" or "LGMD", 5 have had deletions, 3 with a clinical diagnosis of "SMA", 2 with a diagnosis of "LGMD".

Professor Frank L. Mastaglia:
I think this topic is going to be discussed much more in the future, but I feel that it will help us make a lot more sense of those in between cases that clinically have been diagnosed as suffering from Kugelberg-Welander disease or spinal muscular atrophy, where there is clear evidence of a neurogenic process but the biopsy shows both myopathic and neurogenetic changes. It could be that in some of the cases we were dealing with a combined dystrophin deficiency involving not only the muscle but also the motor neurons and I suppose the next question, again to Dr. Sugita, is can he tell us anything more about the distribution of dystrophin in motor neurones and synapses? I think we heard some reference made to that earlier today. Is there anything further that you can tell us about?

Professor Hideo Sugita:
There is a related problem that I have shown this morning with a defect, there was some connection with myasthenia gravis but I do not think that defect was dystrophin related.

Professor Frank L. Mastaglia:
You are saying that there are no dystrophin isoforms as such?

Professor Hideo Sugita:
The neuromuscular junction had the dystrophin. The dystrophin antibody crossed reacted with the surface membrane of the neuromuscular junction. At the same time there was a reaction at the neuromuscular junction which was different from dystrophin.

Professor Allen D. Roses:
We have that experience. I do not find that an ethical problem at all. We just happen to find a minor mutation of this person who is otherwise a fairly normal carrier and we let him go without undue counselling as opposed to the rest of us in the room who have mutations that we don't know about that we may want to counsel.
I think the other argument which was brought up this morning is if you have a deletion or a mutation of the gene, do the subsequent generation of carrier females, have a greater risk of throwing off the mutants. If you look back in the family histories I think in some of the larger pedigrees, there has been this strange phenomenon of an occasionally weak male. In fact, in Lord Walton's original paper about the X-linked nature of Duchenne dystrophy, I think it was in 1957, he had a paper with 22 pedigrees, one of them actually had a transmission through a male between 2 parts of a pedigree. We do not know whether or not they are the same mutation causing Duchenne in either part of the pedigree. But I think that it is quite possible that some of these older individuals who themselves are phenotypically fairly normal but do have a documentable mutation in their dystrophin could pass to their daughters an increased propensity for them to have

children with Duchenne dystrophy. So I feel that it is their daughters which should be counselled and maybe their daughters who should have chorionic screening.

Professor John McC. Howell:
There is also phenotypic variation in the dog. The literature tells us that the symptoms first appear at about 8 weeks of age and that the phenotypic characteristics differ from litter to litter. Today we have heard of additional variations. Even within a litter there may be significant variations and we were also told of animals showing distinct signs before 8 weeks of age. I wonder whether Dr. Cooper or Dr. Kornegay could expand on that.

Dr. Barry J. Cooper:
It is true that one can see some variation in severity of the disease from animal to animal, and that can be within the litter or between litters. Most certainly they are similar clinical signs. There is no doubt that dogs are born with severe lesions already present in some muscles, particularly the tongue. If you look at the tongue of animals at birth, and we have done this a couple of times when animals are stillborn for some other reason, for example a dystotia, it is very severely affected. I think that is related to the fact that the tongue is used in sucking motions in utero and so is subjected to an "exercise" challenge, if you like. The basis of between animal variation, assuming the mutation is consistent and is not complicated by other secondary mutational events, is not clear at all. We have been inclined to believe, and this is a very subjective thing, that larger animals tend to have somewhat more severe clinical disease than the smaller stature animals. We have also been inclined to believe that affected females, which we do generate when we breed carrier females to affected males, also tend on average to have a somewhat less severe phenotype. However there are some exceptions to that, as Joe pointed out. There are sometimes animals that do very poorly and one does not know why. However, they are qualitatively the same. The variation is in just how severely this otherwise identical syndrome is manifested. This does not worry me too much, but it would be absolutely naive to think that every animal with the same molecular defect, given all of the other environmental and inherent differences between animals, would express an exactly identical syndrome.

Professor Joe N. Kornegay:
I would like to make an additional comment regarding other forms of X-linked muscular dystrophy that have been characterized in dogs. Neither Barry nor I discussed these conditions in depth in our earlier discussions; however, they are relevant to the questions relating to variable phenotype. An analogous disease was described in the Irish terrier breed in 1972. This of course predated recognition of dystrophin as the defective protein in Duchenne muscular dystrophy. Affected dogs had dramatic creatine kinase changes and other phenotypic features that are similar to those seen in golden retriever muscular dystrophy. Barry has mentioned the syndrome in Rottweiler dogs, and recently a similar condition has also been described in the Samoyed breed in Norway. Several forms of X-linked dystrophy have therefore been characterized in dogs. If we are patient, John, we may therefore eventually have the opportunity to study differing phenotypes in breeds with considerable size variation, as with Chihuahuas versus Saint Bernards. However I do not know whether size or gender actually are significant variables with regard to phenotype. As discussed and illustrated earlier, we do

see severely affected homozygous females. Variation of phenotype could, of course, relate to the relative percentage of so-called revertant fibers. The potential for alternative splicing subsequent to exon skipping, as was discussed this morning is also an intriguing explanation for phenotypic variation. The bottom line though, is that we do not really have an explanation at this time.

Dr. Miranda D. Grounds:
The similarities and differences between the animal models are very interesting and I would just like to consider a point that Terry Partridge made this morning. He suggested that if the animal survives the major growth phase of its development, then the dystrophic process may plateau. Therefore perhaps differences between individual animals reflects, not so much the actual size of the animal, but the rate of growth (combined with muscle activity). Perhaps one experiment that you might be able to do is to immobilize one limb of a dog while it is growing and when it has reached almost adult size, remove the immobilization: the muscles in that leg would then be subjected to the dystrophic process having been protected through what was essentially its growth phase.

Dr. Barry J. Cooper:
You are suggesting, perhaps, to put a cast on the limb, or some such thing. The problem with that is you introduce more than one variable. The animal would not be using the leg, as well as not growing. One could staple growth plates and try to inhibit growth. Those experiments are not kindly looked upon by animal care committees, and I would be reluctant to attempt them.

Dr. Miranda D. Grounds:
If you immobilize the animal you still get effective growth.

Dr. Barry J. Cooper:
You are thinking that the bones will still grow with the muscle. Our experience in growing animals with neuropathic conditions, in which animals are immobilized because of their inability to use the limb, is that the condition leads very quickly to fixation in extension, so it ends up very messy.

Dr. Terence A. Partridge:
On the last experiment - instead of stapling the growth plates, it would be possible to stop them growing by irradiating them.

Professor Byron A. Kakulas:
I will open it a little broader. In answer to Miranda's question it would be desirable theoretically to sort out the question. There has been quite a large body of thought being given to the idea that the dystrophic process is not so much harmed by the workload during the period of rapid body growth but that the bone lengthening process itself aggravates the lesion. This has been well worked out in the Fukuyama type of congenital muscular dystrophy in Japan. There is a Japanese colleague, Dr. Totsuka, who would like to extend this concept to all of the muscular dystrophies. It seems possible that the mechanisms which are responsible for the growth of the muscle in relation to its increasing length as growth occurs in the bones may be disturbed and thus aggravate the lesion. But again we may come back to the mechanical role of dystrophin I suppose.

Dr. Miranda D. Grounds:
The interesting thing about the increase in length is that it involves proliferation of the muscle precursor cells. As long as the muscles are growing in length the muscle precursor cells probably proliferate in order to maintain the ratio of muscle nuclei to sarcoplasm. Once the adult length is reached and muscle precursor proliferation ceases and these cells become quiescent, the muscles may be more resistant to the lack of dystrophin.

Professor Byron A. Kakulas:
We have all the work of Dr. Ole Sola concerning stretch hypertorphy. There is not just stretch hypertrophy but there is also stretch hyperplasia. Stretch is a very powerful stimulus of muscle growth and hyperplasia. I do not know if satellite cells have been looked at specifically when individual muscle fibres have been counted after stretch experiments.

Professor Allen D. Roses:
There is a natural experiment which occurs in boys with Duchenne dystrophy. They do break their arms, they do break their legs, and they do become immobilized and it is well known phenomenon by anyone who takes care of these kids for any length of time, in that immobilization creates a very rapid progression of the apparent disease. Taking a kid off his feet even for the tendon stretching operations which used to be done for a matter of 3 days, worsens the disease before there are fixed contractures or anything like that. So I suspect that the experiment that you might do if you immobilize would have just the opposite result.

Professor Joe N. Kornegay:
I would like to comment on the question of exercise. I believe we have also potentially seen deleterious effects with exercise restriction. At least, with some animals, daily exercise appears to improve function. One could approach the problem from a different tack. Instead of intentionally immobilizing a limb, one could study the effects of augmented exercise, not by leash walking a dog, but instead by selectively electrically stimulating a muscle on a regular basis, perhaps daily or weekly. One could then objectively assess function of the stimulated muscle and compare results obtained to those from the contralateral unstimulated muscle. Both pathological and functional studies could be done. I am inclined to believe that the stimulation might actually have improved, rather than lessened, muscle function.

Dr. Barry J. Cooper:
We have done that in a very limited way and on a very informal basis. If you stimulate the craniotibial muscle, for example, it is fairly clear that you get more necrotic fibres. I think the problem in this type of experiment is what is meant by more rapid progression or less rapid progression of the disease. If you completely immobilize a patient (or a dog) then you end up with clinical progression because the patient develops contractures and so on, and is actually less able to function then they were before this procedure. On the other hand, it is clear from some of the things that we have done both by electrical stimulation and forced exercise that exercise does cause increased muscle necrosis. So I think that you have counter balancing clinical pathological events going on that contribute to some type of clinical end point. So I think it is really difficult to

answer this question. But I am sure that exercise actually injures the muscle fibres. Lack of exercise injures the patient, if you like.

Professor Joe N. Kornegay:
What rate of stimulation was used and how often were you stimulating?

Dr. Barry J. Cooper:
I can't answer details Joe, because the work was done by some colleagues at the University of Pennsylvania.

Professor Joe N. Kornegay:
Let me just conclude with one additional comment. It seems clear that, depending on the rate and perhaps frequency of stimulation, either a protective or adverse effect could be gained. It is well known that periodic nerve stimulation lessens the severity of neurogenic atrophy. Limited exercise might have protective effects, whereas extreme exercise would probably be deleterious.

Professor George Karpati:
One of the most fascinating aspects of dystrophin deficiency is that there are certain categories of muscle fibres or certain situations of muscle fibres in which dystrophin deficiency is not deleterious and does not cause any morphological or functional disturbance. We know these situations in the mdx mouse and DMD and I think that we should take advantage of the fact that we have the dog experts here and try to find out from them whether the same situations apply to the dog. From this comparison something might emerge. Dystrophin-deficient fibres that seem to be resistant to necrosis include, intrafusal muscle fibres, extraocular muscles, denervated and severely disused muscle fibres. Also in very early life we know both in the mdx, before 15 days and in DMD certainly within the first month or so, no necrosis occurs. So maybe one of the dog experts can comment as to whether, in these situations, muscle fibres remain intact in the dystrophin-deficient dog or not?

Dr. Barry J. Cooper:
I can comment upon a couple of these questions and Joe can complement this, I hope, because I do not have all the answers. I can say that I have noticed intact spindles, with intact fibres in otherwise damaged muscle and I have never noticed scarring associated with intrafusal fibres or muscle spindles for example, so my guess would be that, yes, they are protected in the dog, just as they are in humans. We have looked quite carefully at extra ocular muscles and they are largely spared. We have not done the denervation experiments and we have not done the disuse experiments. They could be done, but we have just not chosen to do them. I think you also said something about early life. I repeat that in the dog it is quite clear that there is early massive muscle damage.

Professor George Karpati:
How about intra-uterine life? Do you see necrotic fibres in dystrophic foetuses?

Professor Joe N. Kornegay:
We have not looked, but I can tell you that some animals, have well-developed lesions at birth. So one assumes that they must have had, in some muscles, particularly the tongue, lesions during intra-uterine development. But I am not sure what stage those first occur.

Professor George Karpati:
It would be very interesting if you found muscle fibre necrosis in the dystrophic dog foetuses, which would be almost unique because it would not occur in either DMD or mdx.

Professor Allen D. Roses:
I do not think that is true George, because in DMD you have no measure of the foetuses which die very early, and I think, from the sex ratio of counselled individuals that there is a foetal wastage which occurs very early in humans. Perhaps the difference is that dogs can carry though and the difficulty you have with keeping the pups alive is that the wastage occurs a little bit later.

Professor George Karpati:
I am talking about aborted foetuses which are known to have the disease and, to my knowledge, no one has ever seen a necrotic muscle fibre in a DMD foetus.

Professor Allen D. Roses:
The basic post natal lesion which you described has not been shown in the foetus.

Professor George Karpati:
My point is that the basic post natal lesion might be rampant in the dog foetuses.

Professor Byron A. Kakulas:
There is no convincing necrosis demonstrated in the human foetus. That is not to say that it may not be present in some of these abortuses, but it has not been seen.

Professor Joe N. Kornegay:
I share Barry's comments relative to intrafusal fibers. We have observed them, and perhaps very subjectively, they are spared. However, we have not done quantitative studies to support this observation. We have not critically evaluated extraocular muscles, nor have we done denervation experiments. As I commented this morning, relative to early pathologic changes, we have looked somwhat systematically at young puppies. Assuming that changes seen at 1 day of age reflect what is present during the late stages of gestation, we can assume that dramatic pathologic changes are present in certain muscles. One feature that has always intrigued me, and I believe you as well Dr. Karpati, is the type 1 predominance that occurs in Duchenne patients. In morphometric studies of the original two dogs that we studies, certain muscles had significant type 1 predominance. This has been supported by additional unpublished studies. In my mind, reasons for selective type 2 myofiber involvement in both Duchenne patients and dogs with golden retriever muscular dystrophy have not been fully clarified.

Professor Allen D. Roses:
Nick described this exon skipping mutation and we have a third of the boys which do not have deletions and obviously the way of clinically approaching that third, is to get muscle biopsies. Another way would be, I believe, is to look at either skin fibroblasts or lymphoblasts in cultures which make messenger RNA, in order to do the PCR work which is necessary to detect similar mutations occurring in this one third of boys who do not have deletions present. I think that this is something that we ought to be thinking about at least clinically in screening the population, as we are talking about a lot of people.

Professor Frank L. Mastaglia:

Perhaps I could follow up by asking Allen if there is some reason why this has not already been done. We heard in 1989, or even before, that at least about a third of cases do not have deletions and are therefore likely to have point mutations and there have been quite a number of other conditions where single base substitutions have been identified in leukocytes or fibroblasts, for example Leber's optic neuropathy.

Professor Allen D. Roses:

I think it is hard to put yourself in the position where Lou Kunkel was 6 years ago. It is hard to look at the body of a boy with the disease that did not have a deletion and start looking for something which you are not quite sure is there. From my point of view we came at it in a different way, with Nick describing this exon deletion, and I think with PCR technology, even since 1989, becoming much more sophisticated and it is now quite possible to either do it by kit or just to do it by using the right primers, to look at different pieces of the messenger RNA. But now it is certainly possible to do it and we are going to be doing it on our population. The reason we have been held up is because the workers have been looking at the dog.

Assist. Professor Richard J. Bartlett:

We have actually begun looking at some of the patients which do not have deletions and the original strategy which we tried relies on what we have designed for the dog. This utilizes very large segments for the PCR amplification. I have since determined that the pieces may have been too large to start with. We were looking at 2-3kb segments, and that was really biting off more than we could chew. We have now gone back to looking at 1KD segment in patients and have been successful.

Dr. Manfred W. Beilharz:

Further to the comment concerning the issue which just came out. The Rottweiler model clearly demonstrates a progressive disease. What is the actual gene defect in the Rottweiler model as demonstrated by Western blot or other procedures?

Dr. Barry J. Cooper:

No we do not know what the mutation is. We have only had the Rottweiler for a year and we only have a very limited number of them so far. They clearly completely lack dystrophin within the fairly sensitive limitations of the Western blots that we use. We can detect a very small amount of protein in the retrievers and I am not sure what the explanation of that is, except that they may be revertant fibres. We can't detect any signal at all in the Rottweiler. I am willing to say that they completely lack dystrophin but I am not sure what the mutation is.

Professor George Karpati:

I think that we should address the often raised question: "Is exercise good or bad for Duchenne dystrophy" I think you have to look at it in a pragmatic way. There are two opposing forces operating here. It appears that reduction in contractile activity, by keeping muscle fibres of small calibre and possibly of shorter length, would be beneficial for the protection of muscle fibres from necrosis; on the other hand, no one would seriously suggest that you should cast the limbs of Duchenne boys because that would cause severe disuse atrophy, an even worse negative effect. Thus, what would be gained by the avoidance of necrosis due to dystrophin deficiency, would be lost by the even worse aggravation to the muscle or disuse atrophy. In our clinic, we recommend just enough exercise for the activities of daily living and to try stretching the muscle to avoid contracture as much as possible.

Professor Byron A. Kakulas:
I would like to talk about the heart. Barry has raised a number of questions. He asked about myocardiopathy and life expectancy in human carriers and so on. As far as I know there have not been any autopsies on carriers reported so we don't know anything about that. In any event, it would be extremely difficult to distinguish the type of fibrosis you see due to the dystrophic fibrosis in the heart and from ischaemic replacement fibrosis. I do have some relevant clinical experience, very limited, just two cases of female carriers who have had cardiac arrhythmias, whom I believed did have a myocardiopathy. I think that it has been documented that ECG changes have been found in female carriers.

Professor Allen D. Roses:
There are definitely studies of carriers in the literature and a certain proportion of the them had a particular characteristic R wave change.

Professor Byron A. Kakulas:
Yes, including heart block. We have been talking about the heart in logitudinal sections in the dog. Did you observe that there was a very clear line of demarcation at the intercalated disc between those cell lines with dystrophin and those without?

Dr. Barry J. Cooper:
I have seen that. You can recognise the junction of adjoining fibres at the intercollated disc and I think you have seen the same, Terry, in the mosaicized mouse heart. It is quite clear that one cell has the protein associated with the membrane and the adjacent side has none. Just to comment a little further on cardiac dysfunction in carriers, I know that ECG abnormalities in humans have been reported, and I did not mention in the dog that you can fairly clearly demonstrate lesions using fairly sophisticated echocardiography techniques. I know that workers in France are looking quite closely at this now so I think that we will see some imaging information come out to suggest that the same kind of thing goes on in humans. I think that if you had the opportunity to obtain heart from a known carrier you can certainly document that the mosaicism persists throughout life and if that is associated with multifocal scarring, particularly in the left ventricle, I think that it would be a reasonable assumption to say that they are related.

Professor Byron A. Kakulas:
With the availability of the immunohistochemistry, if we ever do get the opportunity we will most certainly do that. But it will be the immuno-histochemistry which will tell us what is going on.
A comment was made about the lack of satellite cells in the heart and therefore there can be no regeneration. In fact my understanding is that regeneration will occur in the heart. It is found in young animals or young humans. There is very elegant experimental work with an experimental model for rheumatic fever of about 30 years ago. It was very clear from that work that myoblasts were present in the heart after focal necrosis, and that it regenerated. The myoblasts joined

together in the same way as in skeletal muscle regeneation. In relating the experimental work to children who have died of acute rheumatism, the same types of cells are present and one presumes that they were regenerating myocardioblasts. When David Durack was a student he looked at the quokka with vitamin E deficiency. There is a very clear regeneration in the quokka heart within the patchy lesions which occur. These again are very young animals (1).

Dr. Barry J. Cooper:
I do not think there is any doubt that there are no satellite cells in the heart and that in all animals, including humans, necrotic lesions become organized by scars.

Professor Byron A. Kakulas:
I agree with that.

Dr. Barry J. Cooper:
It is also clear that in very young animals, I think in the dog it would be less than 6 weeks of age, that some of the cells are still mitotically capable. I believe that it is the cardiac myocytes that are mitotically capable. I think one group at least, that has shown that fairly clearly is Alan Kelly and some of his co-workers at the University of Pennsylvania.

Professor Byron A. Kakulas:
This is seen in developing or immature heart. What about when the heart is challenged with a lesion, is there an increased number of mitotic cells?

Dr. Barry J. Cooper:
I do not have any information on that. It is potentially possible. The other thing which can occur in the heart is some development of polyploidy; there can be synthesis of DNA without actual cell division. The cardiomyopathic lesions both in carriers and in affected animals do not develop until 9 months or more of age. I think this is an important point.

Professor Byron A. Kakulas:
We are addressing ourselves to two questions, one of which is whether regeneration will occur in the heart and secondly what is the nature of the lesions in the heart? We all agree that regeneration is limited or absent in adults.

Dr. Terence A. Partridge:
The matter of regeneration in the heart is very difficult to address properly. There is nuclear proliferation in the heart as cardiomyocytes develop oligonuclearity, and in rodents at least, this occurs postnatally. A labelling technique with 3H-thymindine would not distinguish between this process and genuine proliferation of cardiomyocytes. Similarly, there is some elegant work in tissue culture by Eppenberger showing that cardiomyocytes will de-differentiate and re-differentiate but not proliferate; this process would be very difficult to distinguish from differentiation of cardiomyocytes derived from some proliferating precursor cell. Because of this, it is hard to be sure that genuine regeneration of heart muscle is occurring.

Professor Byron A. Kakulas:
Fine, that is an approach of an experimentalist. But for a pathologist who has to synthesize his experience with different animals, the lesions heal. They heal not by fibrosis but by myocardial regeneration it seems.

Dr. Terence A. Partridge:
It could be by mobility of cells.

Professor Byron A. Kakulas:
Whatever, the cells are there which look just like myoblasts.

Dr. Terence A. Partridge:
That's right. But they may be cells which have been moved from somewhere else, not necessarily cells which have been formed by proliferation. They may be migrating from nearby sites to fill the gaps.

Professor Byron A. Kakulas:
As reserve cells maybe.

Dr. Terence A. Partridge:
Yes.

Dr. Barry J. Cooper:
Can I just ask Byron a question? You are saying that histologically some of the cells you see, the mononuclear cells, look like myoblasts, as opposed to differentiated cardiac myocytes.

Professor Byron A. Kakulas:
You see single cells which look like myoblasts. Union of these cells occurs and after a time the lesions have healed.

Dr. Barry J. Cooper:
If that is the question I think you can address it these days because they should express Myo-D1 for example.

Professor Byron A. Kakulas:
It would be nice work to do. The quokka is still there. It is still prone to vitamin E deficiency.

Dr. Nicholas J.H. Sharp:
Did you say that dogs under 9 months of age do not show lesions in the heart?

Dr. Barry J. Cooper:
What I am saying is that it is difficult to appreciate very striking cardiomyopathic lesions in dogs younger than about 9 months. However that is an expensive study. If you start killing carriers just to look at their heart at 1,2,3 months and so on.

Dr. Nicholas J.H. Sharp:
No, I was referring to affected dogs.

Dr. Barry J. Cooper:
In affected dogs the onset of convincing lesions in the heart is somewhere between 6-9 months of age, from our experience.

Dr. Nicholas J.H. Sharp:
One potential explanation for that may be there was regeneration going on earlier.

Dr. Barry J. Cooper:
That went through my head when Byron was making the argument. However, some years ago I was involved in studying viral myocarditis, caused by parvovirus in dogs. Actual nuclear proliferation and probably cell division goes on until about 6 weeks of age in the dog. I cannot quote the literature but I think it has been documented in the dog. They are susceptible to infection with that virus, which requires DNA synthesis, only in the first few days of life. So I think that I would be fairly confident that there would be not much capacity to produce new cardiac muscle tissue after a few days of age or certainly a few weeks of age in the dog. I think that it is possibly part of the explanation, but I do not think we know the explanation. There are other peculiarities; why are the subepicardial myocytes in the heart susceptible in the human and in the dog? They seem to be because the fibrosis is concentrated there. Have you noticed that in the mouse at all, Terry?

Dr. Terence A. Partridge:
Yes, in little bands underneath the epicardium.

Dr. Barry J. Cooper:
It is a very intriguing question. I wish I knew how to approach it. Incidentally I am not at liberty to share all of this data, but we are collaborating with people to look at cardiac function and I willing to say that there are electrically measurable differences between dystrophic heart and normal heart which may be very intriguing to pursue. One of the reasons that I tried to push that project is that in the heart there is a calcium mediated component to the action potential that I thought might be very interesting to look at. I am able to say at this point that there are differences in the action potential between dystrophic cardiac myocytes and normal ones, but we do not know how they are mediated yet.

Dr. Nicholas J.H. Sharp:
It is true that parvovirus only causes cardiomyopathy up until six weeks of age in puppies, presumably because the bulk of cardiac cell division finishes around this time. But this fact does not mean that a smaller population of cells are not capable of division and regeneration on a small scale for a longer period of time, and that such cells might possibly delay in cardiac lesions in affected golden retrievers until 6 months of age or so.

REFERENCES

1. Kakulas B.A., Owen, C.G., Papadimitriou, J.M., Durack, D.T. (1968): The myocardial lesions in the Rottnest Quokka with nutritional myopathy. Proc. Aust. Assn. Neurol., 5:79-85.

Part II

Myoblast Transfer

DUCHENNE MUSCULAR DYSTROPHY: Animal Models and Genetic Manipulation, edited by Byron A. Kakulas, John McC. Howell, and Allen D. Roses. Raven Press, Ltd., New York © 1992.

12

Necrosis and Regeneration in Dystrophic and Normal Skeletal Muscle

Miranda D. Grounds, Terry A. Robertson, Christopher A. Mitchell, John M. Papadimitriou

Department of Pathology, University of Western Australia, Queen Elizabeth II Medical Centre, Nedlands, Western Australia. 6009

INTRODUCTION

Since a striking feature of the X-linked human myopathy Duchenne muscular dystrophy (and the equivalent dog model) is persistent necrosis and failed regeneration of skeletal muscles, these topics need to be thoroughly considered. The absence of the subsarcolemmal protein dystrophin in Duchenne muscular dystrophy and the mdx mouse and golden-retriever dog models (15) is associated with membrane defects which can result in small lesions in the plasmalemma of myofibres (6,19,26). Very small lesions can presumably be repaired locally, but where this does not happen rapidly, leakage of ions such as calcium into the sarcoplasm will disturb the metabolism of the myofibre to the point where the cell can no longer maintain homeostasis (11) and necrosis results (8). Whether the calcium influx is a consequence of such plasmalemmal lesions, or instead produces the ultrastructually visible membrane defects is difficult to determine. In some instances the area of necrotic sarcoplasm might be relatively superficial and not extend across the diameter of the myofibre, whereas more extensive segmental necrosis would disrupt the myofibre longitudinally. Furthermore, necrosis occurs in small groups of adjacent myofibres in these dystrophies. Such damage to the myofibres probably triggers the activation, proliferation and fusion of muscle precursor cells (mpc), among other regenerative events.

In this paper I will discuss the resealing of damaged myofibres after segmental necrosis, and the factors which might account for the species-specific difference in regenerative capacity seen between dystrophic mice, and dogs and humans.

141

RESEALING OF DAMAGED MYOFIBRES

1.   New Plasmalemma Formation

An electron microscopic study of early events after injury to mature skeletal muscle of SJL/J mice described the rapid formation of new plasmalemmal membranes (20). At three hours after segmental injury (induced by painting with aldehyde fixative), the viable stump of injured myofibres was separated from the necrotic segment by a zone of supercontracted myofibrils. It has been proposed (7) that such hypercontracted myofilaments and accumulated cell organelles on either side of the injury site stabilise the internal environement of the myofibre and limit the extent of necrosis. No demarcating membrane was evident at this time, although occasionally collapsed segments of plasmalemma partially covered the viable stump. By 12 hours after injury numerous whorls of membrane material appeared in the vicinity of the Golgi apparatus, and a convoluted, tortuous membrane had apparently sealed the structurally normal part of the injured fibre (Fig. 1). The myoplasm immediately within this demarcating membrane possessed few myofilaments but numerous vesicles and tubules, several of which were continuous with the demarcating membrane; most degraded sarcoplasmic organelles remained external to the demarcating membrane (Fig. 1) and leukocytes were observed internalizing the debris. These observations indicate that after segmental injury to skeletal muscle fibres, active production of new sarcoplasmic membranes occurs, which contributes to the formation of the part of the plasmalemma that demarcates the viable portion of the muscle fibre from the injured area.

Although complete new plasmalemma appears to be formed in some myofibres by 12 hours after injury, ultrastructural studies cannot reveal whether such membranes represent effective barriers to reseal the damaged myofibre. To test the effectiveness of resealing, and to investigate experimentally factors which might influence the speed of resealing, the small molecular size enzyme horse radish peroxidase (HRP) was infused into damaged areas of myofibres and the diffusion of HRP into unsealed myofibres was demonstrated histochemically (24).

2.   Infusion of HRP into unsealed myofibres

A precise small cut injury was inflicted transversely across the mid-region of tibialis anterior muscle of mature SJL/J mice. Horse radish peroxidase was injected subcutaneously over the cut site at various times after injury. Twenty four hours was selected as a time when resealing should be completed, because discontinuities of the plasmalemma at the ends of damaged myofibres were not apparent ultrastructurally by 12 hours after injury (20). Animals were sacrificed 30 minutes after HRP injection, as this represents adequate time for HRP to enter unsealed damaged myofibres, and travel a significant distance into the sarcoplasm (18). The muscles were removed and cut in half transversely through the injury site. Frozen transverse sections (5 μm in thickness) were taken at least 300 μm beyond the cut face of the lesion, and stained using a modified 3-3' diaminobenzidine (DAB) technique to demonstrate HRP activity (24). The stained sections were examined under a light microscope and fibres which did not contain HRP reaction product were considered to have been sealed at the time of HRP injection.

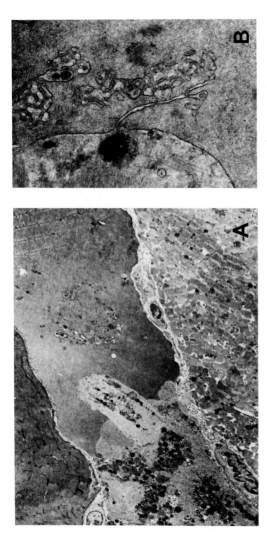

FIG. 1. **Electron Micrographs showing the demarcating membrane of a resealed myofibre 12 hours after injury.**

FIG. 1A. A finger-like process of necrotic tissue (on the left) is indenting the myoplasm at the end of the resealed myofibre (on the right) x 2000.

FIG. 1B. High power view of a zone of myofibrillar-free myoplasm from a serial section of the area depicted in A. Various membraneous structures are continuous with an irregular demarcating membrane. Necrotic myofilaments and debris can be seen at the end of the finger-like process (on the left) x 25,000.

(i)   **Time Course**
This technique was used to quantitate the resealing process after injury over a 24 hour period. The results of the HRP infusion experiment are summarised in Table 1. They show that myofibre resealing is seen by 8 hours and the majority of fibres are resealed by 24 hours after injury. Equivalent samples of cut injured muscles where HRP had not been infused, were taken as controls to test for endogenous myoglobin present in all myofibres which has peroxidase activity.

TABLE 1.   The time sequence of myofibre resealing using the cut injury/HRP infusion technique

Time after injury (hours)	Myofibres resealed (%)
4	0
8	40 ± 5
12	58 ± 6
16	79 ± 4
24	95 ± 5

The HRP/cut injury technique can be employed to test a range of factors that might influence resealing of damaged myofibres. In experimental situations where resealing might be delayed it would be of interest to see if the extent of necrosis is more pronounced along the length of the myofibre. This technique has been used to examine the role of local and circulating cells in the myofibre resealing process, in a series of irradiation experiments.

(ii)   **Irradiation Experiments**
These studies were designed to investigate the relative contribution of the myofibre and of blood-borne cells to the resealing process (24). A dose of 1600 rads was used in all experiments. Irradiation of muscles which are to be injured, eliminates the replicative capacity of local cells, and also affects cellular functions such as protein synthesis. Local irradiation was carried out by protecting the animal with a 2 mm lead sheet, except for one leg which was exposed. Whole body irradiation was carried out to remove the source of bone-marrow derived blood-borne leukocytes, which enter regenerating muscle. In addition some animals had one leg protected with lead sheeting before whole body irradiation.
Muscles of all mice were cut injured either at one hour after injury (at a time when blood-borne cells had not decreased significantly as a result of irradiation) or after 48 hours (when blood-borne cells had essentially disappeared as a result of irradiation). The results from a series of experiments are summarised in Table 2.

TABLE 2.   The extent of myofibre resealing using the cut injury/HRP diffusion technique with a variety of irradiation protocols.

Irradiation protocol	Time of injury after irradiation	Time of HRP injection after injury	% of resealed myofibres
Unirradiated control	-	24	95%
Local irradiation	within 1h	24	72%
Local irradiation	after 48h	24	5%
Whole body irradiation	within 1h	24	65%
Whole body irradiation	after 48h	24	6%
Whole body irradiation	after 48h	48	60%
Whole body irradiation with 1 leg protected	after 48h	24	80%

The greatly reduced numbers of resealed fibres seen when muscles were injured 48 hours after local irradiation can probably be accounted for by impaired function of the injured myofibres. The observation that many fibres were resealed when the injury was inflicted immediately after local irradiation, indicates that the damage resulting from irradiation increases with time. Similarly resealing of myofibres was impaired when muscles were injured 48 hours after whole body irradiation (when circulating leukocyte numbers are essentially zero). However, successful resealing was seen in protected legs injured at 48 hours after whole body irradiation: in these animals there were no peripheral leukocytes at the time of injury yet resealing was unimpaired in the protected leg. The results indicate that new plasmalemmal formation is purely a function of local cells, and is not dependent upon infiltrating leukocytes.

Although resealing was almost totally absent in animals which were injured 24 hours after whole body irradiation and sampled 24 hours later, significant resealing of damaged myofibres was seen when animals were sampled after 48 hours. This shows that the resealing process is slowed but not prevented by irradiation, and again supports the proposal that myofibre function is impaired as a result of irradiation damage.

The formation of new plasmalemma occurs between the zone of hypercontracted myofilaments and the myoplasm of the relatively intact myofibre segment (20). The excluded hypercontracted myofilaments and other necrotic material are then phagocytosed by infiltrating leukocytes. Muscle precursor cells proliferate and fuse with each other and with the new plasmalemmal membranes of the resealed myofibres (25) to repair the injured segment. It was noted that mpc activation and myotube formation can occur in the absence of infiltrating leukocytes: this was observed in muscles of a protected leg injured 48 hours after whole body irradiation, and sampled 4 days later (24). Successful muscle regeneration depends upon the proliferation and fusion of mpc and subsequent maturation into myofibres. Possible reasons for impairment of new muscle formation are examined in the following section.

FACTORS INFLUENCING THE SUCCESS OF
MUSCLE REGENERATION

1.   Species specific differences

It is well recognised that the limb muscles remain relatively healthy in mdx mice, although the diaphragm muscles do not (27). However in the dog model which more closely resembles Duchenne muscular dystrophy (see other chapters this volume), muscles become progressively weaker and are replaced by fat and connective tissue. Although skeletal muscles in all three X-linked myopathies undergo repeated cycles of necrosis, the reasons for the apparently successful regeneration in mdx limb muscles compared with the impaired regeneration in the other species are not clear. Observations that muscle regeneration after experimental injury is similar in mdx and the control parental mouse strain (12,28) emphasise that the different regenerative capacity does not reflect some unique property of mdx mice, but is species-specific (12,28).

There is no conclusive evidence as to whether such species-specific differences might be due to; (i) a fundamental difference in the proliferative capacity of satellite cells related to the size and relative postnatal growth of muscles; (ii) the different life spans and an ageing phenomenon; (iii) the result of the lower metabolic rate in dogs and humans as compared with mice; (iv) more vigorous connective tissue (fibrous and adipose) formation in the larger species which may also directly inhibit myogenesis; or (v) differences in the availability of factors (produced either by mpc or their environment) which favour mpc replication and new muscle formation. The potential importance of these possibilities is discussed in detail in Grounds and Yablonka-Reuveni (14). The first two possibilities are related to proposals that the proliferative capacity of mpc is exhausted with time and that failed regeneration is essentially an inherent failure of mpc replication; and that the dystrophic process might be influenced by development. The other three possibilities emphasise the potential importance of the host environment.

2.   Extracellular matrix

The greater "thickness" of connective tissues in the larger species (presumably attributable to mechanical factors), combined with increased fibrosis consistently reported in regenerating muscles of older host animals, may adversely influence the capacity for new muscle formation (14). This may result, not only from more vigorous production of extracellular matrix components, but also from a change in the balance of the extracellular matrix composition favouring the proliferation of fibroblasts and adipocytes at the expense of mpc (17).

The roles of various extracellular matrix components, growth factors and hormones in the activation, proliferation, differentiation and fusion of mpc have been investigated in tissue culture, and the main effects of some of these factors are summarised in Table 3 (reviewed 13,14). Of the growth factors the most extensively studied are the fibroblast growth factors (FGF), platelet-derived growth factor, insulin-like growth factor and transforming growth factor-beta. In this paper recent information on basic FGF (bFGF) will be presented, as bFGF (or an FGF-like protein) is implicated in mpc activation, and it is the only growth factor that has been examined in dystrophic muscles of mdx mice.

TABLE 3.   **Effects of various factors on muscle precursor cells**
            in vitro

	PROLIFERATION	DIFFERENTIATION AND FUSION
EXTRACELLULAR MATRIX COMPONENTS		
Laminin	↑	-
Fibronectin	↑	↓
Hyaluronic acid	-	↓
Heparin	↓	-
Heparin sulphate Proteoglycans	↓	-
Collagen	-	↑
Glycoproteins (high mannose type)	-	↑
GROWTH FACTORS (GF)		
Fibroblast GF	↑	↓
Platelet derived GF	↑	↓
Bischoff muscle GF	↑	-
Insulin GF	↑	↑
Adrenocorticotrophin	↑	-
Prostaglandin	-	↑
Transforming GF-ß	↓	↓
Interferon	-	↓

3.   FGF-like growth factors

Studies by Bischoff using isolated muscle fibres in tissue culture, implicate bFGF (3,5) or FGF-like growth factors produced by the muscle cells (4,5), in the activation of mpc of mature muscle (widely referred to as satellite cells); however, an additional serum-derived factor is required for proliferation to occur (5). Studies in our laboratories with both transplanted muscles (22,23) and irradiated animals (24), also support the idea that a factor derived from the circulation is necessary for mpc to proceed through the cell cycle to DNA synthesis and replication. The nature of this serum-factor is as yet unknown.

With the recent availability of antibodies and riboprobes to growth factors, it is possible to examine the distribution and expression of bFGF in tissues *in vivo*. It is well documented that bFGF is bound to heparin sulphate proteoglycans and glycosaminoglycans (16,21) in the extracellular matrix surrounding myofibres, and immunofluorescent studies by Di Mario *et al* (10), indicate that bFGF is increased in the extracellular matrix of mdx muscles. This did not appear to be related only to a general regenerative response, as elevated bFGF was also apparent 14 days postnatally (10), before the main onset of necrosis and regeneration which occurs around 19 to 21 days (see paper by McGeachie *et al,* this volume): however, it may reflect some sub-clinical disturbance. In addition, tissue culture studies showed that satellite cells from mdx muscle display a heightened sensitivity to bFGF (i.e. they respond to lower levels of bFGF) compared with controls, and that the threshold response of mdx mpc occurs at lower levels of bFGF compared with fibroblasts from both mdx and control muscles (9). It was proposed that this might permit high rates of mpc proliferation without a parallel hyperplasia in the muscle fibroblast population of mdx mice. While this is an attractive hypothesis, it is difficult to substantiate *in vivo*, and examination of muscle regeneration after severe crush injury reveals no difference in the amount of fibrous and cellular connective tissue formed, or in the pattern of mpc replication in mdx and control mice (12).

More recently, studies with bFGF antibodies have shown binding within muscle cells. It should be noted that antibody preparations from different laboratories may recognise different epitopes and even different members of the family of structurally closely-related, bFGF-like molecules. Immunofluorescent studies by Anderson et al. (2) showed that bFGF was localised to the periphery of undamaged mature myofibres, and that it was associated with myonuclei, satellite cells and possibly the external lamina. The immunostaining was more intense in slow twitch fibres. In contrast with the studies of DiMario *et al.* (10), undamaged areas of mdx muscles showed similar immunostaining to control muscles and there was also greater pericellular and cytoplasmic bFGF accumulation in slow twitch compared with fast twitch mdx muscles (2). Increased amounts of bFGF in damaged muscles was accounted for by foci of degenerating myofibres in mdx muscles and enhanced binding around the nuclei of small regenerating fibres. The production of bFGF by mpc has been confirmed by the detection of bFGF mRNA in these cells in culture (1).

Since bFGF, or FGF-like peptides are so closely associated with the activation of mpc, it would be of great interest to compare the pattern of expression of these growth factors in dystrophic muscles of mice, dogs and humans to see whether there is a correlation with the different capacity for muscle regeneration in these species. It would be particularly valuable to examine muscles from very young dogs and humans, before replacement by fibrous tissue and fat is pronounced. The application of a range of antibodies and nuclei acid probes (which are now becoming available for various growth factors and extracellular matrix components) to such dystrophic muscle specimens, should yield much pertinent information about the biology of skeletal muscle regeneration in the different species.

ACKNOWLEDGEMENTS

The consistent research support for Miranda D. Grounds by the National Health and Medical Research Council of Australia is gratefully acknowledged.

REFERENCES

1. Alterio, J., Courtois, Y., Robelin, J., Dechet, D., Martelly, I. (1990): Acid and basic fibroblast growth factor mRN As are expressed by skeletal muscle cells. *Biochem. Biophys. Res. Commun.,* 166:1205-1212.
2. Anderson, J.E., Liu, L. Kardami, E. (1991): Distinctive patterns of bFGF distribution in degenerating and regenerating areas of dystrophic (mdx) striated muscles. *Dev. Biol.,* 147:96-109.
3. Bischoff, R. (1986a): Proliferation of muscle satellite cells on intact myofibres in culture. *Dev. Biol.,* 115:129-13 39.

4.   Bischoff, R. (1986b): A satellite cell mitogen from crushed adult muscle.
     Dev. Biol., 115:140-147.
5.   Bischoff, R. (1990): Cell cycle commitment of rat muscle satellite cells.
     J. Cell Biol., 111:201-207.
6.   Carpenter, S. Karpati, G. (1979): Duchenne muscular dystrophy. Plasma
     membrane loss initiates muscle cell necrosis unless it is repaired. *Brain,*
     102:147-161.
7.   Carpenter, S. Karpati, G. (1989): Segmental necrosis and its demarcation
     in experimental micropuncture injury of skeletal muscle fibres. *J.
     Neuropathol. Exp. Neurol.*, 48:154-170.
8.   Cullen, M.J., Fulthorpe, J.J. (1975). Stages in fibre breakdown in
     Duchenne muscular dystrophy. *J. Neurol. Sci.*, 24:179-200.
9.   DiMario, J. Strohman, R.C. (1988): Satellite cells from dystrophic (mdx)
     mouse muscle are stimulated by fibroblast growth factor *in vitro.
     Differentiation*, 39:42-49.
10. DiMario, J., Buffinger, N., Yamada, S. Strohman, R.C. (1989):
     Fibroblast growth factor in the extracellulatr matrix of dystrophic (mdx)
     mouse muscle. *Science*, 244, 688-690.
11. Engel, A.G., Biesecker, G. (1982): Universal involvement of complement
     in muscle fibre necrosis. In: Disorders of the Motor Unit. edited by D.L.
     Schotland, pp535-546. John Wiley and Sons, New York, pp535-546.
12. Grounds, M.D. McGeachie, J.K. (1992): Skeletal muscle regeneration
     after crush injury in dystrophic mdx mice: an autoradiographic study.
     Muscle and Nerve, In press.
13. Grounds, M.D. (1991): Towards understanding skeletal muscle
     regeneration. *Pathol. Res. Pract.*, 118:1-22.
14. Grounds, M.D. and Yablonka-Reuveni, Z. (1992): Molecular and Cell
     Biology of Skeletal Muscle Regeneration. In: Molecular and Cell Biology
     of Muscle Regeneration, edited by T.A. Partridge. Chapman and Hall. In
     press.
15. Hoffman, E.P., Gorospe, J.R. (1991): The animal models of Duchenne
     muscular dystrophy: windows on the pathophysiological consequences of
     dystrophin deficiency. In: Topics in Membranes, edited by Morrow, J. and
     Mooseker, M. Academic Press, New York, In Press.
16. Klagsbrun, M. (1989): The fibroblast growth factor family: structural and
     biological properties. *Prog. Growth Factor Res.*, 11:207-235.
17. Lipton, B.H. (1979): Skeletal muscle regeneration in muscular dystrophy.
     In: *Muscle Regeneration*, edited by Mauro, A., et al. pp 101-114, Raven
     Press, New York.
18. Mesulam, M. (1982): Principles of horse radish peroxidase neuro-
     histochemistry and their applications for tracing neural pathways, axonal
     transport, enzyme histochemistry, and light microscopic analysis: In:
     Tracing Neural Connections, edited by Mesulam, M. John Wiley and
     Sons, New York, pp 3-152.
19. Mokri, B., Engel, A.G. (1975): Duchenne dystrophy: electronmicroscopy
     findings pointing to a basic or early abnormality in the plasma membrane
     of the muscle fibre. *Neurol.*, 25:1111-1120.
20. Papadimitriou J.M., Robertson T.A., Mitchell C.A., Grounds, M.G.
     (1990): The process of new plasmalemma formation in focally injured
     skeletal muscle fibres. *J. Struct. Biol.*, 103:124-134.
21. Rifkin, D.B. Moscatelli, D. (1989): Recent developments in the cell
     biology of basic fibroblast growth factor. *J. Cell Biol.*, 109:1-6.

22. Roberts, P. McGeachie, J.K. (1990): Endothelial cell activation during angiogenesis in freely translanted skeletal muscles in mice and its relationship to the onset of myogenesis. *J. Anat.*, 169:197- 207.
23. Roberts, P., McGeachie, J.K., Smith, E.R. Grounds, M.D. (1989): The initiation and duration of myogenesis in transplants of intact skeletal muscles: an autoradiographic study in mice. *Anat. Rec.*, 224:1-6.
24. Robertson, T.A., Grounds, M.D. Papadimitriou, J.M. (1992): Elucidation of aspects of murine skeletal muscle regeneration using local and whole body irradiation. Submitted for publication.
25. Robertson, T., Papadimitriou, J.M., Mitchell, C.A. Grounds, M.D. (1990): Fusion of myogenic cell *in vivo*: an ultrastructural study of regenerating murine skeletal muscle. *J. Struct. Biol.,* 105:170-182.
26. Schmalbruch, H. (1975). Segmental fibre breakdown and defects of the plasmalemma in diseased human muscles. *Acta. Neuropath.,* 33:129-141.
27. Stedman, H.H. Sweeney, H.L., Shrager, J.B., Maguire, H.C., Panettieri, R.A., Petrov, B., Narusawa, M., Leferovich, J.M., Sladky, J.T., Kelly, M. (1991): The mdx mouse diaphragm reproduces the degenerative changes of Duchenne muscular dystrophy. *Nature*, 352: 536-539.
28. Zacharias, J.M. Anderson, J.E. (1991): Muscle regeneration after imposed injury is better in younger than older mdx mice. *J. Neurol. Sci.,* 104:190-196.

DISCUSSION

Professor George Karpati:
Two comments concerning those elegant studies of segmental necrosis and the formation of the delineating membrane. As you know we have done similar experiments where we have inflicted a tiny hole in the muscle fibre by an approximately 10 micron Tungston needle and produced very similar results. The point I wish to make is that one phenomenon I did not see on your picture is the appearance of enormously dilated T tubules in the stump region which persists for sometime, even after the delineating membrane forms. We have shown that the pathophysiology of this phenomenon is due to excess sodium which comes from the extracellular space and is pumped into the intra T tubules by the sodium pump, the sodium cannot escape but it draws in water and these enormously dilated spaces form. This is of practical significance because in many fibres where segmental necrosis occurs you see what myopathologists call "vacuolization". They try to make it out to be a mysterious phenomenon, actually what they see is a stump in cross section.

Dr. Miranda D. Grounds:
The stump is considered to be resealed at this stage?

Professor George Karpati:
That's right. You have seen these dilated spaces I assume, as well.

Dr. Miranda D. Grounds:
I would really have to refer that question to Terry Robertson.

Dr. Terry A. Robertson:
Yes, but not commonly.

Professor George Karpati:
In our model, it was like swiss-cheese in many stumps. It was so remarkable. The second point is that the delineating membrane as it forms with a free edge is a unique phenomenon, and when we have looked at the literature there is no comparible occurrence. The second point about that membrane is that initially it contains no protein. It is simply a protein-free lipid bilayer. It has no channels, no receptors, nothing. All it does is form a ionic barrier between the necrotic segment and the surviving stump. That is what it is designed for.

Dr. Miranda D. Grounds:
In your work you suggest that it forms from the free-edges, whereas we consider that it forms by vesicle accumulation.

Professor George Karpati:
No, I think that it probably forms as you represent.

Dr. Allen D. Roses:
Is there any direct evidence about the loss of proliferative capacity in humans? I am thinking about the possibility of activating myoblasts by genetic therapy. Are they all likely to be worn out and not going to function?

Dr. Miranda D. Grounds:
The proliferative capacity of precursors from dystrophic and normal human muscles of different ages has been studied. However, conflicting results are often obtained from such tissue culture studies when the proliferative capacity of old vs. young muscles is compared in humans and also in rats. Some people say that there is no difference; other people say that there is a difference (1). It is interesting to note that a detailed study of human muscle, in which an age related difference was reported, concluded that the limited proliferative capacity of DMD + muscle precursor cells was secondary to the expression of the disease (5). The extent to which such results accurately reflect the situation in vivo is difficult to determine. The efficiency of extracting all muscle precursors may vary with age, or sub-populations may be more susceptible to extraction, particularly as there is increased fibrosis and collagen in older and dystrophic muscles (2,4).
Secondly, there may be something in the environment which they have just came out of which influences their behaviour in vivo. When such extracted cells are grown in tissue culture the particular standard conditions may favour the replication of precursors derived from young compared with old muscles. The in vivo evidence derived from rats and mice where muscles were isografted between animals of different ages consistently indicates no difference in the proliferative capacity of precursors from old or young muscles in these species. In contrast, in vivo studies with injured or transplanted muscles invariably show that the host environment influences muscle regeneration and that regeneration is impaired in older host animals (1).

Professor Byron A. Kakulas:
For the record, I wish to refer to the work of Dr. Pitsa Manda, a neurologist who was on sabbatical leave from Athens some years ago. Her project was to discover whether or not, as you have also questioned, regeneration could be

exhausted in normal mice. For a period of more than a year she injected mice with a strong myotoxin, iodoacetate. At the end of that period there seemed to be absolutely no difference, between say a week and a year's treatment, regeneration was almost complete even after a year. In fact the animal seemed to become resistant to it. Therefore as a second experiment she injected iodoacetate into the dystrophic mice 129/Re. She was thus able to accelerate the dystrophic lesion in this way (3).

While I am speaking I wish to address George. Do you remember a few years ago when we were discussing the micropuncture lesions? Once you had ruptured the membrane causing the focal necrosis similar to that which Miranda has shown, it may be expected that calcium will diffuse and destroy the muscle fibre from end to end. Now this does not happen. Are you satisfied that this limiting membrane which develops over 4 hours or so, accounts for the cessation, or should there be some other explanation?

Professor George Karpati:
Yes, I am quite happy to say that two factors actually might be responsible for the lateral diffusion of this lethal executor which is the calcium ion and to some extent sodium as well. One is the hypercontracted myofibril segment at the edge which probably soaks up a lot of the calcium, as you can see if you stain for them, which they are encrusted with calcium salts. The main factor is the delineating membrane. If this membrane does not form, the whole necrotic wave would go from end to end and it has relevance to Duchenne dystrophy because if the segmental necrosis can be limited to a very short segment that would be so much better then if a long segment was involved.

Professor Byron A. Kakulas:
I wish to ask Prof. Papadimitriou, whether the Golgi system has anything to do with reconstituted membrane?

Professor John M Papadimitriou:
Our studies show, structurally at least, that large phospholipid accumulations do appear in the area of the stump region. Initially these changes in the muscle fibre are prominent in the vicinity of the Golgi and reflect most likely increasing phospholipid synthesis. It seems therefore, that sealing of the stump is an active process.

Dr. Terence A. Partridge:
I would like to comment on the resealing question. I suspect that there may be descriptions of large-scale resealing of plasmalemmal lesions in the embryological literature. The amphibian egg has been the object of many micro-surgical experiments and the resealing process must surely have been studied in this system.

REFERENCES

1.   Grounds, M.D., Yablonka-Reuveni, Z. (1992): Molecular and Cell Biology of Skeletal Muscle Regeneration. In: Molecular and Cell Biology of Muscle Regeneration, edited by T.A. Partridge. Chapman and Hall. In press.

2. Lipton B.H. (1979): Skeletal muscle regeneration in muscular dystrophy. In: Muscle Regeneration, eds. Mauro, A et al, Raven Press, New York 101-114

3. Manda P, Kakulas, B.A. (1986): The effect of the myotoxic agent idoacetate on dystrophic mice 129/Re. *J. of Neurol. Sci.*, 75:23-32

4. Marshall, P.A., Williams, P.E., Goldspink,.G. (1989): Accumulation of collagen and altered fibre-type ratios as indicators of abnormal muscle gene expression in the mdx dystrophic mouse. *Muscle and Nerve*, 12:528-537.

5. Webster, C., Filippi, G., Rinaldi, A., Mastropada, C., Tondi, M., Siniscalco, M., Blau, H.M. (1986): The myoblast defect identified in Duchenne muscular dystrophy is not a primary expression of the DMD mutation. *Human Genetics*, 74:74-80.

DUCHENNE MUSCULAR DYSTROPHY: Animal Models
and Genetic Manipulation, edited by Byron A. Kakulas,
John McC. Howell, and Allen D. Roses.
Raven Press, Ltd., New York © 1992.

13

Fusion of Myogenic Cells *In Vivo*

Terry A. Robertson, Miranda D. Grounds,
John M. Papadimitriou

*Department of Pathology, University of Western Australia,
Queen Elizabeth II Medical Centre,
Nedlands, Western Australia. 6009*

After injury to skeletal muscle, effective regeneration is said to depend upon the direct fusion of mononuclear myogenic cells (myoblasts) with the damaged muscle fibres, or fusion between myogenic cells to form multinucleated young muscle cells (myotubes) which subsequently fuse with myofibres (2). The majority of studies on myogenic fusion have been carried out on embryonic tissue culture preparations which do not adequately mimic the vascular responses and the complex three-dimensional cellular interactions between various cell types that occur *in vivo*. There is also increasing evidence to suggest that the behaviour of myogenic cells derived from embryonic muscle may not be equivalent to that of myogenic precursor cells derived from mature muscle (3). In addition the critical fusion events between myogenic cells and damaged, mature myofibres in regenerating injured muscle cannot be studied because mature fibres cannot be sustained for long in tissue culture. Finally, apart from its relevance in normal muscle regeneration the appreciation of fusion in myogenic cells *in vivo* has important implications to the current interest in myoblast transfer therapy as a potential treatment for Duchenne Muscular dystrophy (DMD) (4).

In this study electron microscopy was used to investigate myogenic fusion *in vivo* in adult murine SLJ/J skeletal muscle regenerating after three different types of injury to the tibialis anterior (TA) muscle, including superficial focal injuries inflicted either by local application of aldehyde, or a cold probe, or the more severe trauma of a crush lesion. All of these have been described in detail in a previous paper (5).

In this report the following terminology for the various myogenic cell types will be adopted: The term "presumptive myoblast" refers to a suspected muscle precursor cell which lacks evidence of cytoplasmic filamentous muscle proteins. A "myoblast" is a muscle precursor cell confirmed by the presence of thick and thin filaments in the cytoplasm. "Mononuclear muscle precursor cell" is a general term which includes satellite cells, presumptive myoblasts and myoblasts. "Myogenic cells" includes both mononuclear muscle precursor cells, multinucleated myotubes and myofibres.

In any ultrastructural identification of small fusion sites, a major problem is difficulty in resolving plasma membranes that are not perpendicular to the plane of section. Although apparent membrane discontinuities in the region of close apposition between myogenic cells may represent actual areas of cytoplasmic continuity, often such appearances merely represent areas where membranes are oblique to the plane of section, and therefore appear as amorphous fuzzy material. Indeed, many of the published electron micrographs, supposedly demonstrating membranes of fusing myogenic cells, fall into this category. A goniometer stage with a rotational holder is essential for adequate manipulation of the specimen to reduce the possibility of misinterpretation. The minimum criteria that should be met for identification of fusion sites are the presence of clearly resolved membrane continuity at either edge of proposed fusion sites (described by Bischoff as "U" shaped membranes) and the complete absence of amorphous material in the area of cytoplasmic confluence (1).

We have carefully documented instances of fusion of myoblast to myoblast, myoblast to myotube and myotube to myotube in a previous paper (5). In summary fusion of these myogenic cells probably begins with intimate apposition of the plasma membranes of the cells, while the appearance of numerous vesicles near the site of cytoplasmic confluence (Fig. 1), often associated with elements of the Golgi apparatus (Fig. 2) suggests that these also play a role. The foci of confluence are often multiple between the two apposed myogenic cells, while persistence near the fusion site of cell membranes, sometimes with remnants of intermediate junctions between them, (Fig. 3) is a frequent feature.

Sarcoplasmic extensions or buds containing variable numbers of myonuclei were often seen at the ends of resealed myofibres as illustrated in Figure 4. An external lamina was absent at the resealed site while the plasmalemmal membrane of myoblasts and myotubes was consistently closely apposed to the sarcolemma of these protrusions. In instances where the bud had acquired a slender finger-like form (Fig. 5 & 7), myotubes were often closely apposed to it (Fig. 6), and often various myogenic cells displayed cytoplasmic confluence with such stumps (Fig. 8).

An extremely important observation in this study was the fusion of a myogenic cell located beneath the external lamina with an apparently undamaged segment of parent myofibre at a considerable distance from the site of injury (Fig. 9). This myogenic cell contained evidence of sarcomere production and cytoplasmic continuity was evident at multiple sites between it and the adjacent myofibre (Fig. 10 & 11).

All the observations indicate that the fusion of myogenic cells with each other, with the stump site of resealed fibres and with the undamaged parts of the injured fibre are the means by which the zones of necrosis are bridged, resulting eventually in the reconstitution of the myofibre.

For myoblast transfer therapy to be effective, donor myoblasts need to incorporate into myofibres. Detailed knowledge of myogenic fusion is therefore critical in understanding the efficiency that can be expected from fusion of injected donor myoblasts and regenerating myofibres. The observations that fusion of mononuclear and multinuclear myogenic cells occurs at the end and periphery of sarcoplasmic stumps indicates that this will be an important site of incorporation of injected donor myoblasts. Furthermore at such sites of segmental necrosis the donor myoblasts can probably traverse the damaged external lamina. It is not known, however, whether donor myoblasts can traverse the intact external lamina and occupy a satellite cell position in the undamaged areas of host myofibres. However if they can, then fusion of normal donor myoblasts might also occur at several sites along the length of damaged or undamaged segments of host myofibres (as documented in this report) resulting in a much more widespread introduction of donor myoblasts into dystrophic myofibres than would otherwise occur.

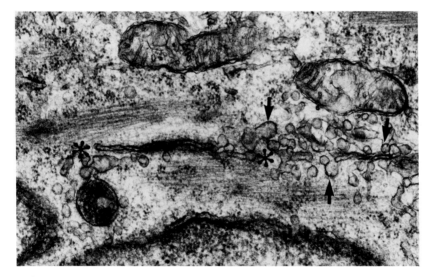

FIG.1. Numerous vesicles (arrows) in and area of close apposition of two myotubes from a 4 day chemically injured animal. Several fusion sites can be observed (asterisk), x 31,200.

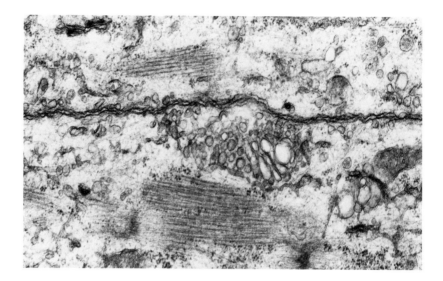

FIG. 2. A Golgi region near the closely apposed membranes of two myotubes (4 day chemically treated animal), x 26,000.

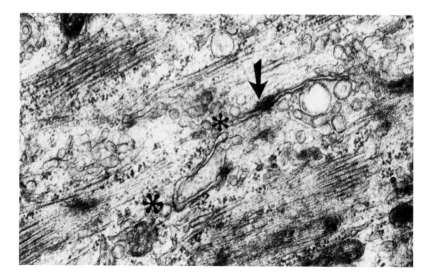

FIG. 3. Electron micrograph of two fused myotubes in muscle sampled 4 days after chemical injury. An intermediate junction (arrow) can be seen and cytoplasmic confluence can be observed between the fused myotubes (asterisk), x 36,000.

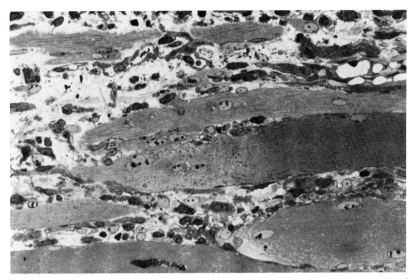

FIG. 4. Light micrograph of a sarcoplasmic stump from a 4 day chemical
induced injury. Organeles are sparse and a 5 myonuclei can be
observed in the sarcoplasm, x 612.

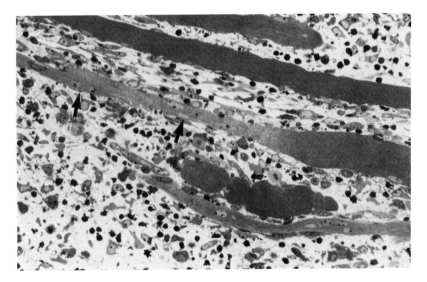

FIG. 5. A elongated sarcoplasmic stump from a 4 day chemically injured animal.
Myotubes and myoblasts can be observed in close apposition to the
process in this light micrograph (arrow), x 372.

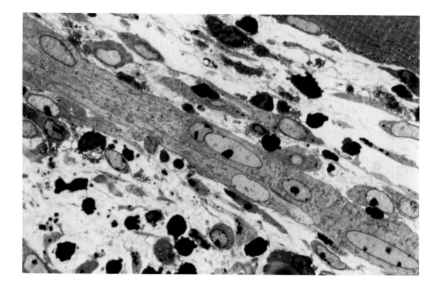

FIG. 6. Myogenic cells can be seen in close apposition to the sarcoplasmic stump from figure 5, x 660.

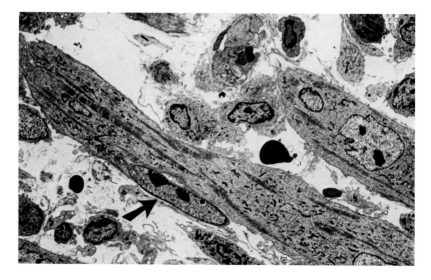

FIG. 7. An electron micrograph of a sarcoplasmic stump similar to that shown in figure 5. A myoblast can be seen in close apposition to the plasma membrane of the bud (arrow), x 1,600.

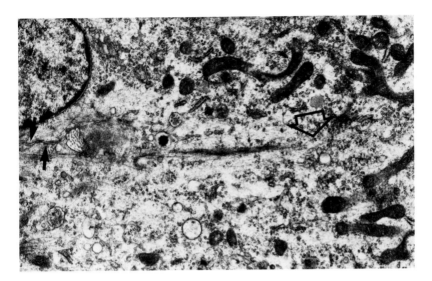

FIG. 8. A high power electron micrograph of a region of possible fusion from figure 7. Although plasma membranes of stump and myoblast can be observed in one area (solid arrows) cytoplasmic confluence can be seen in another region (hollow arrows), x 13,200.

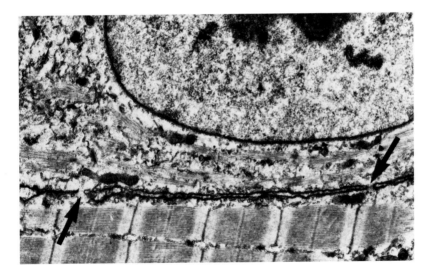

FIG. 9. A myogenic cell located between the external lamina and plasmalemma of a myofibre (i.e. in the satellite cell position). Two areas of cytoplasmic confluence between these two opposed cells were seen (arrows), x 13,200.

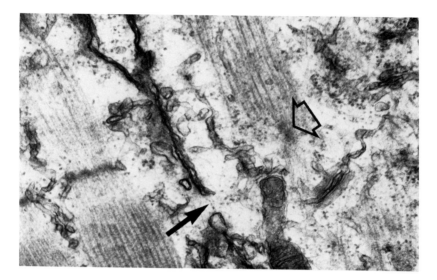

FIG. 10.   High magnification of an area of cytoplasmic continuity between the
opposing cells in figure 9. Sarcomeric structures can be seen in the
cytoplasm of this cell (hollow arrow). Cytoplasmic confluence
indicative of fusion can be observed between the two cells (solid
arrow), x 42,000.

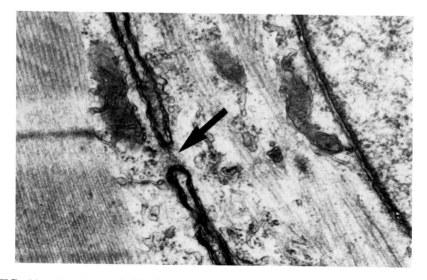

FIG. 11.   Another probable fusion site of cells in figure 9 where cytoplasmic
confluence is apparent and the opposing membranes are distinctive
(arrow). x 43,000.

ACKNOWLEDGEMENTS

Part of this work was supported by the National Health and Medical Research Council of Australia (MDG) and the University of Western Australia.

REFERENCES

1. Bischoff, R. (1978): Myoblast fusion. In: Membrane Fusion,.Poste, G. and Nicholson, G.L. (Eds). Elsievier, North-Holland. *Biomedical Press.* pp.127-179.
2. Carlson, B.M. (1973): The regeneration of skeletal muscle: A review. *Am. J. Anat.*, 137:119-149
3. Grounds, M.D. (1991): Towards understanding skeletal muscle regeneration. *Pathol. Res. Pract.*, 187:1-22
4. Partridge, T.A., Morgan, J.E., Coulton, G.R. Hoffman, E.P. Kunkel, L.M. (1989): Conversion of mdx myofibres from dystrophin-negative to positive by injection of normal myoblasts. *Nature*, 337:176-179.
5. Robertson, T.A., Grounds, M.D., Mitchell, C.A. Papadimitriou, J.M. (1990): Fusion between myogenic cells *in vivo*: An ultrastructural study in regenerating murine skeletal muscle. J. *Struct. Biol.*, 105:170-182.

DISCUSSION

Professor George Karpati:
Henning Schmalbruch of Copenhagen has found that one of the prerequisites for the fusion of intracellular vesicles with the surface membrance from within, during exocytosis, was that a patch of the membrane be clear at the site of intramembranous particles. If the intramembranous protein particles are sticking out, the 2 membranes cannot come together. He used a chemical, chlorpheterine which has enhanced the formation of these "bare" patches that were clear of intramembranous proteins which enhanced exocytosis. Do you think that in the fusion process, which you have described in the various cell types, it is a prerequisite too?

Dr. Terry A. Robertson:
I am very sure that is the case. I have read that article mentioned. I have not looked at intramembranous particles in my work, but I would assume they certainly would be cleared at the site of fusion.

Professor George Karpati:
Have you got any speculations on the mechanism of the disposal of all that membrane. Does it just go away?

Dr. Terry A. Robertson:
The vesicles?

Professor George Karpati:
That the redundant membrane is ejected.

Dr. Terry A. Robertson:
With vesicles travelling backward and forward to the outside, I am sure that both the vesicles and redundant plasma membranes of the cells following fusion would be recycled through the Golgi region. Cytoplasmic movement is occurring continuously and I am sure that there would not be any problems of clearing these structures. Once fusion has occurred these structures disappear.

Dr. Edna C. Hardeman:
In the last illustration how do you know that the cell in the satellite cell position is not separating from the myofibre, and not the other way around?

Dr. Terry A. Robertson:
I am sure this is not the case. I have read an article by Schultz (1976) where he looked at growing muscle from ice and he presented an electron micrograph (Fig 8) which he interpreted as fusion of a satellite cell with a myofibre. Very large vacuoles separated the two cells and I would not interpret this as satellite cell fusion. To me fusion only occurs when two plasma membranes are in extremely close apposition. The cell I have described displayed sarcomeric differentiation and fusion where the myofibre would contribute new myonuclei and myofilaments to the sarcoplasma of the myofibre.

Professor Byron A. Kakulas:
Terry, in foetal development there is splitting off, of populations of muscle fibres, and this is one way hyperplasia develops. The same thing happens in mature animals under conditions of stretch, that is splitting off occurs and new fibres form. I think you have mentioned everything except fusion of myofibres to myofibres. Is it true that that doesn't happen?

Dr. Terry A. Robertson:
I certainly have not seen fusion of myofibres to myofibres. I have stated before, that myogenic fusion occurs within minutes. I am certain that the reason that a thorough study of myogenic fusion has not been carried out is that it needs patience and conciderable time to cut the hundreds of blocks and examine hundreds of grids to find each particular fusion event or each myogenic cell and even then there is no guarantee that you will find it. It may happen but I certainly have not seen it yet. The cell in the satellite cell position fusing with the myofibre was only photographed 4 weeks ago. It is an exciting find when viewing the screen of an electron microscope to view such an event. To my knowledge this has certainly not been reported in the literature before.

Dr. Terence A. Partridge:
You showed a myoblast and a cell which was fusing. Are you sure that it was a single cell and not a myotube?

Dr. Terry A. Robertson:
No, I do not think that it was a myoblast. If we compare its size with that of an activated satellite cell next to it, it is a much larger cell. I think that it is an odd cut through a myotube as I have often seen myotubes containing 4 o 5 nuclei in an identical position. I think that satellite cells can be stimulated in normal areas of a myofibre to proliferate and fuse with each other. The resulting myotube can then be induced to fuse with the myofibre.

DUCHENNE MUSCULAR DYSTROPHY: Animal Models
and Genetic Manipulation, edited by Byron A. Kakulas,
John McC. Howell, and Allen D. Roses.
Raven Press, Ltd., New York © 1992.

14

Genetic Probes for Tracking Muscle Precursor Cells *In Vivo*: Technical Aspects

Manfred Beilharz*, Kerryn Garrett*, Ying Fan◻,
Sue Fletcher◻, Ricardo Lareu*, Moira Maley+,
Marilyn Vague+, Alan Harvey°, Miranda Grounds+

*Departments of Microbiology, +Pathology, °Anatomy and Human Biology,
The University of Western Australia.
◻The Australian Neuromuscular Research Institute ,
Queen Elizabeth II Medical Centre,
Nedlands, Western Australia 6009

INTRODUCTION

Myoblast Transfer Therapy (MTT) is a radical procedure which has aroused enormous interest as a potential treatment for various myopathies, in particular the human X-linked condition Duchenne muscular dystrophy (DMD). MTT involves the transfer of healthy muscle precursor cells into dystrophic muscle. The healthy donor cells are then required to fuse with regenerating dystrophic muscle, thus providing a genetic and phenotypic rescue of the condition (11,16). The apparent simplicity of this concept and the experimental demonstration that genetically different nuclei can function within the one muscle cell (17) have led to considerable activity in this area. However, the ability of researchers to monitor the details of this process has been hampered by a lack of suitable cell markers.

Various applied cell markers such as vital dyes, tritiated thymidine, soluble gold and polystyrene microspheres suffer from the drawbacks of loss, dilution or transfer *in vivo*. Furthermore the ability to localise such markers at the level of individual cells is limited. Muscle cell specific genetic markers, as a group, constitute a more useful approach. Although individual genetic markers may vary their level of expression during the life-span of a cell, they will not be lost, diluted or transferred. A further requirement of a suitable genetic marker is that it be endogenous to either the donor or host cells. Non-endogenous genetic markers, such as those introduced by retroviral or other transfection techniques, may alter the behaviour of the cells under study. In this paper the development of two new genetic markers is described for application to MTT.

MYOD1 AND MYOGENIN RIBOPROBES

In the last 4 years several related skeletal muscle specific genes involved in muscle determination and differentiation have been described in mammals (2,3,5,6,13,18,19,22). The structural features and in vivo activities of the gene products suggests them to be transcriptional activators of genes expressed along the muscle lineage. The most extensively studied of the genes have been MyoD1 (5,6) and myogenin (6,22). Cardiac α-actin was previously considered to be the earliest genetic marker expressed by muscle precursor cells during differentiation (10,12,20); however, myogenin mRNA has been demonstrated to occur somewhat earlier and at higher levels than that of cardiac α-actin in the mouse embryo (21). It was therefore reasoned in this laboratory that MyoD1 and myogenin might be useful genetic markers for the very early identification of muscle cell precursors *in vivo* (8).

In situ hybridization with MyoD1 (or myogenin) riboprobes labelled with ^{35}S or ^{125}I showed clear hybridization of muscle precursor cells as soon as 6 hours after muscle injury in the mouse (8). The expression of these genes peaked 24-48 hours after injury and was rapidly down-regulated by 120-192 hours post injury. Figure 1 shows strongly hybridizing muscle precursor cells in the tibialis anterior muscle of the mouse, four days after injury. It is presently considered that this use of MyoD1 and myogenin as a cell marker *in situ* is the only known way to positively distinguish early muscle cell precursors from other mononuclear cells present in regenerating tissue at the light microscope level (7). The application of this approach to MTT in the mouse mdx model will clearly assist in delineating the survival and movement of active donor muscle precursor cells.

The radioisotopically labelled nucleic acid riboprobes showed little or no mRNA in multinucleated young muscle cells (myotubes), see Figure 1, indicating rapid downregulation of these genes around the time of fusion of precursor cells (8); however more recent observation in our laboratory indicates the persistance of low levels of myogenin mRNA in newly formed myotubes. Several technological improvements to the *in situ* procedure have allowed this progress: predominant is the use of a non-radioactive detection system based on the steroid molecule digoxigenin (Boehringer Mannheim). In this system the final image-producing chromophore is deposited in the plane of the section by an alkaline phosphatase catalysed reaction. This contrasts with the radioactive approach where silver grains are deposited in an overlying photographic emulsion which reduces resolution at the cellular level. In addition, multiple cycles of the enzymatic reaction result in accumulation or amplification of the signal.

Y-CHROMOSOME SPECIFIC PROBES

The preceding section has discussed the use of MyoD1 and myogenin as suitable markers for tracking muscle precursor cells *in vivo*. However, whilst a low level of expression of these genes is seen in newly formed myotubes it appears to be down regulated around the time of fusion (8). An endogenous genetic marker which allows tracking of muscle precursor cells beyond the fusion stage, with no loss of signal intensity, is the Y-chromosome specific probe. This

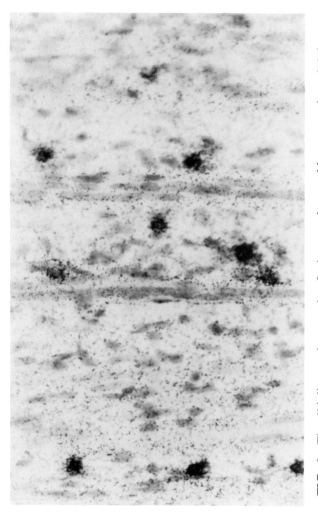

FIG. 1. The tibialis anterior muscle of mice was damaged by a central crush injury. Sections were taken 4 days post-injury and hybridised to 35S labelled MyoD1 riboprobe. Strong hybridization of apparently mononuclear muscle precursor cells is clearly visible, although little evidence of signal in newly formed myotubes is evident.

probe is a powerful tool for identifying all donor male cells introduced into female hosts and is applicable to all cell types. Development of this cell marker system for transplantation studies in the mouse model has been achieved in this laboratory (1,9) and by another laboratory (4). The advantages of a Y-chromosome specific probe lie chiefly in the fact that expression of the marker is not required and that nuclear localization is possible. The latter point is particularly suited to the study of multinucleated syncytia such as muscle cells.

A selection of available Y-chromosome probes were evaluated for their suitability for *in situ* studies in the mouse. The probe 145SC5 proved the most suitable as this sequence is repeated on the mouse Y-chromosome some 250 times (15 and Y. Nishioka, personal communication). Labelling of the probe with the non-radioactive digoxigenin system and methanol/acetic acid perfusion of the muscle tissue gave the best results. Figure 2 shows hybridizing male nuclei derived from injected male muscle precursor cells 10 days after injection. The same Y-chromosome specific mouse probe, 145SC5, has been used to demonstrate the survival and movement of male astrocytes transplanted into female mouse brains: the results of a typical experiment showing the preferential location of the donor cells in the white matter of the brain and their extensive movement from the site of injection is shown on Figure 3. It should be noted that no evidence of immunological rejection of the transexually isografted tissue has been observed. The transplants have all been performed between male and female animals of the same inbred strain and detection of the marker DNA does not require gene transcription.

CONCLUDING COMMENTS

The development of MyoD1 (and myogenin) and Y-chromosome probes for the *in situ* tracking of muscle precursor cells *in vivo* represents a significant technical advance on previously available approaches. Details of the survival, movement and fusion of donor cells during MTT may now be studied *in vivo* at the cellular level.

The two main animal models for such studies are the mdx mouse and the x-linked dystrophic golden retriever dog. Whilst the mouse model studies are presently underway in this and other laboratories, the dog model awaits the characterization of a suitable Y-chromosome specific probe. The species specificity of MyoD1 and myogenin probes appears low as cross-hybridization between species has been common. Clearly the evolution of these skeletal muscle specific regulators occurred a long time before the mammalian divergence (14). Therefore the MyoD1/myogenin probes should be directly applicable to dog model studies. In contrast the Y-chromosome specific probes show very high levels of species specificity. For example, the 145SC5 murine probe shows very poor sex specificity in the rat, and none of the Y-chromosome specific sequences examined in this laboratory showed any useful sex specificity on dog tissue (1). The value of several dog Y-chromosome specific probes, derived in this laboratory by subtractive hybridization, is presently being evaluated (unpublished data). As the dog model phenotypically resembles the human DMD situation more than the mouse model, the outcome of the evaluation is keenly awaited.

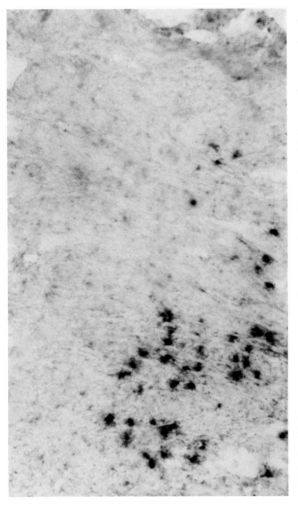

FIG. 2. Male muscle precursor cells were injected into the tibialis anterior muscle of mice 24 hours after a central crush injury. Sections were taken 10 days post-injury and hybridized to digoxigenin labelled 145SC5 probe. Strongly hybridizing male nuclei are apparent against the background of unlabelled female host muscle.

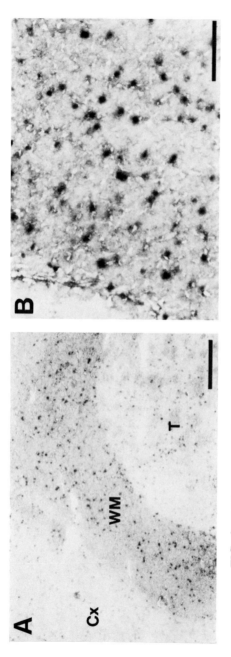

FIG. 3. Male astrocytes isografted into female host brains.
A. 7 days after transplantation. Transplanted cells are found predominantly in the white matter (WM). Scattered cells labelled with the Y-chromosome specific probe can also be seen in the thalamus (T).
B. Male donor astrocytes present in the fornix of a female host, 14 days post-transplantation.

Scales, A=250 μm; B=50 μm.

REFERENCES

1. Beilharz, M.W. Garrett, K.L., Fan, Y., Harvey, A.R., Lai, M.C., Codling, J.C. Grounds, M.D. (1991): Use of the Y-chromosome as a marker in transplantation studies. *Proc. Aust. Physiological and Pharm. Soc.*, 22(2):168-77.

2. Braun, T., Bober, E., Winter, B., Rosenthal, N. Arnold, H.H. (1990): Myf-6, a new member of the human gene family of myogenic determination factors: evidence for a gene cluster on chromosome 12. *EMBO J.,* 9:821-831.

3. Braun, T., Buschlausen-Denker, E., Bober, E., Tannich, H. and Arnold, H. (1989): A novel human muscle factor related to but distinct from MyoD1 induces myogenic conversion of 10T1/2 fibrobasts. *EMBO J.*, 8:701-709 (1989).

4. Coulton, G.R., Skynner, M.J., Smith, T., Pagel, C.N. Partridge, T.A. (1991): Localisation of donor nuclei in skeletal muscle grafts by in situ hybridisation to a cDNA probe. *Histochem., J.* 23:323-327.

5. Davis, R.L., Weintraub, H. Laser, A.B. (1987): Expression of a single transfected cDNA converts fibroblasts to myoblasts. *Cell*, 51:987-1000.

6. Edmondson, D.G. Olsen, E.N. (1989): A gene with homology to the myc similarity region of MyoD, is expressed during myogenesis and is sufficient to activate the muscle differentiation program. *Genes and Dev.*, 3: 628-640.

7. Grounds, M.D. (1991): Towards understanding skeletal muscle regeneration. *Pathol. Res. Pract.*, 187:1-22.

8. Grounds, M.D., Garrett, K.L., Lai, M.C., Wright, W.E. and Beilharz, M.W. (1991). Identification of skeletal muscle precursor cells *in vivo* by use of MyoD1 and myogenin probes. *Cell and Tissue Res.*, 267:99-104.

9. Grounds, M.D., Lai, M.C., Fan, Y., Codling, J.C. Beilharz, M.W. (1991): Transplantation in the mouse model: the use of Y-chromosome specific DNA clone to identify donor cells in situ. *Transplantation,* 52(6):1101-1105

10. Gunning, P., Hardeman, E., Wade, R., Ponte, P., Bains, W., Blau, H.M. and Kedes, L. (1987): Differential patterns of transcript accumulation during human myogenesis. *Mol. Cell Biol.*, 7:4100-4114.

11. Karpati, G. (1991). Myoblast transfer in Duchenne Muscular Dystrophy: a perspective. In: Muscular Dystropy Research. Edited by Angelini, C et al. Elsevier Science (Biomedical Division) pp 101-107.

12. Lawrence, J.B., Taneja, K. Singer, R.H. (1989): Temporal resolution and sequential expression of muscle-specific genes revealed by in situ hybridisation. *Dev. Biol.*, 133:235-246.

13. Miner, J.M. Wold, B. (1990): Herculin a fourth member of the MyoD family of myogenic regulatory genes. *Proc. Natl. Acad. Sci. USA,* 87:1089-1093.

14. Murre, C., McCaw, P.S. Baltimore, P. (1989): A new DNA binding and dimerisation motif in immunoglobulin enhancer binding, daughterless, MyoD, and myc proteins. *Cell*, 58: 777-783.

15. Nishioka, Y. (1988): Application of Y-chromosomal repetitive sequences to sexing mouse embryos. *Teratology*, 38:181-185.

16. Partridge, T.A. (1991): Myoblast transplantation: a possible therapy for inherited myopathics. *Muscle and Nerve,* 14:197-212.

17. Partridge, T.A., Grounds, M.D. Sloper, J.C. (1978): Evidence of fusion

between host and donor myoblasts in skeletal muscle grafts. *Nature*, 273:306-308.

18. Pinney, D.F., Pearson-White, S.H., Konieczny, S.F., Latham, K.E. & Emerson, C.P. (1988). Myogenic lineage determination and differentiation: evidence for a regulatory gene pathway. *Cell*, 53:781-793.

19. Rhodes, S.J. Konieczny, S.F. (1989): Identification of MRF4: a new member of the muscle regulatory factor gene family. *Genes and Devel.*, 3:2050-2061.

20. Sassoon, D.A., Garner, I. Buckingham, M. (1988): Transcripts of a-cardiac and α-skeletal actins are early markers for myogenesis in the mouse embryo. Dev., 104:155-164.

21. Sassoon, D. Lyons, G., Wright, W.E., Lin, V., Lassar, A., Weintraub, H. and Buckingham, M. (1989): Expression of two myogenic regulatory factors myogenin and MyoD, during mouse embryogenesis. *Nature*, 341:303-307.

22. Wright, W.E., Sassoon, D.A. Lin, V.K. (1989): Myogenin, a factor regulating myogenesis, has a domain homologous to MyoD1. *Cell*, 56:607-617.

DISCUSSION

Assist. Professor Richard J. Bartlett:
Manfred, have you considered using a RNA PCR method for measuring the RNA in the whole muscle studies you have been doing.

Dr. Manfred W. Beilharz:
We considered using a PCR method and discussed it at length. The reason we pulled back from doing this was the quantitation of the PCR. One of the things we think is going to be quite important for our biological in vivo studies is that we be able to monitor the up regulation and down regulation in the expression of these genes in some detail. I feel that the quantitation with Northern and RNA protection experiments is well established as opposed to the PCR methodology where the quantitation of the actual message is semi-quantitative at best.

Assist. Professor Richard J. Bartlett:
I was actually thinking of potentially doing an analysis where you have your injury location, doing a segmental analysis moving out from the injury and using the periphery as a normalization to actually attempt quantiation. Do you presume that the MyoD1 would be elevated like you see in your experiments and would you use different segments to compare this to each other?

Dr. Manfred W. Beilharz:
Yes, such experiments should be possible.

Dr. Terence A. Partridge:
You should be able to see a gradient there.

Dr. Manfred W. Beilharz:
Sure.

Professor Joe N. Kornegay:
Manfred, with regard to the myoblast transfer studies you showed briefly, were those mixed cultures or were the cultures enriched for myoblasts?

Dr. Manfred W. Beilharz:
Those initial cultures which we used for transfer were in fact mixed cultures. We also took them through to the fusion stage in vitro, so we were reasonably confident that muscle precursor cells were there.

Professor George Karpati:
These were very elegant studies which showed the activitation of myogenic cells at a distance from the actual damage sites. This is a more elegant way of showing what Edward Schulz already showed by demonstrating that satellite cells undergo mitosis at a fair distance from the actual damaged segment. You showed the same in a much more "hightech" way. My question is; what happened in the regenerated segment itself where the fibres actually regenerated after the crush? When do you lose the MyoD signal in the regenerating myotubes and myofibres.

Dr. Manfred W. Beilharz:
The answer to that is that our experimental process goes to the point where the signal can still be observed. At day 19 post crush, we essentially have lost the signal from the probes. Am I understanding your question George?

Professor George Karpati:
In the actual crushed zone where regeneration will occur. You never see MyoD signal in that zone at all? Or if so, why not?

Dr. Manfred W. Beilharz:
Not much but maybe I will hand this over to Miranda because in fairly severe crush injuries, I am not sure if the muscle regenerates all that well.

Dr. Miranda D. Grounds:
These experiments were carried out in Swiss mice which regenerate very well. In contrast with strains such as BALB/C, the Swiss (SJL/J) mice don't get extensive scar tissue in the centre of the injury zone. New muscle formation starts at the outside and progressively moves towards the centre of the lesion. The mononuclear muscle precursors fuse to form multinucleated myotubes until the entire lesion, including the central area, is occupied by new muscle cells.

Professor George Karpati:
Why do you think that the non-radioactive detection system is more sensitive?

Dr. Manfred W. Beilharz:
This is a speculative explanation. In the case of the digoxigenin probes the deposition of the insoluble colour marker is at the actual site of hybridization, right away you are getting a much better localization of your signal compared to the radioactive one, which is some distance away from where you want it to be. The other factor is, I think, that methyl green counter staining technique which is used. The dark brown and black signal seems to contrast well with the counterstain.

Dr. Terence A. Partridge:

There is probably one other explanation too, that you are using an enzyme as a marker, you have amplification of your signal so that it is more apparent .

Dr. Manfred W. Beilharz:

Yes, that is almost certainly true. We have used quite long reaction times of twenty four hours for some of the *in situ* results you have seen.

Assist. Professor Richard J. Bartlett:

I would like to comment on that. When you do any radioactive studies you are only actually detecting about 1/3 of your emissions because your emulsion is present in a thin layer above the sample and you have a sphere of disintegration events which are occurring so that you can only detect roughly about 1/3 of the total emissions passing through the plane above the point source.

Dr. Manfred W. Beilharz:

Again, what Richard has said is certainly a factor. The results speak for themselves.

DUCHENNE MUSCULAR DYSTROPHY: Animal Models
and Genetic Manipulation, edited by Byron A. Kakulas,
John McC. Howell, and Allen D. Roses.
Raven Press, Ltd., New York © 1992.

15

Myoblast Transplantation

T.A. Partridge, J. E. Morgan, C.N. Pagel, G.R. Coulton*,
M.F. Skynner*, M. Coleman†, D.J. Watt†

*Departments of Histopathology, *Biochemistry and †Anatomy,
Charing Cross & Westminster Medical School,
Fulham Palace Road, London W6 8RF, U.K.*

It is the therapeutic application of myoblast transfer which has dominated research on the topic. In the course of such goal-directed research, however, it has become evident that the technique will be of use for investigating the basic molecular and cell biology of muscles, both diseased and normal, thus providing information which may lead to a more comprehensive approach to the treatment of inherited and acquired myopathies (26). Here we consider the constraints on research into this topic and ways of overcoming them, together with the information that has emerged from such studies to date.

Beneficial effects of myoblast transplantation in genetic muscle disease may arise from two processes. First, the implanted cells may construct new muscle at sites of muscle damage. This could be an important contribution where the endogenous myogenic cells are inadequate in number or vigour, as appears to be the case in the later stages of Duchenne muscular dystrophy (DMD) (40);. Second, because myogenic cells contribute their nuclei to muscle fibres during growth and during regeneration after damage, normal myogenic cells can be used to introduce copies of the normal genome into muscle fibres whose endogenous nuclei are genetically defective. As an extension of this second idea, it is possible to introduce copies of particular genes into the donor myogenic cells prior to implantation. This may be used to boost the number of gene copies carried into muscle fibres by a given number of myogenic cells. Alternatively, if sufficient control can be obtained over the proliferation and differentiation of myogenic cells, then normal copies of the defective gene might be introduced into a patient's own cells prior to re-implantation of these cells into his muscles. This would have the advantage of avoiding rejection problems arising from histocompatibility differences between donor and recipient.

Experiments on the mdx mouse have demonstrated the feasibility, in principle, of each of these possibilities. Ultimately, their practicability for therapeutic purposes must be assessed on man but it is rarely possible to perform satisfactory experiments on man and detailed investigation requires the degree of control over experimental design which is most easily achieved in the mouse. Information gathered from the mouse will not necessarily be applicable directly to man but it can be used to test basic principles and to gain general guidance on possible problems and on ways of overcoming them.

CRITERIA OF SUCCESS IN MYOBLAST TRANSFER THERAPY

For the clinician, the definitive criterion of success in myoblast transfer is, clinical improvement, a halt in the clinical decline or, minimally, a slowing of the rate of decline. However, the progressive loss of function in skeletal muscle of DMD patients is almost certainly not a simple and direct result of the lack of dystrophin, since there is little physiological deficit in the muscles of the mdx mouse (2, 4). Rather, the delayed onset suggests that it is the result of the cumulative disruptive effects of secondary, tertiary or yet more remote consequences of chronic degeneration, inflammation and repair processes, driven by the lack of dystrophin (8, 27). Some of the changes produced by these processes, such as the exhaustion of myogenic cells (40) seem likely to be remediable by myoblast transplantation. Other components, seem unlikely to be susceptible to improvement by this approach. This applies particularly to the fibrotic changes (35) which may, it has been suggested (19), play an active part in the pathogenesis of the final decline in muscle physiology, particularly in a mechnically active and highly vascularized tissue like skeletal muscle.

To avoid missing any beneficial effects of myoblast transplantation, we must be able to distinguish those elements of the disease which may be amenable to improvement by this technique from those which are not. Such an analytical approach requires careful and controlled studies of myoblast transplantation, taking in data of two major types: first, we need to know how successfully the transplanted myogenic cells have been introduced into the muscle and, second, we want to know what effect these myogenic cells have had on the clinico-pathological process. For the latter, ideally, we would look for objective measures of biochemical rectification, methods of determining changes in pathology of individual muscle fibres, measures of improvement of physiological function, and measures of improvement of gross muscle function at a clinical level. This, combined with one or more unbiased markers of the extent of survival of donor cells and of their contribution to the host muscle in the form of mosaic fibres and totally donor-derived fibres, would give detailed data for assessment of the therapeutic effect of any particular variant of myoblast transplantation technique. Histologically visualizable markers of donor cells are also of great potential use in determining the physical extent of the contribution of these cells to the donor muscle.

CELL MARKERS

A variety of markers exist for following the fate of injected cells but none is perfect. Use has been made of persistent markers which are added to cells prior to their injection, such as carbocyanin dyes or fluorescent beads (1), and semi conserved markers, such as ^{3}H-thymidine (14, 20), but these are diluted below the level of detectability in rapidly dividing cells and can be reutilized on death of the originally labelled cell, so their usefulness is restricted.

Genetic markers, detected in the form of their expressed gene products, such as allotypic isoenzymes, have proven useful as estimators of donor genome. The isoforms of glucose-6-phosphate isomerase (GPI) we have commonly used as tracers in grafting experiments have been particularly informative in this respect and their capacity to form heterodimer enzyme in mosaic muscle cells has provided the most unequivocal evidence of the existence of this class of cell in after myoblast transplantation (17, 18, 21, 22, 29, 38, 39). A further useful property of these cytosolic enzyme markers, is that the isoforms have been shown to equilibrate within mosaic fibres (5). This means that for a simple muscle like the extensor digitorum longus, a single mid-belly section, will provide a sample of the GPI isoform composition of the entire muscle.

Much the same is true of exogenous genetic markers such as bacterial b-galactosidase, which can be introduced into myogenic cells by transfection or by infection with replication-defective retroviral vectors (10). Here again the expressed enzyme diffuses along the muscle fibre, away from the nucleus containing the β-galactosidase gene (32) and it has the additional advantage that it can be visualized cytochemically or immunocytochemically. Although the diffusion is useful in some ways, it does mean that the β-galactosidase gene cannot be used as a nuclear marker in muscle fibres, for even the nuclear-localizing form stains nuclei other than that containing the gene for it. If properly standardized and controlled, these enzymic markers can be used to obtain unbiased estimates of the genomic contribution of donor myogenic cells to the muscle into which they have been grafted.

The dystrophin gene, which produces a clear signal of its presence in the contribution of normal myogenic cells to mdx or DMD muscle, also has the advantage of being a sign of biochemical rectification of the genetic defect. Unlike the cytosolic enyme products of marker genes, it seems to display a limited diffusion from the nucleus which carries the gene for it (14, 29), and in mosaic normal/dystrophic fibres it is present in disproportionately large amounts compared with the amount of normal genome present (15, 36), suggesting a degree of bias arising from excessive expression or reduced degradation of dystrophin under conditions of low concentration of this protein.

At first sight, revelation of marker DNA sequences such as the Y-chromosome repeat sequences (3, 6, 25), by *in situ* labelling, seems to provide a perfect marker system for transplanted myonuclei. Quantitation on blots can be standardized to give good semi-quantitative, unbiased estimates of donor genomic contribution. In addition these markers can be demonstrated in individual nuclei in tissue sections by *in situ* hybridization with labelled probes. In the latter instance however, this type of label does present unexpected difficulties if precise identification or quantitation is attempted.

The difficulty arises because the commonly used range of tissue section thicknesses and the dimensions of the average nucleus are very similar to one another. Thus many of the nuclei are themselves sliced during sectioning and are represented as nuclear profiles on more than one section. Since there is only one Y-chromosome repeat sequence per nucleus, a proportion of these sectioned nuclear profiles will therefore not contain this sequence and the proportion of labelled nuclear profiles will always be an underestimate of the true number.

A. Transverse section   **B.** Longitudinal section

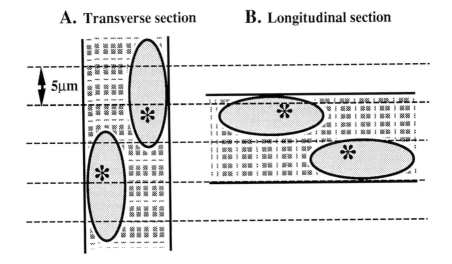

Fig 1.   This illustrates the influence of angle of section on the frequency
with which a punctate nuclear marker is found in nuclear profiles in
sections of skeletal muscle. A muscle containing a punctate marker,
e.g. Y-chromosome repeat sequence * is shown being transected, A,
transversely and B, longitudinally, by horizontal 5μm sections. In
transverse section, each myonucleus, 12-15μm long, is cut into 3-4
portions, each represented in adjacent sections, only one of which
contains the marker. Thus the proportion of labelled nuclear profiles
is about 30%. In longitudinal section, the same nuclei, 4-6μm in
width, are represented in only 1-2 sections, giving approximately
75% labelled profiles.

More seriously for comparative studies, the extent of this underestimate is
highly dependent on section thickness and on the nuclear dimension at right
angles to the plane of section, and this has a major impact on measurements
made on a highly anisotropic tissue like skeletal muscle. As shown in figure 1,
even a male muscle, in which each nucleus bears a Y-chromosome, will give
very different incidences of marking, depending on whether the muscle is
sectioned transversely or longitudinally. This effect also raises difficulties when
comparing nuclei of different size, e.g. mature muscle nuclei with those in
young myotubes.

The inevitable consequence of a proportion of false-negative nuclear
profiles, also complicates any attempt to relate donor nuclei as, recognized by
such a marker, to the distribution of dystrophin. This problem can be minimized
by use of two distinguishable positive markers, one for host nuclei, one for
donor nuclei but, even here, a small proportion of nuclei within any given
section will remain unassignable.

Each of the cell markers therefore has its own limitations which determine
its most effective use and a comprehensive picture can be obtained only by use
of a combination of markers of different properties.

CLINICAL CRITERIA OF SUCCESS

Current experiments on myoblast transplanation in man (16) are being conducted mainly in children of 5 years or older, whose muscles would usually be expected to have already undergone a degree of myopathic change. The main value of such experiments is in demonstrating that injected normal myoblasts survive, that they do not provoke immune rejection by the recipient, that they do not form neoplasms and that they produce dystrophin which becomes correctly located within muscle fibres in the recipient muscle.

In an attempt to gain more information, Karpati and colleagues (this volume) have selected their patients and donors such that they can use exons deleted from the dystrophin gene of the recipient, but present in the donor, as an indication of the presence of donor cells, independently of the detection of dystrophin. It is important to have such markers because of the presence of the so-called 'revertant' dystrophin-positive fibres (9) found sporadically in many DMD muscle biopsies (24).

Because of the limited numbers of patients and the ethical and practical constraints on access to their muscles, it will be difficult to make more detailed studies than this on myoblast transfer experiments in man. Further advance is likely to be made by experimenting on younger patients where there is more prospect that the procedure will arrest the secondary pathological changes.

In these studies, the X-linked dystrophic mouse and dog dystrophies play a complementary rôle, making it possible to examine critically those points which are difficult to address in man. Observations of a more detailed and more extensive nature can be made and individual variables can be studied systematically. In the dystrophic dog, it is possible to make clinico-pathological assessments which closely parallel those one would make on DMD patients. In the mdx mouse, it has only been possible to use the primary pathological changes as criteria of clinical status, but the recent description of more typical dystrophic changes in the diaphragm (33) may extend the usefulness of this animal somewhat.

It should be mentioned, that studies of myoblast transplantation on the mdx mouse call into question two of the more obvious criteria of functional success. In the short term at least, the muscle bulk of pre-irradiated mdx muscles is preserved at least as well by transplantation of mdx myoblasts as by normal myoblasts (22). In as far as the irradiated mdx muscle can be regarded as a simulation of the exhaustion of myogenic cells in DMD muscles, these results show that the mere replenishment of satellite cells may have a temporary beneficial effect on muscle without necessarily remedying the biochemical defect. Second, in these pre-irradiated muscles of the mdx mouse, implantation of myogenic cells gives rise initially to an almost normal histological appearance to the muscle, notably by forming peripherally rather than centrally nucleated fibres. Since this occurs with both normal and mdx cells and only later do the mdx-implanted muscles become abnormal, this initial change is again not attributable to biochemical rectification of the disease. Care should be taken not to make equivalent mistakes when judging the clinical effectiveness of myoblast transplantation in human subjects.

MYOBLAST TRANSPLANTATION EXPERIMENTS
IN THE MOUSE

Although the first myoblast transplantation experiments were performed on the rat and the quail (13, 20), the majority have been conducted on the mouse. Our particular reasons for using this animal was the availability in this species of genetic markers with which to follow the fate of transplanted cells and the extensive knowledge of transplantion immunology in the mouse, which enabled us to minimize rejection problems, and to put such problems as did occur into perspective.

The combined usefulness of these two properties was demonstrated in our early studies, where we used strain-specific isoforms of the enzyme glucose-6-phosphate isomerase (GPI) to study the survival of allografted minced muscle and the extent of mixing of myogenic cells within these grafts by their ability to form mosaic muscle fibres in which the two allotypic isoenzyme subunits were able to form heterdimer GPI composed of one subunit of each type. These grafts were made between strains of animal which were matched at the major histocompatibility complex (MHC) locus (7, 28). To our surprise, we found that , despite MHC matching, minced muscle allografts were freqently rejected unless the host animal was tolerized to the donor strain. Furthermore, mixtures of minced muscle fragments of the two strains only rarely formed mosaic muscle fibres when implanted into tolerized hosts of either strain, whereas the same mixture implanted into a nude mouse host almost always formed mosaic fibres. Thus, even when there was no actual rejection of the implanted muscle, there seemed to be some inhibition of fusion of myoblasts except in highly immunocompromised hosts. A similar unexplained inhibition of formation of mosaic muscle fibres was noted in myoblast transplantion experiments on the dy^{2J} mouse (17). Such phenomena may be significant factors in determining the success of therapeutic myoblast transplantation and would be missed in the absence of the powerful marker system provided by these allelic enzyme isoforms.

These markers were also invaluable as accessory evidence of successful myoblast transplantation in the phosphorylase kinase-deficient mouse and the mdx mouse. The former was the first available animal model of a known genetic deficiency of an identifiable protein in skeletal muscle and was thus the first to be used to show that transplantation of normal myogenic cells could lead to synthesis of this protein (23). However, the production of significant amounts of phosphorylase kinase required the transplantation of very large numbers of normal myogenic cells into phosphorylase kinase-deficient muscle which had been induced to regenerate by mincing and autotransplantation. The difficulty seemed to be both that there was inefficient introduction of normal genome into the host muscles and that expression of phosphorylase kinase was not proportional to the amount of normal genome present.

By contrast, the mdx mouse has proven a relatively simple animal in which to elicit expression of the missing gene product, dystrophin, by transplantation of normal mouse myogenic cells (29). Indeed, in the short-term at least, transplantation of human myogenic cells into mdx mouse muscles has led to the production of dystrophin (14). By immunostaining with specific antibody, it is possible to demonstrate that dystrophin introduced into mdx muscles by myoblast transplantation is widely distributed in the host muscle, is correctly located in the juxtasarcolemmal position and has a patchy distribution within some individual fibres, suggesting that in mosaic muscle fibres, each normal myonucleus has a territory within which it is able to distribute this protein. By immunoblotting, it has been shown that the dystrophin is of the correct molecular size and is present at up to 30-40% of normal levels.

Although a most convenient animal for demonstrating biochemical correction of the mdx myopathy, the mdx mouse is not well suited to a study of the clinicopathological benefits of this procedure because it does not develop the severe fibro-fatty degenerative changes seen in DMD, except in the diaphragm (33). It is possible, however, to examine the effects of myoblast transfer on the primary pathological consequence of the lack of dystrophin, namely the higher than normal frequency of muscle fibre necrosis. This effect is seen most dramatically in muscle which has been irradiated to prevent endogenous regeneration (34). In such a muscle, regeneration can occur only from the introduced myogenic cells and the course of this process can be followed by means of the GPI isoenzyme markers of host and donor tissues.

Where the transplanted cells are of normal genotype, dystrophin also serves as a marker of these cells in the mdx host muscle. Immunochemical staining for dystrophin shows that these cells permeate the entire muscle in a matter of a few weeks and are often found in muscles adjacent to the injected muscle too (22). By 4 weeks, individual muscles often contained 70-80% dystrophin-positive fibre profiles. In parallel, the proportion of donor and heterodimer GPI rose to 50-60% of the total. Histologically, both dystrophin-negative fibres, which we assume had survived since birth, and the dystrophin-posititive fibres, which we suspect had regenerated from the injected myogenic cells, were of normal appearance, with peripherally located nuclei. This latter finding was surprising because murine muscle normally retains its myonuclei in a central position for long periods after regeneration.

Many of the same initial changes, in terms of GPI isoform composition and peripheral nucleation were seen when mdx myogenic cells were injected into pre-irradiated mdx muscles, although, of course, dystrophin-positive muscle fibres did not increase in number beyond their normal sporadic incidence. By 7-10 weeks however, marked differences were noted, depending on whether the injected cells were normal or mdx in origin. In both cases, the injected cells prevented the progressive loss of muscle fibres from pre-irradiated muscles but the total content of normal myogenic cells seemed to remain at a stable level of about 50%, as assessed by GPI isoform composition, whereas mdx myoblasts progressively replaced the host muscle fibre segments as they continued to degenerate.

We are now analysing experiments designed to examine the longer-term fates of normal myoblasts in mdx muscle. These cells were injected as a pellet in a minimum of fluid into the two tibialis anterior muscles of each mouse, the right leg having been pre-irradiated. After 50 days or 250 days the mice were killed and the tibialis anterior, extensor digitorum longus and peroneus muscles of both legs were removed for analysis. At 50 days, dystrophin-positive fibres, accompanied by host, donor and heterodimer GPI were found in the tibialis anterior muscles only. By 250 days, these markers are present in significant amounts in several of the extensor digitorum longus and peroneus muscles of the pre-irradiated leg but still only in the tibialis anterior muscle of the non-irradiated leg. Thus, in the irradiated leg, the injected cells must have continued to proliferate and migrate into fresh areas of host muscle, even between individual muscles - a process involving penetration of epi- peri- and endo-mysial barriers. These properties are valuable for the therapeutic application of myoblast transfer; what it is about irradiated muscle which promotes them, is a subject of our present research.

USE OF MYOBLAST TRANSFER AS A TOOL FOR STUDYING BEHAVIOUR AND MOLECULAR BIOLOGY OF SKELETAL MUSCLE FIBRES AND MYOGENIC CELLS

Interest in transplantation of myogenic cells has been directed largely at its application to therapy of primary myopathies such as DMD. But this technique may eventually prove to be of even greater value as a tool for investigation of the molecular and cell biology of normal and diseased skeletal muscle. Insights gained from these studies may, in turn, lead to new ideas for dealing with muscle dysfunctions.

In essence, myoblast transplantation presents us with the opportunity to construct skeletal muscles in vivo wholly or partially from transplanted cells. These cells may be derived from a selected source or may be genetically altered in tissue culture prior to transplantation. The advantage of in vivo studies is that the muscles so-formed are vascularized, innervated, and capable of performing mechanical work; conditions which permit a more extensive and physiologically relevant expression of muscle genes.

Myoblasts extracted from neonatal mouse muscle can be implanted into freeze-killed mouse muscles or into an innert substratum such as woven Vicryl suture thread and implanted into the anterior tibial compartment of a mouse leg, after removal of the host muscles. In such a site they will form up to a few milligrams of new muscle fibre, but there is always a slight danger of contamination by invading myogenic cells from surrounding host muscle (21). This invasion process is, in itself, an interesting demonstration of the motility of myogenic cells and seems to occur more markedly when no cells have been transplanted into the freeze-killed muscle.

Larger amounts of muscle can be produced by transplanting cells of the C2C12 myogenic cell line. On occasion, some tens of milligrams of muscle can be grown from a transplant of a few thousand such cells, but in dead muscle sites, tumours eventually form, infiltrating and eventually replacing the muscle fibres. Prior to this point however, the muscle formed from C2C12 cells is often quite well organised and forms motor-end-plates with invading axons(30). Muscle formed from this cell-line however, never seems to stabilize totally and even prior to the appearance of tumours, the muscle continues to grow.

In search of a more normal source of purified myogenic cells, Jones *et al.* (12)have used an antibody-affinity method to extract myogenic cells from the mixed cell preparations obtained by enzymatic digestion of neonatal mouse muscle. Myogenic cells are panned onto antibody-coated Petri dishes by means of a monoclonal antibody specific to mouse muscle N-CAM, and separated from the non-myogenic population which are removed in the supernatant.

Myogenic cells prepared in this way proliferate vigorously in culture and can be cloned for short periods. Recently, we have infected cells prepared in this way with a replication-deficient retrovirus carrying the bacterial β-galactosidase gene and the neomycin-resistance gene. By subsequent selection in G418 we have obtained almost pure populations of myogenic cells expressing bacterial β-galactosidase. These, on transplantation into the muscles of a nude/mdx mouse, form muscle fibres expressing the β-galactosidase gene. This strategy can be used as a marker of transplanted cells and is currently being used by Watt &

England to determine whether myogenic cells can move across micropore filters placed between adjacent muscles (37).

A current example of the usefulness of this gene is illustrated by its application to the identification of a population of cells in regenerating mdx skeletal muscle which are susceptible to a particular marking technique, and which are suspected of being myogenic cells. Gary Coulton, in our Department of Biochemistry, has found that some cells present in frozen sections of the lesions of mdx mouse muscle are able to incorporate labelled deoxynucleotides into their DNA in the presence of DNA polymerases. Unfortunately, it has not been possible to combine this marking process with immunolabels which might identify the cells concerned as myogenic. However, this category of cells is removed from the lesions by high dose X-ray treatment administered 1 week previously,as are myogenic cells (34) and it is now possible to test empirically whether these cells which incorporate labelled deoxynucleotides are myogenic by seeing whether they are replaced by the re-implantation of cloned myogenic cells into such pre-irradiated muscles.

To increase the usefulness of this type of approach we need to have reproducible sources of implantable cells and so our interest has turned to the matter of trying to determine whether there are any sources of myogenic stem cells, i.e. a self-renewing population of cells which can give rise to committed lineages of myogenic cells. Such cells, if they can be identified and isolated, would be of value from the point of view of myoblast transplantation therapy, for they could provide a source of myogenic cells within the muscle long after the initial transplantation.

Because they could be cloned, these cells would also be of use for studies involving genetic alteration with, for example, the dystrophin gene, which are too large to be inserted by efficient retroviral vectors. If the gene is inserted by a relatively inefficient method, like transfection, it is necessary to select and expand the few clones which have integrated and are expressing the gene.

Our main approach to the identification of such cells employs a similar strategy to that used to detect multipotential haematopoeitic stem cells in bone marrow. Myogenic cells are injected into mdx mouse muscles which have been pre-irradiated to block proliferation of endogenous myogenic cells (34). Here, the injected cells constitute the only source of myogenic cells to repair the spontaneously degenerating host muscle fibres and any committed cells should be rapidly consumed in this process, leaving non-committed proliferating muscle precursors as a highly enriched population to be re-extracted from the muscle and cloned in tissue culture. Confirmation that any extracted myogenic clones are derived from the originally injected cell population can be obtained by analysis of donor-specific markers. Being derived from normal muscle, these cells will give rise to dystrophin-positive muscle fibres; they are also chosen to be of a different Glucose-6-phosphate Isomerase allotype from the host animal.

Using this approach, we have failed to find any myogenic stem cells in the population of cells extractable from neonatal skeletal muscle, although these cells rapidly infiltrate and repair the pre-irradiated host muscle. We have however found such cells in a non-transformed line of myogenic satellite cells derived form adult mouse skeletal muscle (Morgan & Partridge, in prep.). This line proliferates slowly and only at low density in tissue culture and gives rise to only small patches of dystrophin-positive muscle fibres in irradiated mdx muscle. This suggests that not all myogenic cells are equivalent in respect of their ability to proliferate and to form new muscle fibres.

Recently, we have had collaborative access to a transgenic mouse which looks likely to be exceptionally useful as a source of myogenic cells. This animal, the H-2ts6 mouse carries the SV40 thermolabile large T gene (A58) driven by the 5′ promoter of the K allele of the murine Major Histocompatibility Complex (11). This promoter is activated in many cell types in the presence of murine γ-interferon. Clearly the transgene is not expressed to any significant extent in the mouse where the concentration of γ-interferon is too low and where the temperature is too high for this mutant form of the large T antigen to activate cell proliferation. However under 'permissive conditions' in tissue culture at 33°C and, in the presence of γ-interferon, the large T protein expressed and is active as a proliferative agent, driving cells into continuous proliferation; the switch to differentiation is achieved by removing the interferon and raising the temperature to 39°C, the conditions prevailing in the mouse.

With this animal, we have been able to re-design the experiments in search of the stem cell. First, the cells injected into the pre-irradiated mdx muscles are distinct myogenic clones, obtained from a variety of sites and from animals of various ages. Second, the cells re-extracted from the muscles after several weeks can be cloned very efficiently in the presence of γ-interferon at 33°C, providing sufficiently large numbers of cells to attempt further rounds of passage though irradiated mdx muscles.

The most effective use of these conditionally immortalizable cells however, will be in experiments where genetic alterations are made prior to reimplantation of the cells into suitable sites in a host mouse. By transfection of new or altered genes or by disruption of endogenous genes by homologous recombination, it will be possible to dissect and study discrete aspects of expression and interaction of given proteins. Application of this technology to the creation of transgenic mice, is limited to those genetic alterations which are compatible with survival of the whole animal; for individual cells the constraint is less severe, requiring only the survival of the cell in question. For example, one of the more powerful approaches to the study of growth and differentiation control would be by study of the effects of ablation of the genes for candidate growth/ differentiation factors or for their receptors, combined with the reversal of these effects by retransfection of the gene concerned. Such strategies are in current use in tissue-culture studies of cell/cell interactions and should prove equally important when applied to transplantable myogenic cells, in the study of such interactions in normal and diseased muscle.

ACKNOWLEDGEMENTS

Our work in this field, over a number of years, has been supported by the Muscular Dystrophy Group of Great Britain and Northern Ireland and Action Research for the Crippled Child.

REFERENCES

1.   Allameddine, H.S., Dehaupas, M. Fardeau, M. (1989): Regeneration of skeletal muscle fibers from autologous satellite cells multiplied in vitro. *Muscle and Nerve,* 12: 544-555.

2. Coulton, G.R, Curtin,N.A., Morgan, J. Partridge, T.A. (1988): The mdx mouse skeletal muscle myopathy: II, contractile properties. *Neuropath. Appl. Neurobiol.*, 14:299-314.
3. Coulton, G.R., Skynner, M.J., Smith, T., Pagel, C.N. and Partridge, T.A. (1991): Localization of donor nuclei in skeletal muscle grafts by *in situ* hybridization to a cDNA probe. *Histochem. J.*, 23:323-327.
4. Dangain, J. Vrbova, G. (1984): Muscle development in mdx mutant mice. *Muscle and Nerve,* 7:700-704.
5. Frair, P.M., Peterson, A.C. (1983): The nuclear-cytoplasmic relationship in 'mosaic' skeletal muscle fibres from mouse chimaeras. *Exp. Cell Res.*, 145:167-178.
6. Grounds, M.D., Lai, M.C., Fan, Y., Codling, J.C. Beilharz, M.W. (1991): Transplantation in the mouse model: the use of a Y-chromosome specific clone to identify donor cells *in situ. Transplantation,* in press.
7. Grounds,M.D., Partridge, T.A. and Sloper, J.C. (1980): The contribution of exogenous cells to regenerating skeletal muscle: an isoenzyme study of muscle allografts in mice. *J. Path.* , 132:325-341.
8. Hoffman E.P. Gorospe J.R. (1991) The animal models of Duchenne muscular dystrophy: windows on the pathophysiological consequences of dystrophin deficiency. In: Topics in Membranes, edited by J. Morrow & M. Mooseker, Academic Press, New York, in press.
9. Hoffman,E.P., Morgan, J.E., Watkins, S.C., Slayter, H.S. Partridge, T.A. (1990): Somatic suppression/reversion of the mouse mdx phenotype *in vivo. J. Neurol. Sci.*, 99, 9-25.
10. Hughes, S.M., Blau, H.M. (1990): Migration of myoblasts across basal lamina during skeletal muscle development. *Nature,* 345-350-353.
11. Jat, P.S., Noble, M.D., Ataliotis, P., Tanaka, Y., Yannoutsos, N., Larsson, L, Kioussis, D. (1991): Direct derivation of conditionally immortal cell lines from an H-2K^{b}ts58 transgenic mouse. *Proc. Natl. Acad. Sci. U.S.A.*, in press.
12. Jones, G.E., Murphy, S.J. Watt D.J. (1990): Segregation of the myogenic lineage in mouse muscle development. *J. Cell Sci.*, 97:659-667.
13. Jones, P.H. (1979): Implantation of cultured regenerate muscle cells into adult rat muscle. *Exp. Neurol.*, 66:602-610.
14. Karpati, G., Pouilot, Y., Zubrzycka-Gaarn, E., Carpenter, S., Ray, P.N., Worton, R.G. Holland, P. (1989): Dystrophin is expressed in mdx skeletal muscle fibers after normal myoblast implantation. *Am. J. Pathol.*, 135:27-32.
15. Karpati, G., Zubrzycka-Gaarn, E.E., Carpenter, S., Bulman, D.E., Ray. P.N. Worton, R.G. (1990): Age related conversion of dystrophin-negative to -positive fibre segments of skeletal muscle but not cardiac muscle fibres in heterozygote mdx mice. *J. Neuropath. Exp. Neurol.* , 49: 96-105.
16. Law, P.K., Bertorini, T.E., Goodwin, T.G., Chen, M., Fang, Q., Li, H-J., Kirby, D.S., Florendo, J.A., Herrod, H.G. and Golden, G.S. (1990): Dystrophin production induced by myoblast transfer therapy in duchenne muscular dystrophy. *Lancet* ii, 14:114-115.
17. Law, P.K., Goodwin, T.G. Li, J. (1988): Histoincompatible myoblast injection improves muscle structure and function of dystrophic mice. *Transplant. Proc.*, 20:1114-1119.
18. Law, P.K., Goodwin, T.G. Wang, M.G. (1988): Normal myoblst injections provide genetic treatment for murine dystrophy. *Muscle and Nerve,* 11:525-533.

19. Lipton, B.H. (1979): Skeletal muscle regeneration in muscular dystrophy. In: Muscle Regeneration, edited by A. Mauro, pp.101-114, Raven Press, New York.
20. Lipton, B.H., Schultz, E (1979): Developmental fate of skeletal muscle satellite cells. *Science*, 205:1292-1294.
21. Morgan, J.E., Coulton, G.R., Partridge, T.A.(1987): Muscle precursor cells invade and repopulate freeze-killed muscle grafts. *J. Muscle Res. Cell Motil.*, 8:386-396.
22. Morgan, J.E., Hoffman, E.P. Partridge, T.A. (1990): Normal myogenic cells from newborn mice restore normal histology to regenerating muscles of the mdx mouse. *J. Cell Biol. 111*: 2437-2449.
23. Morgan, J.E., Watt, D.J., Sloper, J.C. Partridge, T.A. (1988): Partial correction of an inherited defect of skeletal muscle by grafts of normal muscle precursor cells. *J. Neurol. Sci.*, 86:137-147.
24. Nicholson, L.V.B., Johnson, M.A., Gardner-Medwin, D., Bhattacharya, S., Harris, J.B. (1990): Heterogeneity of dystrophin expression in patients with Duchenne and Becker muscular dystrophy. *Act. Neuropathol.*, 80:239-250.
25. Palmer, S.J., Burgoyne, P.S. (1991): XY follicle cells in the ovaries of XO/XY and XO/XY/XYY mosaic mice. *Development*, 111:1017-1019.
26. Partridge, T.A. (1991): Myoblast transfer: a possible therapy for inherited myopathies. *Muscle and Nerve*, 14:197-212.
27. Partridge, T.A. (1991): Animal models of muscular dystrophy - what use are they? *Neuropath. Appl. Neurobiol.*, in press
28. Partridge, T.A., Grounds, M.D. Sloper, J.C. (1978): Evidence of fusion between host and donor myoblasts in skeletal muscle grafts. *Nature,* 273:306-308.
29. Partridge, T.A., Morgan, J.E., Coulton, G.R., Hoffman, E.P., Kunkel, L.M. (1989): Conversion of mdx myofibres from dystrophin-negative to positive by injection of normal myoblasts. *Nature,* 337:176-179.
30. Partridge, T.A., Morgan, J.E., Moore, S.E., Walsh, F.S. (1988): Myogenesis in vivo from the mouse C2 muscle cell-line. *J. Cell. Biochem.,* Suppl. 12C:331.
31. Pavlath, G.K., Rich, K., Webster, S.G. Blau, H.M. (1989): Localization of muscle gene products in nuclear domains. *Nature,* 337:570-573.
32. Ralston, E, Hall, Z.W. (1989): Transfer of a protein encoded by a single nucleus to nearby nuclei in multinucleated myotubes. *Science*, 244:1066-1069.
33. Stedman, H.H., Sweeney, H.L., Shrager, J.B., Maguire, H.C., Panettieri, R.A., Petrof, B., Narusawa, M., Leferovich, J.M., Sladky, J.T., Kelly, A.M. (1991): The mdx mouse diaphragm reproduced the degenerative changes of Duchenne muscular dystrophy. *Nature,* in press.
34. Wakeford, S., Watt, D.J., Partridge, T.A. (1991): X-irradiation improves mdx mouse as a model of muscle fibre loss in DMD. *Muscle and Nerve*, 14:42-50.
35. Watkins, S.C., Cullen, M.J. (1985): Histochemical fibre typing and ultrastucture of the small fibres in Duchenne muscular dystrophy. *Neuropath. Appl. Neurobiol.*, 11:447-460.
36. Watkins, S.C., Hoffman, E.P., Slayter, H.S., Kunkel, L.M. (1989): Dystrophin distribution in heterozygote mdx mice. *Muscle and Nerve,* 12:861-868.

37. Watt, D.J. England, M.A. (1991): Extent of migration of donor precursor cells introduced into recipient myopathic muscle. *J.Cell. Biochem.*, Suppl. 15C:46.
38. Watt, D.J., Lambert, K., Morgan, J.E., Partridge, T.A., Sloper, J.C. (1982): Incorporation of donor muscle precursor cells into an area of muscle regeneration in the host mouse. *J. Neurol. Sci.*, 57: 319-331.
39. Watt, D.J., Morgan, J.E., Partridge, T.A. (1984): Use of muscle precursor cells to insert allogeneic genes into growing mouse muscles. *Muscle and Nerve*, 7:741-750.
40. Webster, C., Filippi, G., Rinaldi, A., Mastropaolo, C., Tondi, M., Siniscalco, M. Blau, H.M. (1986): The myoblast defect identified in Duchenne muscular dystrophy is not a primary expression of the DMD mutation. *Hum. Genet.*, 74:74-80.
41. Webster, C., Pavlath, G.K., Parks, D.R., Walsh, F.S., Blau, H.M. (1988): Isolation of human myoblasts with the fluorescence-activated cell sorter. *Exp. Cell Res.*, 174:252-265.

DISCUSSION

Professor Joe N. Kornegay:
You mentioned that you have been successful in getting implantation of transplanted cells only during times of active regeneration. This would suggest that you have performed transplants at other stages of the disease. Have you implanted cells into normal muscle and noted whether they implant. I am assuming that they would not.

Dr. Terence A. Partridge:
We have no really good histological markers when we implant myoblasts into normal muscle. Using the GPI isoenzyme markers we have shown that we can get myoblast fusion into regenerating or growing normal muscles, the latter at low levels of efficiency. In fact the type of nuclear marker which Manfred described is the best way of looking at this type of graft.

Professor Joe N. Kornegay:
My comments in this area relate to whether myoblasts transplanted into normal or relatively normal, nonregenerating muscle would implant. Fibrosis would apparently have deleterious effects on the transplant, but I wonder whether cells injected into relatively mildly affected muscles, as perhaps would be the case with Duchenne patients early in the disease, would actually fuse and implant.

Dr. Terence A. Partridge:
I imagine that regeneration is going on quite early in DMD muscle, long before the fibrosis becomes severely obstructive. We have begun working on the question of whether fibrosis in mouse muscle has any effect on the success of myoblast transplantation.

DUCHENNE MUSCULAR DYSTROPHY: Animal Models
and Genetic Manipulation, edited by Byron A. Kakulas,
John McC. Howell, and Allen D. Roses.
Raven Press, Ltd., New York © 1992.

16

Replication of Myogenic Cells with Age, and Myogenesis after Experimental Injury in mdx Mouse Muscle: Quantitative Autoradiographic Studies

John K. McGeachie*, Miranda D. Grounds+,
Terence A. Partridge°, Jennifer E. Morgan°

Department of Anatomy and Human Biology, and Pathology+,
The University of Western Australia, Nedlands, 6009 Australia,
Department of Histopathology°, Charing Cross & Westminster
Medical School, Fulham Palace Road, London W68RF, U.K.*

Two studies were designed for the following purposes:

1. **CELL REPLICATION WITH AGE**
   To examine the replication of myogenic cells in mdx muscle at different ages, (McGeachie, Morgan, Partridge, Grounds - to be published.)

2. **MYOGENESIS AFTER INJURY**
   To compare the pattern of myogenic precursor cell replication in mdx muscle after traumatic injury with that in the control strain (9).

1. CELL REPLICATION WITH AGE

Introduction

The mdx mouse (3) has been used extensively as a model for x-linked muscular dystrophy. There is now great interest in its application as a model for myoblast replacement therapy for Duchenne Muscular Dystrophy (DMD) and other related myopathies (15,16). In the mdx mouse, muscle regeneration is effective and in the long term there is no permanent muscle weakness, although it has been reported that there is ultimately a change in distribution of muscle fibre types and an increase in muscle collagen content (14). It is noteworthy that muscle necrosis and regeneration in mdx mice does not appear to occur consistently throughout the age of the animal. It has been reported that the most active phase is around 3 to 4 weeks of age and is substantially reduced in older animals (5,10). Conversely it has also been reported that after the onset, muscle necrosis and regeneration occur constantly, or are only slightly diminished throughout the life of mdx mice (2,4,14,17).

Because of the importance of the mdx mouse as a model for the understanding of the disease processes involved in DMD, and also as a model system for testing potential therapies (such as myoblast transfer therapy), it is crucially important to determine the degree of necrosis and regeneration, and specifically the replication of myogenic precursor cells in mdx muscles with age. Thus the time of maximal myogenic precursor cell replication can be revealed. With these data the most appropriate time to conduct experimental myoblast transfer procedures can be determined.

Materials and Methods

Forty eight inbred mdx mice aged between 15 days (2 weeks) to 300 days (43 weeks) were injected intraperitoneally with tritiated thymidine (^{3}H-TdR: specific activity 5 Ci/m.mol, Amersham, U.K.) at the dosage of 1 uCi/gram body weight; 3 mice at each of the following 16 time periods: 15, 17, 19, 20, 21, 22, 23, 24, 25, 31, 50, 60, 80, 100, 149 and 300 days of age (Fig. 1).

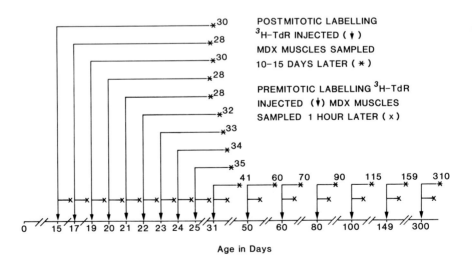

FIG. 1. Injection times for ^{3}H-TdR and muscle sampling times for premitotic and postmitotic nuclear labelling in mdx mouse muscle.

One hour after injection with ^{3}H-TdR one of the three mice injected at each of the above time periods was sacrificed by anaesthetisation with ether followed by cervical dislocation. Muscle samples from these 16 mice would be analysed later for the presence of premitotically labelled nuclei, because all labelled nuclei would have insufficient time to pass from the DNA synthesis phase of the cell cycle (S), through the G2 premitotic phase to mitosis, M phase.

The remaining 2 mice for each injection time (total of 32 mice) were left for times varying from 10-15 days after injection before being sacrificed, as above (Fig. 1). Muscle nuclei labelled in samples from these mice would be postmitotic because they had sufficient time to pass through mitosis and either become incorporated into myoblasts and myotubes, or to continue to replicate as myogenic precursor cells.

After sacrifice samples of the following muscles were taken from both left and right legs of all 16 premitotic mice, and the left legs only of the 32 postmitotic mice: tibialis anterior, extensor digitorum longus, peroneus, gastrocnemius and soleus. All samples were immerse fixed in 2% glutaraldehyde in 0.1m phosphate buffer (ph 7.2) overnight, post-fixed in 1% osmium tetroxide in 0.1m buffer for 1 hour, washed in 70% ethanol and block stained in 1% Paraphenylenediamine in 70% ethanol for 1 hour (6). Samples were embedded in Araldite: Epon, 1:1, and 1um thick transverse sections cut for autoradiography. Sections were placed on glass slides and coated with Kodak ARIO stripping film, exposed in light-tight boxes at -20°C, developed in Kodak D19b, fixed in acid hardener fixer, washed and dried.

For the analysis of each sample of dystrophic muscle at least 300 muscle nuclei (within the contour of the muscle fibre) were counted and labelled and unlabelled nuclei recorded. Muscle nuclei included both myonuclei and satellite cell nuclei because the latter cannot be distinguished at the light microscopic level. In addition the numbers of myotube nuclei (centrally located) associated with regenerating mdx muscle, were counted. The percentages of labelled muscle nuclei and myotube nuclei were calculated. The number of grains per labelled nucleus were also recorded. Labelled nuclei of connective tissue cells (fibroblasts, macrophages, etc.) in the same region as the "normal", regenerating and necrotic muscle were recorded.

Results

Premitotic Labelling

It is important to emphasise that labelled "muscle" nuclei within the contour of intact muscle fibres were probably satellite cell nuclei, because myonuclei are post-mitotic and do not synthesise DNA, and therefore do not incorporate ^{3}H-TdR. Examples of labelled muscle nuclei are shown in Fig. 2A.

At 15 to 22 days of age there were few labelled muscle nuclei (Fig. 3). The labelling was scattered throughout the various 5 muscles analysed from each of both legs of the 16 mdx mice. From 23 to 50 days the uptake of ^{3}H-TdR was maximal (Fig. 3) and was also roughly evenly distributed amongst all the muscles. Fewer labelled nuclei were evident at 60 to 300 days where the uptake was even lower than in the first 15-22 days (Fig. 3).

In addition to calculating the percentages of labelled premitotic muscle nuclei in mdx muscles, the ratios (percentages) of myotube nuclei to muscle nuclei were recorded to give some indication of the degree of muscle regeneration at different times after birth. Typical myotube nuclei are shown in Fig. 2B and the percentages of myotube nuclei are indicated in Fig. 3.

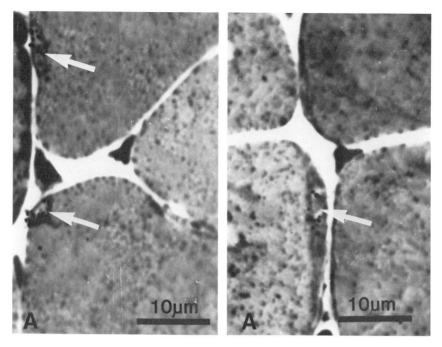

FIG. 2A.   Labelled premitotic muscle nuclei (arrows) in an mdx mouse.

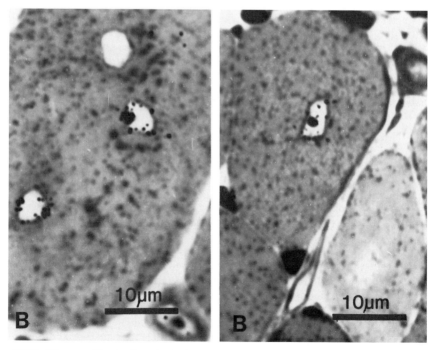

FIG. 2B.   Typically labelled postmitotic, myotube nuclei in mdx muscle.

Postmitotic Labelling

In these muscles both peripheral and non-peripheral nuclei were labelled with ^{3}H-TdR because the premitotically labelled muscle precursor cells had sufficient time to pass through mitosis and become incorporated into myotubes or muscle fibres. In fact there was time for labelled myoblasts to divide a number of times before becoming fused into myotubes.

Data from the analysis of labelled myotubes and muscle nuclei are summarized in Fig. 3. The majority of labelled nuclei were in myotubes, often in focal clusters.

Of the 30 mdx mice (2 for each of the 15 time periods) where a total of 150 individual muscles were analysed, only 52 samples (35%) had any labelled myotube or muscle nuclei labelled. Each sample had 300 muscle nuclei, and variable numbers of associated myotube nuclei counted in adjacent areas. Therefore the incidence of labelling was low (0.1-6.0%) but it was evident that the maximal labelling was from 15-50 days of age (2-7 weeks).

Discussion

At 15 days of age the existence of necrosis in mdx muscle fibres with little or no premitotic labelling of muscle precursor (satellite) cells was quite striking. Even more striking was the rapid onset of satellite cell proliferation at 21 to 25 days where individual values for some muscles were as high as 3 to 4% of muscle nuclei. These are very high levels when considering that at a point in time (a one hour window) there are that many satellite cells proliferating in mdx muscle. It is important to re-state that counts for muscle nuclei included myonuclei and satellite cell nuclei. Myonuclei are postmitotic and do not incorporate DNA, therefore these premitotic labelling levels are much higher in cell proliferative terms when one considers that satellite cells constitute 1-5% of the cell population of muscle (1). To emphasise this high level of cell replication measured premitotically in these mdx muscles, if ^{3}H-TdR is injected into normal healthy mice it is extremely rare to find any labelled premitotic nuclei at all. Even if mice are labelled every day for 7 days it is rare to find 1% of nuclei labelled postmitotically (11). Therefore the levels of premitotic replicative activity in mdx muscle measured in this present study at 21-30 days of age are comparatively very high indeed.

With such levels of premitotic labelling it was predicted that these muscle precursor cells would go through mitosis and pass the ^{3}H-TdR on to daughter cells; most of the progeny would become incorporated into myoblasts and myotubes. Therefore it would be expected that much higher numbers of labelled nuclei would be seen in postmitotic muscles; numbers which would amplify the premitotic levels. Such was not really the case because mean postmitotic levels were similar to those of premitotic samples (Fig. 3). The unexpected result of no major increase in postmitotic labelling may have been due to two possible factors. Firstly, many of the satellite cells labelled premitotically may have undergone a number of subsequent mitotic divisions as either satellite cells or myoblasts, before becoming incorporated into postmitotic myotube nuclei. Because there was a 10-15 day difference between the premitotic and postmitotic sampling (Fig. 1), the number of cell divisions may have diluted out the ^{3}H-TdR label beyond the sensitivity of the autoradiographic analysis.

Alternatively, as a second possible explanation, labelled premitotic cells may have been located in areas of muscle more prone to necrosis immediately following regeneration. Thus the labelled cells passed through a cycle of regeneration and became necrotic again, such that they were phagocytosed by the

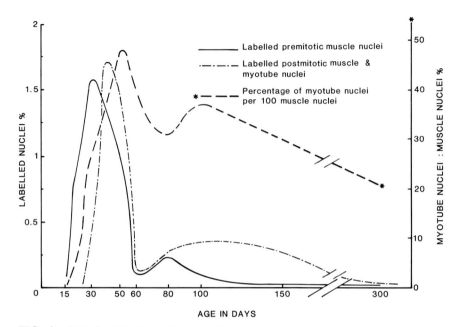

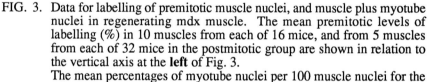

FIG. 3. Data for labelling of premitotic muscle nuclei, and muscle plus myotube nuclei in regenerating mdx muscle. The mean premitotic levels of labelling (%) in 10 muscles from each of 16 mice, and from 5 muscles from each of 32 mice in the postmitotic group are shown in relation to the vertical axis at the **left** of Fig. 3.

The mean percentages of myotube nuclei per 100 muscle nuclei for the 16 premitotic mice at different ages are plotted relative to the vertical axis at the **right** of Fig. 3.

time the postmitotic samples were taken for analysis, 10-15 days later. This alternative explanation is less likely because mdx muscles progressively become replaced by regenerated fibres, as evidenced by the existence and persistence of centrally located nuclei. Therefore these are progeny of myoblasts which have gone through regeneration and have survived in the "regenerated" condition.

Data presented in Figure 3 show that the numbers of centrally nucleated fibres rise rapidly from 4-5 weeks and stay high, declining slowly through to 150 and 300 days of age. The reasons for this are unclear but it is likely that as the regenerated fibres matured, central nuclei in myotubes migrated peripherally.

In summary, myogenic cell proliferation in mdx muscle commences rapidly at 3-4 weeks of age and declines equally as rapidly at 7-8 weeks. This premitotic cell proliferative activity is associated later with the appearance of labelled myotube nuclei, particularly in the 3-8 week period, followed by comparatively low levels of cell proliferation (regeneration) from 8 to 50 weeks of age.

2. MYOGENESIS AFTER INJURY

Introduction
Data from the previous study on Cell Replication With Age in mdx mouse muscle reveal that there is substantial replication of myogenic cells, which is maximal at 3-8 weeks of age. These data have been compared with other published studies which also show that there is constant necrosis and regeneration in mdx muscle.

As a result of this myogenic cell replication it was hypothesised that mdx mice might have inherently more effective muscle regeneration than in non-dystrophic mice. In addition it was considered that since myogenic precursor cells in mdx mice were "primed" that they could possibly react more rapidly to a traumatic injury.

To test this hypothesis, the timing of muscle precursor cell replication after a crush injury in mdx mice was compared with that in non-dystrophic parental control mouse strain (C57B1/10Sn). These experiments were based upon autoradiographic techniques developed by McGeachie and Grounds (12) and used in a number of related studies (7,8,13).

Materials and Methods
Thirty mice were used in this experiment: 15 inbred male mdx mice aged between 42-50 days, and 15 male C57B1/10Sn matched controls (35-49 days old).

Each mouse received a small single crush injury to the tibialis anterior muscle (TA) of the right leg by the technique described in detail in McGeachie & Grounds (12). All experimental procedures were officially approved by the Animal Welfare Committee of the University of Western Australia and the National Health and Medical Research Council of Australia. Replicating muscle precursor cells were labelled with ^{3}H-TdR injected into each mouse (1uCi/g body weight) at times from 24-120 hours after crush injury. One injection of ^{3}H-TdR was given to each mouse. Ten days after injury all mice (mdx and control) were anaesthetised with ether and sacrificed by cervical dislocation. TA muscles from the regenerated lesions and from the contralateral, uninjured legs of the same mice were removed, and prepared for autoradiography, as described in Part 1 (Cell Replication With Age) of this paper.

Regenerated muscle lesions 10 days after injury were analysed in transverse sections, by counting the numbers of labelled and unlabelled myotube nuclei and the data were expressed as the percentages of labelled myonuclei. These were the progeny of myogenic precursor cells labelled at the time of ^{3}H-TdR injection. The scheme of injections and sampling for this experiment is shown in Fig. 4.

In each muscle sample removed 10 days after injury 200 myotube nuclei were counted. In uninjured muscles of control non-dystrophic C57B1/10Sn mice where no myotubes were present, 200 muscle nuclei were counted.

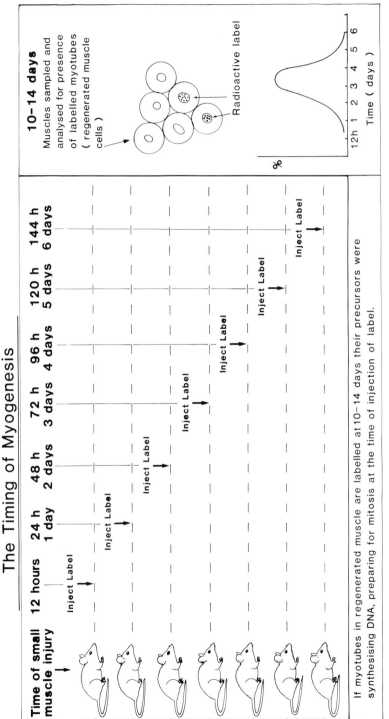

FIG. 4. A diagrammatic scheme of the ^{3}H-TdR injection and sampling schedule for the mdx muscle injury experiment

Results

Microscopically, in 10 day old crush lesions there was a central zone of fibrous scar tissue with a few myotubes. Adjacent to this was a region of well developed myotubes. This appearance was slightly complicated in mdx muscles because additional myotubes were spread unevenly throughout the muscle, as a consequence of continued necrosis and regeneration inherent in dystrophic muscle. This was also evident in uninjured mdx muscle, where the levels of myotube nuclear labelling were indicative of turnover of myogenic cells. (These latter data are complimentary to those presented in the postmitotic section of the first part of this paper). By comparison muscle fibres from the uninjured non-dystrophic strain matched controls were healthy with typical peripheral myonuclei.

Autoradiographically, in 10 day old regenerated lesions, labelled myotube nuclei and muscle nuclei were similar to those shown in Fig. 2.

In mdx mice injected with ^{3}H-TdR at 24 hours after injury there was effectively no labelling of myotube nuclei 10 days after injury, indicating that myogenic precursor cells were not synthesising DNA at 24 hours (Fig. 5). By contrast significant proportions (5-26%) of myotube nuclei were labelled in regenerated muscles from mdx mice which had been injected with ^{3}H-TdR between 30-120 hours after injury. It is important to emphasise that a small proportion of this labelling was attributable to the ongoing regenerative turnover of myogenic cells in dystrophic mdx muscle and was not the direct result of the crush injury. The level of this background labelling was revealed by data from uninjured control legs on the other side of the mdx mice, where 1-6% of myotube nuclei were labelled, although the average level was 2%.

Control, non dystrophic mice had similar levels of myotube labelling at 10 days after injury, to those in the mdx regenerated lesions. The highest level (33%) was from a mouse injected with ^{3}H-TdR at 72 hours after injury. In noninjured muscles from the other legs from these same control animals there was essentially no labelling of muscle nuclei.

Graphic comparisons of labelling in mdx lesions and controls, together with non mdx control lesions are shown in Fig. 5.

Discussion

It was hypothesised that injured mdx muscle would respond more rapidly to traumatic injury than control "quiescent" muscle. This was based upon the fact that mdx muscle has a substantial amount of satellite cell replication during the 3-8 weeks of age, the age of the mdx mice used in this experiment. Moreover, with the continual necrosis and regeneration of mdx muscle during this age span it was considered that the muscle would be "primed" to react rapidly to injury.

Such was not the case because mdx muscle regenerating after injury had the same timing and pattern of myogenic cell replication as in control C57B1/10Sn mice. Myogenic cells started to synthesise DNA at 24 hours after injury, maximal replication was at 72 hours, and declined rapidly thereafter, in both mdx and control muscle.

One factor worthy of mention was the continual level of satellite cell proliferation in mdx muscle. Although this has been discussed in Part 1 of this paper (Cell Replication With Age) it is important to emphasise that this "background" had to be taken into account when analysing the mdx regenerating muscle. In Figure 5 the labelling levels of myotube nuclei in the non-injured contra-lateral legs of mdx mice revealed the extent of this background labelling.

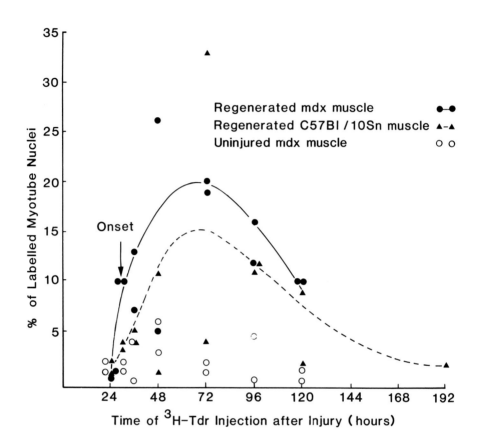

FIG. 5.   Labelling of myotube nuclei in regenerated muscles 10 days after crush injury to mdx and control muscles

In fact, these control data are comparable with those for postmitotic labelling in Part 1 of this paper (Fig. 3).

Histologically there was also no discernible difference between regenerating mdx and control muscle, both had a central fibrous connective tissue zone surrounded by myotubes. This is similar to that seen in similar lesions in BALB/c mice (12). By contrast regeneration in Swiss (SJL/J) mice is remarkably efficient with little or no fibrous scar tissue remaining (8). Therefore these collaborative data show that the dystrophic muscles of mdx mice have no special or exceptional capacity for muscle regeneration.

A much more detailed account of these experiments is published in Grounds and McGeachie (9).

ACKNOWLEDGEMENTS

The authors are sincerely grateful to Mrs. Jean Yeomans for typing this manuscript, and to Mr. Martin Thompson for his artistic assistance with the diagrams and graphs.

This research was supported financially by the Nicholas and Eliza McCluskey Memorial Bequest to John McGeachie, and the National Health and Medical Research Council of Australia's grant to Miranda Grounds.

REFERENCES

1.   Allbrook, D.B., Han, M.F. Helmuth, A.E. (1971): Population of muscle satellite cells in relation to age and mitotic cycle. *Pathol.*, 3:233-243.
2.   Anderson, J.E., Ovalle, W.K. Bressler, B.H. (1987):   Electron microscopic and autoradiographic characterisation of hindlimb muscle regeneration in the mdx mouse. *Anat. Rec.*, 219:243-257.
3.   Bulfield, G., Siller, W.G.F., Wight, P.A.L. Moore, K.J. (1984):   X-chromosome-linked muscular dystrophy (mdx) in the mouse. *Proc. Natl. Acid. Sci. U.S.A.*, 81:1189-1192.
4.   Carnwath, J.W., Shotton, D.M. (1987): Muscular dystrophy in the mdx mouse: histopathology of the soleus and extensor digitorum longus muscles. *J. Neurol. Sci.*, 80:39-54.
5.   Dangain, J., Vrobova, G. (1984): Muscle development in mdx mutant mice. *Muscle and Nerve*, 7:700-704.
6.   Dilley, R.J., McGeachie, J.K. (1983):   Block staining with p-phenylenediamine for light microscope autoradiography. *J. Histochem. Cytochem.*, 31:1015-1018.
7.   Grounds, M.D., McGeachie, J.K. (1987): A model of myogenesis in vivo, derived from detailed autoradiographic studies of regenerating skeletal muscle, challenges the concept of quantal mitosis. *Cell Tiss. Res.*, 250:563-569.
8.   Grounds, M.D., McGeachie, J.K. (1989): A comparison of muscle precursor replication in crush injured skeletal muscle of Swiss and BALBc mice. *Cell Tiss. Res.*, 255:385-391.
9.   Grounds, M.D., McGeachie, J.K. (1992): Skeletal muscle regeneration after crush injury in dystrophic mdx mice: an autoradiographic study. *Muscle and Nerve*, in press.
10. Karparti, G., Carpenter, S., Prescott, S. (1988): Small calibre skeletal muscle fibres do not suffer necrosis in mdx mouse dystrophy. *Muscle and Nerve*, 11:795-803.

11. McGeachie, J.K., Allbrook, D.B. (1978): Cell proliferation in skeletal muscle following denervation or tenotomy. *Cell Tiss. Res.*, 193:259-267.

12. McGeachie, J.K. Grounds, M.D. (1987): Initiation and duration of muscle precursor replication after mild and severe injury to skeletal muscle. *Cell Tiss. Res.*, 248:125-130.

13. McGeachie, J.K., Grounds, M.D. (1990): Applications of an autoradiographic model of skeletal muscle myogenesis in vivo. In: Pathogenesis and Therapy of Duchenne and Becker Muscular Dystrophy, edited by B.A. Kakulas and F.L. Mastaglia, Raven Press Ltd., New York, pp 151-170.

14. Marshall, P.A., Williams, P.E., Goldspink, G. (1989): Accumulation of collagen and fibre-type ratios as indicators of abnormal muscle gene expression in the mdx dystrophic mouse. *Muscle and Nerve*, 12:528-537.

15. Morgan, J.E., Hoffman, E.P., Partridge, T.A. (1990): Normal myogenic cells from newborn mice restore normal histology to degenerating muscle of the mdx mouse. *J. Cell Biol.*, 111:2437-2449.

16. Partridge, T.A. (1991): Myoblast transplantation: a possible therapy for inherited myopathies? *Muscle and Nerve*, 14:197-212.

17. Torres, L.F.B., Duchen, L.W. (1987): The mutant mdx: inherited myopathy in the mouse. *Brain*, 110:269-299.

DISCUSSION

Professor George Karpati:
I would like to address the point that you found unexpectedly low labelling in central myonuclei in the natural history of the mdx mouse and I wonder if, at least in part, this could not be due to two factors. One is, that you have a label dilution and secondly, you also have to consider the fact that only about 70% of the myonuclei are central in a regenerated fibre in mdx. So, if you consider these two points your low number may not be as unexpected as it seems now. Is that fair?

Assoc. Professor John K. McGeachie:
Yes that is fair.

Dr. Barry J. Cooper:
John, you often hear when you go to meetings that the mdx is resistant, if you like, to developing progressive clinical disease. Would you people say that the mouse regenerates more efficiency than other species do? I always assumed what other people mean by that is that necrosis and regeneration are going on and that, somehow, the mouse continues to be able to regenerate efficiently or effectively while other species don't. It seems to me that an alternative explanation, and a more appealing one, is that the fibres which are regenerated are stable in the mouse. Would you agree that your data would support that conclusion.

Assoc. Professor John K. McGeachie:
Yes, it would suggest that. We would need to go back and do some more experimental work on mdx mice, but we suggest that this is the case. We have no evidence that muscle regeneration in mice is more rapid than in other species. We have done many things to muscle to try to modify the pattern of regeneration, and generally it conforms to a rigid time frame. However, in very old and very young mice, there is a major difference in the timing of myogenic precursor cell

proliferation. The only other difference we have measured is between two different strains of mice: the Swiss (SJL/J) strain regenerates more rapidly and efficiently than the BALB/C strain.

Dr. Miranda D. Grounds:
I was just going to say that it doesn't necessarily mean that the "apparently resistant" mdx myofibres have regenerated. It may be in fact what Terry Partridge spoke about yesterday, that the muscle fibre population in mice may have come to the end of their major growth phase, and it is this that makes myofibres of older mice less susceptible to the dystrophic process.

Dr. Terence A. Partridge:
There is one experiment which provides evidence as to whether a regenerated mdx muscle fibre can undergo subsequent necrosis. It is the experiment in which we grafted whole EDL muscle between the two strains; from mdx into normal and *vice versa* to investigate whether the myopathy is primary to muscle. Virtually all muscle fibres in such grafts undergo necrosis and regenerate in response to the grafting procedure but, in mdx muscle grafts, we still found continued degeneration and degeneration of muscle fibres for over 100 days after grafting. So muscle fibres that had already undergone one round of regeneration were still susceptible to further bouts of degeneration as a result of the lack of dystrophin.

Professor George Karpati:
My response is, that these two processes are not mutually exclusive and it is likely both are operative to the extent that the resistance to the necrosis is not absolute.

Dr. Manfred W. Beilharz:
I wanted to ask you about the post-mitotic nuclei, a question which came up earlier. You were expressing the number of labelled nuclei as a percentage of total nuclei. I was wondering could you reflect on the number of labelled mononuclear cells seen in the post-mitotic samples.

Assoc. Professor John K. McGeachie:
In the post-mitotic samples the data shown included counts of labelled myotube nuclei and muscle (peripheral) nuclei combined. There were very few of the latter, suggesting that most of the satellite cell nuclei which were labelled premitotically actually divided and became incorporated into myotubes. The few postmitotically labelled peripheral muscle nuclei were either satellite cells or myonucleic that had gone through a myogenic cycle and passed from the central myotube nuclear position to the periphery of the more mature fibre.

DUCHENNE MUSCULAR DYSTROPHY: Animal Models
and Genetic Manipulation, edited by Byron A. Kakulas,
John McC. Howell, and Allen D. Roses.
Raven Press, Ltd., New York © 1992.

17

Results of Myoblast Transplantation in a Canine Model of Muscle Injury

J.N. Kornegay[+], S.M. Prattis[+], D.J. Bogan[+], N.J.H. Sharp[+*],
R.J. Bartlett[+*], H.S. Alameddine[#], M.J. Dykstra[+]

[+]College of Veterinary Medicine, North Carolina State University,
Raleigh, NC, 27606. *Duke University Medical Center, Durham, NC.
#INSERM, Paris France.

In our early studies of myoblast transplantation in dogs with golden retriever muscular dystrophy (GRMD), we used the 60 kd antibody from the spectrin-repeat area of the dystrophin molecule provided by Hoffman and noted positive fibers in both treated and untreated muscles (1). Several groups have subsequently shown that clusters of dystrophin-positive myofibers may be seen in DMD patients (2). We became convinced that a means other than dystrophin was necessary to identify transplanted myoblasts and felt that initial studies of this marker system, as well as certain other experiments, should first be done in a reproducible model of muscle injury. In developing this model system, we were motivated by our desire to ultimately study the potential for systemically administered myoblasts to implant in muscle. Notexin, a phospholipase derived from the Australian tiger snake, selectively affects mature myofibers, while sparing nerves, vessels, and myoblasts (3).

A model of notexin-induced muscle injury has been developed in the dog (4,5). The cranial sartorius muscle was chosen for initial studies, because it is markedly involved in GRMD (1), has a well-defined arterial supply through the femoral artery (6), has known fiber type distribution (7) and is a strap muscle ideally situated superficially over the cranial aspect of the thigh. Preliminary studies indicated that a dose of 0.1µg caused a relatively well defined, grossly evident area of muscle necrosis and consistent elevation of serum creatine kinase.

The sequence of muscle necrosis and regeneration after notexin injury was determined in 3-month-old Beagle dogs (4,5). Muscle regeneration was essentially complete by 21 days. Considering the rapidity and completeness of regeneration, we felt the relative contribution of donor myoblasts in future myoblast transplantation studies could be obscured by those of the recipient. X-irradiation has been shown to inhibit muscle regeneration in other species and was used in our muscle injury system (8). In preliminary studies, we found that doses of 15, 22.5 and 30 Gy given 17 days prior to notexin injection all inhibited regeneration. A dose of 15 Gy was subsequently studied more thoroughly. Muscle necrosis similar to that seen without prior radiation was observed; however, at 3 and 7 days post-injury, there was minimal regeneration. Instead, individual muscle fascicles were essentially devoid of myofibers, with only scattered macrophages being seen at 7 days and only residual fibrosis at the point of injury at 21 days (Prattis, S.M., et al, unpublished observations).

A third experiment using the same model system, irradiation to block host regeneration, and subsequent localized myoblast transplantation is currently underway. Use was made of a modification of Alameddine's culture and fluorescein labelling techniques (9). Previously irradiated, three-month-old, Beagle dogs injured with notexin receive autologous myoblasts labelled with fluorescein microspheres. Our initial transplant schedule was:

Day - 17: The cranial thighs, to include the caudal and cranial sartorius muscles, are irradiated bilaterally.
Day - 10: The lateral head of the triceps brachii is biopsied, removing approximately 2 grams of muscle. Myoblast cultures are established.
Day 1: The cranial and caudal sartorius muscles were injected bilaterally with 0.1 µg of notexin.
Day 5: Myoblasts were injected at the site of notexin injection in both cranial sartorius muscles; the left caudal sartorius muscle received DMEM and the right caudal sartorius muscle was not treated.
Day 12 and 26:
Injected muscles were removed. Multiple histochemical stains were done. Sections for fluorescence microscopy were stained with toluidine blue prior to study.

Thus far, 12 dogs (9 on day 12 and 3 on day 26) have been studied subsequent to this basic schedule. Up to 30 million cells have been injected at sites of notexin injury. Studies of these dogs were disappointing, in that microspheres were confined principally to perimysial connective tissue (Fig. 1). Microspheres were also aggregated in relatively few cells, suggesting that transplanted cells had perhaps lysed and microspheres were then phagocytized by macrophages. Several potential problems were identified.
(1) Although injections were made between sutures placed at the time of notexin injury, we could not definitely identify the actual lesion site in most cases. Therefore, we felt it was possible that myoblasts were injected into non-injured muscle, where they might not be utilized in the regenerative process.
(2) It seemed possible that, given the fact that our cultures were mixed cultures and no specific steps were made to enrich them further for myoblasts, most of the cells were fibroblasts.
(3) Even though we were using autologous cells and given that *in vitro* culture is thought to reduce antigenicity of the cultured cells, we felt it was possible

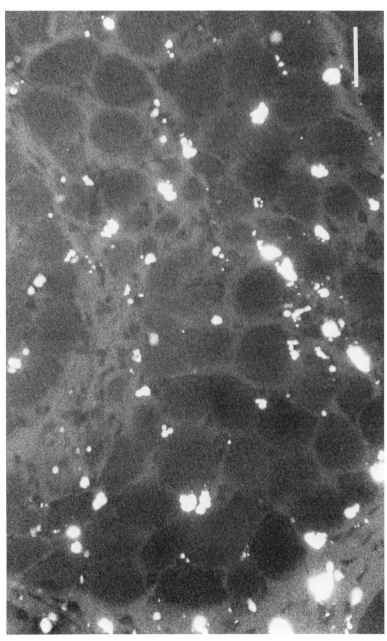

FIG. 1.   Cranial sartorius muscle in which myoblasts were transplanted 4 days after notexin injury.   Fluorescein-microspheres are concentrated in relatively few cells confined to endomysial and perimysial connective tissue.   Toluidine blue; bar = 30 μm.

that an immune-mediated response was being mounted against transplanted myoblasts.

A different injection schedule was developed for the latest transplants. At the suggestion of Dr. John Harris, the notexin and myoblast injections were done concomitantly, thus ensuring that myoblasts would be at the point of injury. Methylene blue was also added to the injectant to allow clearer definition of lesion sites, particularly those produced by percutaneous injections. In addition, the culture technique was modified somewhat, and yielded greater numbers of myoblasts.

Again 3-month-old beagle dogs were transplanted. The cranial and caudal sartorius muscles were injected at surgery, whereas the pectineus and cranial tibialis were injected percutaneously. Cranial sartorius and pectineus muscles received $2\text{-}3 \times 10^7$ myoblasts, and cranial tibialis muscles received $4\text{-}6 \times 10^7$ cells. On gross evaluation of muscles removed 7 days later, a focal area of bluish discoloration was noted in the sartorius muscles (Fig. 2A.); other muscles contained multiple, smaller areas (Fig. 2B.). Microscopically, large aggregates of mononuclear cells arranged in fascicles well demarcated from pre-existing muscle were noted with bright field microscopy (Fig. 3A., 4A.). Cells within these aggregates contained fluorescein microspheres when viewed with fluorescence microscopy (Figs. 3B, 4A.). On further histochemical evaluation, these mononuclear cells stained eosinophilic with H&E, blue with toluidine blue, and were weakly positive with ATPase (Fig. 5.). However, distinct myotube formation was not seen. No cells in these areas stained positive for non-specific esterase, indicating that phagocytosis was not occurring. Sartorius muscles contained far more cells than the others.

We have subsequently studied 6 additional dogs using a similar schedule. In one study, a considerably lesser number of cells (7×10^5 to 2×10^6) were injected into the cranial sartorius muscles. Injected muscles were removed on day 26. Similar, but less prominent microsphere-containing cell aggregates were noted. Staining characteristics of these cells were similar to those of the 7 day group. However, individual cells were larger and often contained multiple microspheres, suggesting that fusion between donor cells had occurred (Fig. 6.). In a final experiment, we increased the amount of notexin injected to 0.3 µg in 1 ml of saline in hopes of producing a more distinct lesion. When muscles were removed on day 26, prominent pale areas were noted at the injection sites. On microscopic examination, there was extensive fibrosis, with little if any evidence of regeneration. Fluorescein microspheres were present in areas of fibrosis and were aggregated in relatively few cells, again suggesting that injected cells had lysed and the microspheres were phagocytized. It is unclear if the injected cells were killed by the notexin itself or by macrophages that invaded subsequent to necrosis.

Concomitant myoblast and notexin injection ensures that myoblasts will be deposited at sites of necrosis. In addition, notexin injury presumably increases host myoblast proliferation, thus potentially augmenting chimeric fiber formation. In future studies, there is a need to more critically determine the optimal dose of notexin, ie. one that causes focal necrosis, while injected myoblasts are spared by the notexin itself and the secondary inflammatory infiltrate. Percutaneous injections of the peroneus longus muscle have been used to lessen fibrosis and serum accumulation that have occurred subsequent to surgery in some of our sartorius injections. This model should be useful in studying myoblast transplantation.

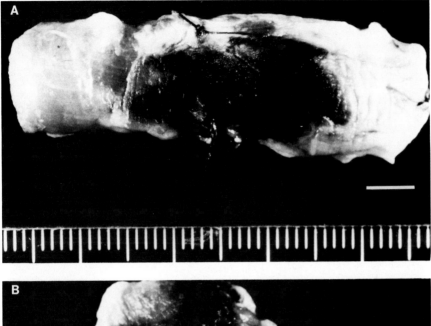

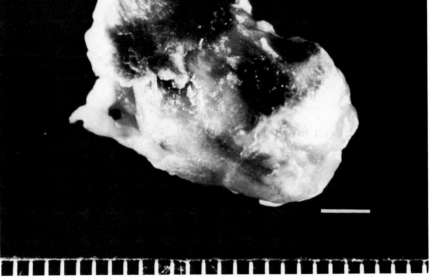

FIG. 2.   Muscles 7 days after surgical (cranial sartorius - A) and percutaneous (pectineus - B) injection with a mixture of myoblasts, notexin, and methylene blue.   Sutures in A flank the single site of injection. Multiple injections led to several discoloured areas in B.   Bar in A = 5 mm; bar in B = 3 mm.

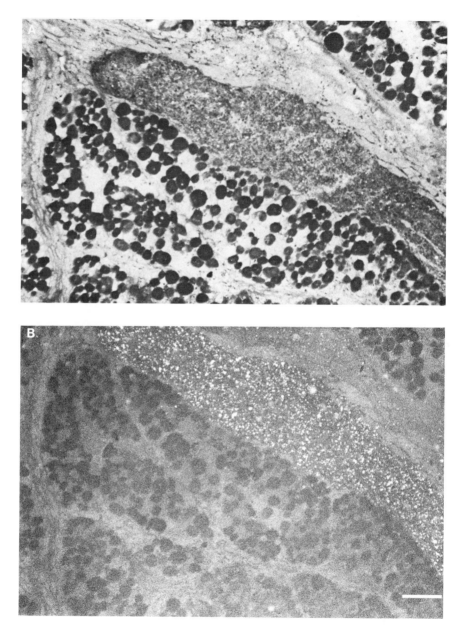

FIG. 3. Cranial sartorius muscle 7 days after concomitant injection of myoblasts, notexin, and methylene blue viewed with bright field (A) and fluorescence (B) microscopy. A large aggregate of fluorescein microsphere-containing cells is seen. Toluidine blue; bar = 120 μm in each.

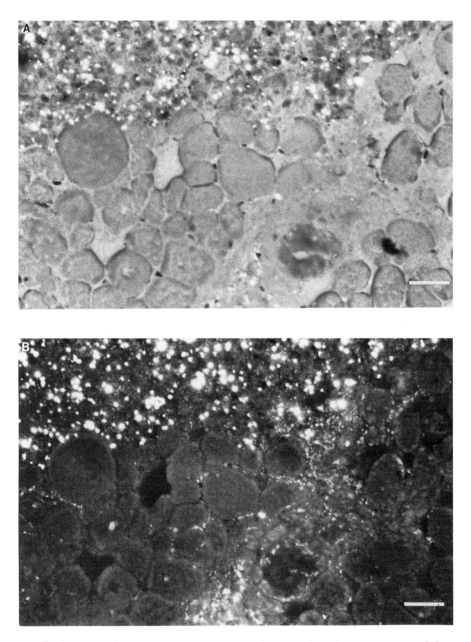

FIG. 4. Interface between transplanted fluorescein-microsphere containing cells and pre-existing host muscle viewed with partial (A) and full (B) fluorescence. Toluidine blue; bar in each = 30 μm.

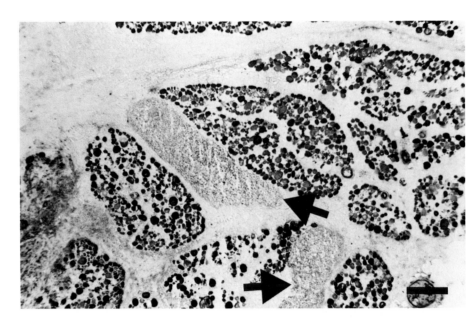

FIG. 5.   Overview of cranial sartorius muscle transplanted concomitantly with myoblasts, notexin, and methylene blue 7 days earlier. Transplanted cells are arranged in distinct clusters resembling fascicles (arrows). ATPase, 9.4 pH; bar = 120 μm.

FIG. 6.   Overview (A,B) and higher power (C,D) of cranial sartorius muscle viewed with bright field (A,C) and fluorescence (B,D) microscopy 21 days after recomitant myoblast, notexin, and methylene blue injection. A distinct cluster of fluorescein-microsphere containing cells is seen in A and B (arrows). On higher magnification in C and D, these cells are larger than those seen at 7 days and often contain multiple microspheres, perhaps indicating fusion of donor cells. Dark pigment seen at the periphery of the cell aggregate is methylene blue. Toluidine blue; bar in A and B = 80 μm; bar in C and D = 20 μm.

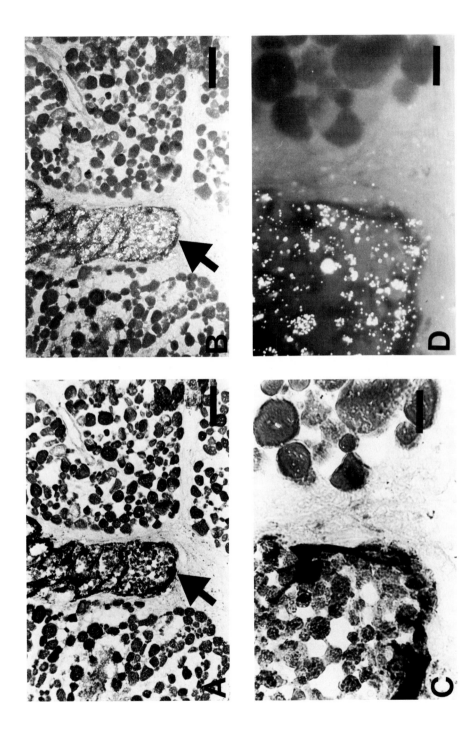

ACKNOWLEDGEMENTS

Supported by the Muscular Dystrophy Association of America, March of Dimes Birth Defects Foundation, Association Francaise Contre les Myopathies, and the State of North Carolina.

REFERENCES

1. Kornegay, J.N., Sharp, N.J.H., Bartlett, R.J., Van Camp, S.D., Burt, C.T., Hung, W.Y., Kwock, L., Roses, A.D. (1990): Golden retriever muscular dystrophy: Monitoring for success. In Eastwood, A.B., Karpati, G., Griggs, R. (eds). Myoblast Transfer Therapy. Plenum Publishing Corp. 267-272.

2. Nicholson, L.V.B., Johnson, M.A., Gardner-Medwin, D., Bhattacharya, S., Harris, J.B. (1990): Heterogeneity of dystrophin expression in patients with Duchenne and Becker muscular dystrophy. *Acta. Neuropathol. (Berl)*, 80:239-250.

3. Harris, J.B., Johnson M.A., Karlsson, E. (1975): Pathological responses of rat skeletal muscle to a single subcutaneous injection of a toxin from the venom of the Australian tiger snake, Notechis scutatus scutatus. *Clin. Exp. Pharm. Phys.,* 2:383-404.

4. Dykstra, M.J., Sharp, N.J.H., Bogan, D.J., Kornegay, J.N. (1990): Notexin-induced muscle injury in dogs. *J. Neurol. Sci. 98, (Suppl)* 127.

5. Sharp, N.J.H., Kornegay, J.N., Bartlett, R.J., Hung, W.Y., Dykstra, M.D.: Notexin-induced muscle injury in the dog. Submitted.

6. Weinstein, M.J., Pavletic M.M., Boudrieau, R.J., Engler, E.J. (1989): Cranial sartorius muscle flap in the dog. *Vet. Surg.,* 18:286-291.

7. Kuzon, W.M., Rosenblatt, J.D., Marchetti, P.J., Plyley, M.J., McKee, N.H. (1989): A comparative histochemical and morphometric study of canine skeletal muscle. *Can. J. Vet. Res.,* 53:125-132.

8. Gulati, A.K. (1987): The effect of X-irradiation on skeletal muscle regeneration in the adult rat. *J. Neurol. Sci.,* 78:111-120.

9. Alameddine, H.S., Dehaupas, M., Fardeau, M. (1989): Regeneration of skeletal muscle fibers from autologous satellite cells multiplied *in vitro*. An experimental model for testing cultured cell myogenicity. *Muscle and Nerve,* 12:544-555.

DISCUSSION

Professor Joe N. Kornegay:
The possibility that radiation might actually impede chimeric fiber formation is a question that has occurred to us, and we are currently doing comparative studies.

Assoc. Professor John K. McGeachie:
One thing I would like to add about markers. We are looking at Evan's blue dye in blood vessels. This has been used as a marker for fascular permeability for many years. When you look closely at the cells by EM, Evan's blue dye is very toxic to endothelial cells, as evidenced by significant changes in cytoplasmic elements, such as rough ER, mitochondria and vesicles.

Dr. Terence A. Partridge:
There is a very good marker of injection sites which we use. It is, if anything slightly antifibrotic, it marks the site well and persists through tissue processing. It is a dye used by tattooists to colour skin blue. It comes from Hoechst who sell it as dye for plastic. (C.I. Pigment Blue 15:3, known in tattooing circles as P.V. Fast Blue B2G Type 808).

DUCHENNE MUSCULAR DYSTROPHY: Animal Models
and Genetic Manipulation, edited by Byron A. Kakulas,
John McC. Howell, and Allen D. Roses.
Raven Press, Ltd., New York © 1992.

18

Production of Chimeric Animals Successes and Limitations

Anna E. Michalska

*The Murdoch Institute for Research into Birth Defects Limited,
10th Floor Royal Children's Hospital,
Flemington Road, Parkville, Victoria 3052, Australia*

The possibility of producing experimental mammalian chimaeras was first demonstrated by Tarkowski (33) and Mintz (21). In these experiments early preimplantation mouse embryos of different phenotypes were aggregated and the resulting mosaic blastocysts when reimplanted into recipient females gave rise to genetically mosaic mice. Subsequently, it was proven that embryo derived pluripotential cells such as teratocarcinoma cells (EC, ref. 22) and more recently, embryonic stem cells (ES, ref. 2) when introduced into blastocysts or aggregated with 4-8 cell embryos can take part in the formation of chimeric mice.

The ability to maintain EC and ES cell lines in culture (8, 19) provides the attractive possibility of introducing foreign DNA into cultured cells. This can be achieved by any of the somatic cell techniques and by selecting the cells for the desirable characteristics prior to manipulating them into embryos. It has been shown that EC cell lines, following their selection *in vitro*, can be used for introducing genes into germ-line of mice (31). These cells however, have been shown to accumulate chromosomal abnormalities during *in vitro* culture and have a low rate of colonisation of the embryo. EC cells also display a restricted pattern of differentiation and few germ lines of chimaeras are formed (38). By contrast, ES cells are genetically more stable in culture and, after introducing into a blastocyst, they participate in the formation of all tissues of the developing foetus, including the germ-line (2). Furthermore blastocysts injected with ES cells, which have been subjected to genetic manipulation, resulted in a high proportion of the produced mice being mosaic with up to one third germ-line chimaeras (10, 25).

The demonstration that homologous recombination between a native target chromosomal gene and exogenous DNA can be used in culture to modify specifically the target locus (29) opened up the possibility of making predetermined alterations in the mouse genome. This technology was applied in

ES cells for the first time in 1987, when it was shown that both gene correction (5) and gene inactivation (34) can be achieved. Soon after the experiments by Thompson *et al.* (36) demonstrated that ES cells targeted by homologous recombination can colonise host blastocysts and give rise to germ-line chimeric mice. To date, quite a number of genes have been modified by homologous recombination in ES cells and transmitted through the germ-line of chimeric mice. These mice should prove invaluable not only for the study of fundamental problems of gene function and gene regulation, but also as model systems for the investigation of early mammalian development and models for some of human inherited diseases.

This article briefly describes the technical aspects of ES cell culture and gene targeting as well as the production and applications of chimeric animals.

EMBRYONIC STEM CELLS (ES)

Embryonic stem cells are derived in culture directly from the inner cell mass (ICM) of a mouse blastocysts (8, 19). During normal development the ICM cells give rise to all tissues of the developing foetus. However, when the cells are first isolated they are still undifferentiated. To preserve this embryonic phenotype *in vitro* the ES cells are co-cultured on a layer of fibroblast cells or in medium conditioned by Buffalo rat liver (BRL) cells (28).

Recently, a factor called LIF (leukemia-inhibiting factor) has been isolated and it is now commercially available (Amrad P/L, Melbourne). It has been shown that the addition of LIF to culture media inhibits the differentiation of ES cells (39). The ability to grow the fully pluripotential ES cells *in vitro* permits their genetic manipulation. DNA can be introduced into the cells and these cells can be selected for the desired genotype. Since the cells multiply rapidly, enough material can be obtained for further analysis before cell cloning and production of chimaeras.

When the ES cells are injected into mouse blastocysts, they participate fully in normal development. By selecting distinguishable coat colour alleles of the donor ES cells and the host blastocysts, chimaeras can be easily identified by their mixture of differentially pigmented hair. Chimeric mice are bred and in the first generation of mice half of the ES-derived offspring will carry the introduced gene as heterozygotes. The interbreeding of heterozygous siblings yields homozygous animals which can then be tested for the effects of the gene alteration.

GENETIC MANIPULATION OF ES CELLS

At present, the main research interest of many laboratories centers on the possibility of performing homologous recombination experiments in ES cells as a means of producing transgenic mice with a desired phenotype. By this method, the genes can be either disrupted or corrected. However in mammalian cells homologous recombination between endogenous chromosomal allele and introduced gene construct is relatively rare. It is also obscured by random gene integration into the genome. When DNA is introduced into the cells, generally 1 in 10^3 cells will integrate the DNA randomly. Of the cells that have undergone the integration, only 1 in 10^3 cells will achieve the gene targeting by homologous recombination. Thus, in total only 1 in 10^6 cells will take up DNA by homologous recombination.

Given the relatively low frequency of homologous recombination, isolation of successfully targeted cell(s) would be almost impossible without a proper selection system. The very elegant and widely applied system has been developed in Capecchi's laboratory and is known as positive - negative selection (PNS, ref. 18). The PNS approach is based on a positive selection for homologous recombination events and a negative selection for random integration.

In this system, two selectable markers are introduced into the gene of interest. The *neo* (neomycin phosphotransferase) gene serves as a positive marker and is generally also introduced to disrupt the gene of interest. The *HSV-tk* (herpes simplex virus thimidine kinase) gene serves as a negative marker and is placed at the end of the homologous region. The *HSV-tk* gene will be retained during random integration but it will be lost during homologous recombination.

After introduction of the DNA into the ES cells by electroporation, the cells are selected in media supplemented with G418 and gancyclovir selection media. G418 is a neomycin analogue and gancyclovir is a nucleoside analogue that is cytotoxic to the cells containing viral thymidine kinase but is not toxic to the cells containing the mammalian enzyme. Thus, cells in which homologous recombination has occurred will express functional *neo* gene and will be resistant to G418. The retaining of the *HSV-tk* gene during random integration will make the cells sensitive to gancyclovir. The use of this approach can provide up to 2000-fold enrichment for the cells that have undergone homologous recombination (18).

APPLICATION OF CHIMERIC MICE

A number of genes have been targeted in ES cells by homologous recombination and numerous chimeric mice have been produced from such ES cells. Mice carrying alterations in specific genes now provide a tool for the study of the expression of these genes and their potential role in development. Introduction of mutations in ES cells has also been exploited for the generation of mouse models for human inherited diseases.

Homeobox genes

Several mouse homeobox gene families related to Drosophila developmental control genes have been cloned and structurally analysed. It has been proposed that, like in Drosophila, these genes are involved in the specification of positional information during embryogenesis. So far three homeobox genes: *Hox 1.1* (42), *Hox 1.3* (17), *en-2* (13) have been targeted and disrupted in ES cells. In experiments involving all three genes chimaeras have been produced and are now being bred to produce heterozygote and homozygote mice. Studying the effect of mutations in these homeobox genes will help to elucidate their involvement in the control of development.

Proto-oncogenes

Another group of genes targeted in ES cells are proto-oncogenes. It is assumed that they play a role in growth, and possibly development, of the embryo. However, details of the expression of these genes are so scant that only mutations made in these genes which result in loss of their functions might help to elucidate their role.

Examples of that have so far been targeted are: *int-1* (20, 35), *c-abl* (26, 37), *c-fos* (12), *N-myc* (3). In experiments with *int-1* and *c-abl* genes germ-line chimaeras were produced and the analysis of transgenic offspring has revealed important properties of these two proto-oncogenes (20, 26, 35, 37). These are briefly summarised below.

int-1 gene

It has been postulated that the *int-1* proto-oncogene plays a role in spermatogenesis and in the development of the central nervous system (27). Mice homozygous for the null mutation exhibit a range of phenotypes from death before birth to survival with severe ataxia. Examination of these mice at various stages of embryogenesis revealed severe abnormalities in the development of the mesencephalon and metencephalon indicating a prominent role of the *int-1* in the determination and/or subsequent development of a specific region of the central nervous system (20, 35).

c-abl gene

This gene encodes for a tyrosine kinase enzyme which is expressed ubiquitously in all mammalian tissues and cell types examined (24). In spite of the wealth of information about the biochemical properties of activated forms of *c-abl*, its normal function remains unclear.

Mice homozygous for *c-abl* mutation are severely affected, displaying increased perinatal mortality, runtedness, abnormal head and eye development and thymic and splenic atrophy. In addition, many of these mice showed specific defects in lymphocyte development (26, 37).

IGF II gene

It has been postulated for a long time that *IGF II* might play a role in the growth of the foetus, but direct evidence was lacking until chimeric mice carrying mutated *IGF II* gene were produced (4). Interestingly, the effect of the inactivation of this gene was observed in heterozygous mice which were about 50% smaller than their wild-type littermates. These growth deficient animals were otherwise normal and fertile. The effect of the mutation was exerted during the embryonic period. These results provide the first direct evidence for a physiological role of *IGF II* in embryonic growth.

HPRT gene

The inherited deficiency in the level of hypoxanthine phosphorybosil transferase causes the Lesch-Nyhan syndrome in males (32). It is a rare neurological and behavioral disorder which is characterised by mental retardation and self-mutilation. To derive an animal model for Lesch-Nyhan syndrome, HPRT gene has been mutated in ES cells and mice carrying *HPRT* null mutation were produced (6, 11, 16, 34). However, these *HPRT* deficient mice were phenotypically normal and showed no behavioral abnormalities. This has been explained by differences in purine related intermediary metabolism between mice and humans (1).

This example raises a concern that genetically engineered mice may not always provide a useful model for at least some of the human inherited diseases.

For this purpose, it may be more useful to establish the ES from species other than mouse. So far ES cells have been isolated and established from hamsters (7). In several cases, hamsters are more suitable than mice. Because of certain metabolic analogies between hamsters and humans, this animal model may be more suitable than mice for the studying of lipid metabolism, atherogenesis and cardiovascular problems (7). Attempts have also been made to isolate ES cell lines from porcine (9, 23), bovine (9) and ovine embryos (23), although it is still unknown if these cells will participate in the formation of chimeric animals.

OTHER GENES

The technique of homologous recombination has been used to introduce mutations in *adipocyte P2* and *adipsin* genes (12). These results demonstrated the feasibility of targeting genes which are not expressed in ES cells in order to study their function at the later stages of mouse development.

Gene targeting has also been used to introduce specific point mutations into an endogenous RP II 215 (RNA polymerase II) gene of ES cells (30). Such subtle alterations, when introduced into coding and regulatory regions, will allow detailed study of gene structure and function.

Another example of gene alteration in ES cells is an inactivation of $ß_2$-microglobulin ($ß_2$-m) gene (15, 41). Studying the effects of the disruption of this gene in homozygous mice should allow better understanding of the function of $ß_2$-macroglobulin and $ß_2$-m dependent proteins during development (14, 40).

In our laboratory at the Murdoch Institute, we are interested in the function of two proteins: metallothionein (MT) and ceruloplasmin (CP). Possible functions of these proteins are homeostasis and detoxification of heavy metals, such as copper, zinc and cadmium. Despite the large body of work which has been done, the biological roles of these proteins still remain to be elucidated. There is no animal or human disease model available for a deficiency of these genes, so we have decided to disrupt these genes by homologous recombination in transgenic mice using the ES cell approach outlined above.

In designing the homologous recombination construct we used the positive-negative selection of Capecchi. Following introduction of our construct into ES cells by electroporation and their selection in G418 and gancyclovir media, we observed a much lower than expected enrichment for homologously targeted cells. On average the enrichment was between 2 to 10-fold instead of 100-1000 fold initially reported. Similar observations have been made by other researchers targeting different genes (20). At this stage we are not able to explain the discrepancy between our results and those reported by Cappecci's group.

In our gene targeting experiments we have encountered additional problems. Some of the targeted cells were spontaneously differentiating into endoderm-like cells or undergoing karyotypic changes (including chromosomal translocations and aneuploidy). The first problem has been overcome by substituting LIF-supplemented media with fibroblast feeder cells, while the second problem has been corrected by using wild-type ES cells of better quality for targeting experiments. We are currently testing the ability of the mutated ES cells to produce chimeric mice.

CONCLUSIONS

Production of chimeric animals by means of genetically modified ES cells certainly provides a unique tool for biological and medical research. In recent years the techniques for the production of ES cells-derived chimaeras, in mouse have been established in many laboratories. A number of genes have already been successfully targeted in the ES cells and transmitted through a germ-line in transgenic animals. Such transgenic animals should provide model systems for developmental and genetic studies, as well as for the study of some of the human inherited diseases.

However, there remain some limitations in the currently available techniques. The efficiency of gene targeting is variable and can be quite low for some genes despite the use of enrichment procedures. Increasing the understanding of the mechanisms involved in homologous recombination itself will certainly improve our ability to target a wider range of genes at a more predictable and satisfactory frequency. Although in general ES cells are pluripotent and karyotypically stable, when cloned and exposed to harsh selection conditions, they can loose their ability to form chimaeras. Thus, it is very important to grow these cells in optimal conditions, minimise handling time and stringently monitor the cells for any phenotypic and karyotypic changes. Lastly, limitations have also been imposed because only mouse ES cells derived chimaeras are available. Clearly, establishment of ES cells from other species would allow the choice of the most suitable experimental animal for any given problem. This will be achieved once more knowledge is gained about embryonic development and the requirements for *in vitro* culture of embryos and, when the appropriate conditions are developed for isolating pluripotent ES cells from other species.

ACKNOWLEDGEMENTS

The author wishes to thank Dr K.H. Choo and Dr W.P. Michalski for helpful comments during preparation of this manuscript.

REFERENCES

1. Ansell, J.D., Samuel, K., Whittingham, D.G., Patek, C.E., Hardy, K., Handyside, A.H., Jones, K.W., Miggleton-Harris, A.L., Taylor, A.H. Hooper, M.L. (1991): Hypoxanthine phosphoribosyl transferase deficiency, haematopoisis and fertility in the mouse. *Development*, 112:489-498.
2. Bradley, A., Evans, M., Kaufman, M.H. Robertson, E. (1984): Formation of germ-line chimaeras from embryo-derived teratocarcinoma cell lines. *Nature*, 309:255-256.
3. Charon, J., Mallyn, B.A., Robertson, E.J., Goff, S.P. Alt, F.W. (1990): High-frequency disruption of the N-myc gene in embryonic stem and pre-B cell lines by homologous recombination. *Mol. Cell Biol.*, 10:1799-1804.
4. DeChiara, T.M., Efstratiadis, A. Robertson, E.J. (1990): A growth-deficiency phenotype in heterozygous mice carrying an insulin-like growth factor II gene disrupted by gene targeting. *Nature,* 345:78-80.

5. Doetschman, T., Gregg, R.G., Medea, N., Hooper, M.L., Melton, D.W., Thompson, S. Smithies, O. (1987): Targeted correction of mutant HPRT gene in mouse embryonic stem cells. *Nature,* 330:576-578.
6. Doetschman, T., Maeda, N. and Smithies, O. (1988). Targeted mutation of the HPRT gene in mouse embryonic stem cells. *Proc. Natl. Acad. Sci. USA,* 85:8583-8587.
7. Deotschman, T., Williams, P. Maeda, N. (1988): Establishment of hamster blastocyst-derived embryonic stem (ES) cells. *Develop. Biol.,* 127:224-227.
8. Evans, M.J. and Kaufman, M.H. (1981). Establishment in culture of pluripotential cells from mouse embryos. *Nature,* 292: 154-156.
9. Evans, M.J., Notarianni, E., Laurie, S. Moor, R.M. (1990): Derivation and preliminary characterisation of pluripotent cell lines from porcine and bovine blastocysts. *Theriogenology,* 33:125-128.
10. Gossler, A., Doetschman, T., Korn, R., Serfling, E. Kemler, R. (1986): Transgenesis by means of blastocyst-derived embryonic stem cell lines. *Proc. Nat. Acad. Sci. USA,* 83:9065-9069.
11. Hooper, M., Hardy, K., Hanyside, A., Hunter, S. Monk, M. (1987): HPRT-deficient (Lesch-Nyhan) mouse embryos derived from germ-line colonization by cultured cells. *Nature,* 326:292-295.
12. Johnson, R.S., Sheng, M., Greenberg, M.E., Kolodner, R.D., Papaioannou, V.E. and Spiegelman, B.M. (1989). Targeting of nonexpressed genes in embryonic stem cells via homologous recombination. *Science,* 245: 1234-1236.
13. Joyner, A.L., Skarnes, W.C. and Rossant, J. (1989): Production of a mutation in mouse En-2 gene by homologous recombinations in embryonic stem cells. *Nature,* 338:153-156.
14. Koller, B.H., Marrack, P., Kappler, J.W. Smithies, O. (1990): Normal development of mice deficient in ß$_2$-m, MHC class I proteins, and CD8$^+$ T cells. *Science,* 248: 1227-1230.
15. Koller, B.H. Smithies, O. (1989): Inactivating the ß$_2$-microtubulin locus in mouse embryonic stem cells by homologous recombination. *Proc. Natl. Acad. Sci. USA,* 86:8932-8935.
16. Kuehn, M.R., Bradley, A. Robertson, E.J. and Evans, M.J. (1987). A potential animal model for Lesch-Nyhan syndrome through introduction of HPRT mutations into mice. *Nature,* 326: 295-298.
17. Le Mouellic, H., Lallemand, Y. Brûlet, P. (1990): Targeted replacement of the homeobox gene Hox 1.3 by the *Escherichia coli* Lac Z in mouse chimeric embryos. *Proc. Natl. Acad. Sci. USA,* 87:4712-4716.
18. Mansour, S.L., Thomas, K.R. Capecchi, M.R. (1988): Disruption of the proto-oncogene int-2 in mouse embryo-derived stem cells: a general strategy for targeting mutations to non-selectable genes. *Nature,* 336:348-352.
19. Martin, G.R. (1981). Isolation of pluripotent cell line from early mouse embryos cultured in medium conditioned by teratocarcinoma stem cells. *Proc. Natl. Acad. Sci. USA,* 78:6314-6317.
20. McMahon, A.P. Bradley, A. (1990): The Wnt-1 (Int-1) proto-oncogene is required for development of large region of mouse brain. *Cell,* 62:1073-1085.
21. Mintz, B. (1962): Formation of genotypically mosaic mouse embryo. *Am. Zool.,* 2:432 (Abstract).

22. Papaioannou, V.E., McBurney, M.E., Gardner, R.L. Evans,M.J. (1975): Fate of teratocarcinoma cells injected into early mouse embryos. *Nature*, 258:70-73.

23. Piedrahita, J.A., Anderson, G.B. BonDurant, R.M. (1990): On the isolation of embryonic stem cells: comparative behaviour of murine, porcine and ovine embryos. *Theriogenology,* 34:879-901.

24. Renshaw, M.W., Capozza, M.A. Wang, J.Y.J. (1988): Differential expression of type-specific c-abl mRNAs in mouse tissue and cell lines. *Mol. Cell Biol.,* 8:4547-4551.

25. Robertson, E., Bradley, A., Kuehn, M. Evans, M. (1986): Germ-line transmission of gene introduced into cultured pluripotential cells by retroviral vectors. *Nature,* 323:445-448.

26. Schwartzberg, P.L., Stall, A.M., Hardin, J.D., Bowdish, K.S., Humaran, T., Boast, S., Harbison, M.L., Robertson, E.J. Goff, S.P. (1991). Mice homozygous for the abl^{m1} mutation show poor viability and depletion of selected B and T cell population. *Cell*, 65:1165-1175.

27. Shackleford, G.H. Varmus, H.E. (1987): Expression of the proto-oncogene int-1 is restricted to postmeiotic germ cells and the neural tube of mid-gestation embryos. *Cell*, 50:89-95.

28. Smith, A.G. Hooper, M.L. (1987): Buffalo rat liver cells produce a diffusible activity which inhibits the differentiation of murine embryonal carcinoma and embryonic stem cells. *Develop. Biol.,* 121:1-9.

29. Smithies, O., Gregg, R.G., Boggs, S.S., Kovalewski, M.A. Kucherlapati, R.S. (1985). Insertion of DNA sequences into the human chromosomal ß-globin locus by homologous recombination. *Nature*, 317:230-234.

30. Steeg, C.M., Ellis, J. and Bernstein, A. (1990). Introduction of specific point mutations into RNA polymerase II by gene targeting in mouse embryonic stem cells: evidence for DNA mismatch repair mechanism. *Proc. Natl. Acad. Sci. USA*, 87:4680-4684.

31. Stewart, C.L., Vanek, M. Wagner, E.F. (1985): Expression of foreign genes from retroviral vectors in mouse teratocarcinoma chimaeras. *EMBO J.*, 4:3701-3709.

32. Stout, J.T. Caskey, C.T. (1989): Hypoxanthine phosphoribosyl transferase deficiency: the Lesch-Nyhan syndrome and gouty arthritis. In: The metabolic basis of inherited disease (ed. C.R. Scriver, A.L. Beaudet, W.S. Sly and D. Valle) 6th ed. Vol. 1. pp. 1007-1028. New York: McGraw-Hill.

33. Tarkowski, A.K. (1961): Mouse chimaeras developed from fused eggs. *Nature,* 190:857-860.

34. Thomas, K.R. Cappecchi, M.R. (1987): Site-directed mutagenesis by gene targeting in mouse embryo-derived stem cells. *Cell*, 51:503-512.

35. Thomas, K.R. Capecchi, M.R. (1990): Targeted disruption of the murine int-1 proto-oncogene resulting in severe abnormalities in midbrain and cerebellar development. *Nature*, 346:847-850.

36. Thompson, S., Clarke, A.R., Pow, A.M., Hooper, M.L. Melton, D.W. (1989): Germ-line transmission and expression of a corrected HPRT gene produced by gene targeting in embryonic stem cells. *Cell*, 56:313-321.

37. Tybulewicz, V.L.J., Crawford, C.E., Jackson, P.K., Bronson, R.T. Mulligan, R.C. (1991). Neonatal lethality and lymphopenia in mice with a homozygous disruption of the c-abl proto-oncogene. *Cell* 65: 1153-1163.

38. Wagner, E.F., Veller, G., Gilbua, E., Ruther, U. Stewart, C.L. (1985): Gene transfer into murine stem cells and mice using retroviral vectors. *Cold Spring Harb. Symp.*, 50:691-700.

39. Williams, R.L., Hilton, D.J., Pease, S., Wilson, T.A., Stewart, C.L., Gearing, D.P., Wagner, E.F., Metcalf, D., Nicola, N.A. Gough, N.M. (1988): Myeloid leukemia inhibitory factor maintains the developmental potential of embryonic stem cells. *Nature,* 336: 684-687.
40. Zijlstra, M., Bix, M. Simister, N.E., Loring, J.M., Raulet, D.H. and Jaenisch, R. (1990): .ß2-microglobulin deficient mice lack CD4⁻8⁺ cytolytic T cells. *Nature,* 344: 742-746.
41. Zijlstra, M., Li, E., Dajjadi, F., Subramani, S. Jaenisch, R. (1989): Germ-line transmission of a disrupted ß2-microtubulin gene produced by homologous recombination in embryonic stem cells. *Nature,* 342:435-438.
42. Zimmer, A., Gruss, P. (1989): Production of chimaeric mice containing embryonic stem (ES) cells carrying a homeobox Hox 1.1 allele mutated by homologous recombination. *Nature,* 338:150-153.

DISCUSSION

Dr. Manfred W. Beilharz:
There are a few questions I wish to ask. This was a good oversight of the area. One of the limitations of this technology, is that your targeting efficiency is very poor and you can only hit a single allele of one gene. There is also the situation which is present in many diseases where there is more than one locus involved. I know Ashley Dunne's Group at the Ludwig just down the road from you are looking at multiple targeting of the stem cells; so I wanted to ask you if you know any progress being made in the areas of improving the hit rate and multiple targeting.

Dr. Anna E. Michalska:
I do not know of any report where more than one gene has been targeted in a single targeting event. The present strategy for multiple gene targeting is to target one gene (or locus) to prove that the ES cells are germ-line competent and then to use these cells in the second targeting experiment. As far as I know this approach has been used in Ashley Dunn's laboratory to inactivate both alleles of a TGFb gene.

Dr. Manfred W. Beilharz:
But then you are facing the problem of keeping them in culture for longer periods and compromising pluripotency?

Dr. Anna E. Michalska:
Yes.

Dr. Manfred W. Beilharz:
One of the recent papers which has been published is the successful breeding of a mouse in which they disrupted the microglobulin gene and then bred for homozygosity. As I recall the immunologists made predictions as to the consequences of not expressing microglobulin in the mouse, in fact it was said that mice wouldn't even get through the embryo stage. Last I heard the mice not only got through the embryonic stage but they breed and are apparently quite normal. Do you have any more information on further experiments which have been carried out similar to this?

Dr. Anna E. Michalska:
As you said, mice homozygous for the disrupted β2-microglobulin gene develop normally, although they show gross deficiency in the major histocompatibility complex (MHC) class I proteins and are lacking the cytotoxic T cells (CD4-8+ T cells). These animals when kept under pathogen-free conditions are healthy and fertile. It cetainly would be very interesting to study them after exposure to infectious agents or carcinogens.

Dr. Manfred W. Beilharz:
So they have not been subjected to viral challenges?

Dr. Anna E. Michalska:
I understand that these experiments are now in progress.

DUCHENNE MUSCULAR DYSTROPHY: Animal Models and Genetic Manipulation, edited by Byron A. Kakulas, John McC. Howell, and Allen D. Roses. Raven Press, Ltd., New York © 1992.

19

Approaches to the Introduction of Normal Alleles into Skeletal Muscle Fibers for Therapeutic Purposes in Duchenne Muscular Dystrophy

George Karpati

*Isaac Walton Killam Chair of Neurology,
Neuromuscular Research Group, Montreal Neurological Institute,
Montreal, Quebec, Canada.*

INTRODUCTION

Therapeutic approaches to diseases caused by single gene mutations may be divided into 3 general categories (Fig. 1).

1. Modification of certain biological characteristics of the relevant cell types and/or the body in order to mitigate or negate the deleterious effects of the absence or a defect of a particular protein produced by mutation of the gene that codes for it.

2. Supplying the relevant cells with the normal protein which is either missing or defective because of a mutation of the gene that codes for that protein. This approach would only be therapeutic if the introduced protein could perform all or most of its expected physiological role(s).

3. Introduction of the normal alleles of the gene which suffered the mutation into relevant cell types. The introduced normal gene, if properly expressed, would negate the deleterious effects of the native defective allele upon the cells and tissues in which it is expressed and has a major physiological role.

223

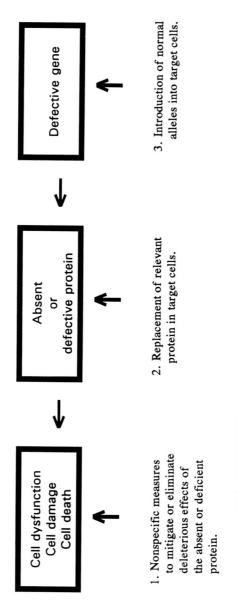

MAJOR TREATMENT STRATEGIES IN INHERITED DISEASES

FIG. 1.   Major treatment strategies in genetically determined diseases.

The foregoing principles may be applied to Duchenne muscular dystrophy (DMD) which is caused by a deficiency of a large sarcolemmal cytoskeletal protein, dystrophin, due to various mutations of a 2.5 kb gene at the Xp.21 locus of the X-chromosome (1,2).

1. Modification of certain aspects of the biology of the organism and/or skeletal muscle cells can be achieved by the administration of glucocorticoids which have proven beneficial effects on DMD without restoring dystrophin in muscle fibers (3,4). The mechanism(s) by which glucocorticoids achieve this effect is still unknown. This approach to the therapy of DMD is less than ideal because of significant side-effects of long-term glucocorticoid administration and because of a probable temporary nature of the beneficial effect.

Another possible therapeutic approach in this category includes an upregulation of certain autosomally coded dystrophin analogue(s) (5,6,7), that may be able to compensate, at least partially, for the dystrophin deficiency. In fact, glucocorticoids may exert their beneficial effect on DMD, at least in part, by such mechanism.

2. Replacement of dystrophin to skeletal muscle fibers by direct administration is not likely to be therapeutically effective. Dystrophin is a large rod-shaped cytoskeletal protein that is believed to form an hexagonal lattice on the cytoplasmic aspect of the plasmalemma of muscle fibers (8,9). In other words, it is a complex structural molecule which probably interacts with other molecules in the cytoplasm (10), and plasmalemma (11), and, as a protein, it has a still unknown turnover rate. Thus, its functional replacement into skeletal muscle fibers by any conceivable route or frequency of administration is likely to fail, even if the production of large amounts of pure dystrophin were attainable.

3. In the light of the above considerations the most promising approach to DMD therapy appears to be the introduction of normal alleles into skeletal muscle fibers that could code for a functionally normal or, at least, an adequate dystrophin. This goal may be attained by 3 possible methods:

A.   Heterologous myoblast transfer (HMT).
B.   Gene therapy.
C.   Autologous myoblast transfer (AMT).

3A. HETEROLOGOUS MYOBLAST TRANSFER (HMT)
(i)   General considerations:

In this technique normal myoblasts derived from satellite cells of a donor are injected into DMD muscles; the injected myoblasts carry the normal dystrophin genes (along with their entire genome) into the DMD host fibers by fusing with them (12,13,14).

Certain distinctive characteristics of skeletal muscle fibers make myoblast transfer possible: a) Multinucleation and large size, b) existence of satellite cells (in association with muscle fibers) which can give rise to a multitude of myogenic mononuclear cells (myoblasts) *in-vitro.* c) Myoblasts under special circumstances can fuse with either each other or with myotubes or with muscle fibers. This creates the possibility that a single muscle fiber may end up with myonuclei of different genotypes (mosaic muscle fibers). When a suspension of normal, viable and fusion- competent myoblasts are injected into a dystrophin-deficient muscle, some of the injected myoblasts will fuse with host muscle cells creating mosaic myofibers. Before such an occurrence, the injected myoblasts may divide once or more. Other myoblasts will probably nonspecifically disintegrate which could evoke an antibody response to various molecules of muscle cells. Other myoblasts may fuse only partially into the host fibers and remain in the satellite position. It is likely that some of the injected myoblasts will fuse with each other. This can be enhanced if the host muscle had received a large dose of ionizing radiation prior to transfer which inactivated the native dystrophin- incompetent satellite cells (12). If the transferred myoblasts are not fully histocompatible with the donor, the myoblasts could be destroyed by immunorejection unless the recipient is sufficiently immunosuppressed. Of the various fates that can befall on the injected myoblasts, from the point of view of efficient myoblast transfer, mosaic muscle fiber formation would be the most desirable outcome.

The most advantageous circumstances that would favor the formation of large numbers of mosaic fibers, containing myonuclei with normal dystrophin gene after HMT, would be that a large number of the viable, fusion-competent and histocompatible myoblasts are deposited in the close proximity of muscle fibers that are in a very early phase of regeneration after having suffered a cycle of segmental necrosis. In this situation, the injected myoblasts could fuse with the host's activated myoblasts in the regenerated segments forming mosaic fibers [In case the native satellite cells are inactivated by prior high-dose ionizing radiation (which can only be contemplated in animal experiments), the regenerated segments of muscle fibers will contain mainly donor, dystrophin-competent myonuclei].

Two additional critical factors must be taken into consideration for the optimization of HMT. Firstly, since the longitudinal cytoplasmic domain of dystrophin appears to be relatively restricted (15), a large number of dystrophin-competent myonuclei must be present in the mosaicized host fibers to generate enough dystrophin to cover a large portion of the inner aspect of the sarcolemma. Furthermore, the dystrophin-competent myonuclei should be well dispersed to avoid large dystrophin-negative patches of the surface membrane. Secondly, myoblasts must traverse the basal lamina of regenerating fibers segments to be in a position to participate in the regeneration and the formation of mosaic fibers. The basal lamina may be compared to a burlap in which there are two major overlapping filamentous networks. The two principal molecules making up these networks are collagen IV and laminin (16). Other components of the basal lamina include fibronectin, proteoglycans, glycoproteins and entactin (17). Some of these molecules ensure that the collagen IV and laminin "backbone" of the basal lamina is linked to the plasma membrane on one side and the extracellular matrix on the other. It has been estimated that the physical pore size of the basal lamina is approximately 40 nm (16) which could represent a considerable impediment to the transit of cells like myoblasts, notwithstanding the fact thatsome migration of myoblasts across the basal almina of muscle fibers has ben demonstrated in developing muscles (17a). Some changes occurring in the chemical composition of the basal lamina during necrosis and regeneration (18) are not expected to alter this pore size, although they may allow transit of macrophages that is very active during the phagocytic phase of necrosis.

3A. (ii) Heterologous myoblast transfer in mdx mice:

The discovery of dystrophin deficiency in mdx mice (19), prompted investigators to use this animal model to test some of the described principles of HMT. Partridge and co-workers (20) reported the conversion of some dystrophin-negative muscle fibers in immune-deficient mdx mice by the injection of normal murine myoblasts. Karpati and co-workers (15) reported similar results by the injection of cloned human myoblasts into nonimmunosuppressed mdx muscles. The number of dystrophin-positive fibers after these procedures were variable and ranged from 5-30% of all fibers. The dystrophin-negative to dystrophin-positive conversion rate was substantially increased by either the creation of an artificial necrosis or by prior X-irradiation of the recipient muscle (21).

More recently we have developed a technique by which a maximum number of dystrophin-positive fibers can be created in mdx muscles by HMT. In order to attain a **spatial coincidence** of all the previously cited desirable circumstances for a maximal number of dystrophin-positive fiber formation, we have added to the injectable myoblast suspension (20 μl medium containing 25,000 myoblasts) Marcaine and collagenase and made multifocal injections to anterior tibialis muscles of mdx mice (Fig. 2). The Marcaine whose concentration in the injectate was adjusted to be 0.75% assured that massive necrosis and rapid regeneration will occur in the **same exact pockets** where the myoblasts were deposited. This is important since mobility of the injected myoblasts in the host muscles is quite limited. Collagenase in the injectate was designed to fenestrate the basal lamina by dissolving one of the key elements of that membrane. This fenestration is expected to facilitate the passage of myoblasts into the regenerating fiber segments. Plasmin-activated collagenase IV seems to be the ideal agent for this purpose (Dr. Paul Holland, personal communication). However, we attained a similar result with clostridial collagenase I at very low concentration in the injectate. Collagenase I may have also helped the dissemination of myoblasts, since it also removes interstitial collagen I. Neither Marcaine nor low concentration of collagenase seem to have an appreciable deleterious effects on myoblasts.

This approach, although it may appear radical at first glance, may be employed to upgrade the efficiency of human myoblast transfer **(vide-infra)**.

3A. (iii) HMT in DMD patients:

Encouraged by early promising results of HMT in mdx mice, in 1990 we have assembled a multidisciplinary team of 12 scientists and physicians for an experimental one-muscle pilot study of HMT in 8 selected Duchenne boys. We have set out to determine the feasibility and safety of the procedure and to gain some idea concerning its therapeutic effectiveness. Approximately 55 million myoblasts (derived from haplotypically HLA-matched fathers' biopsies and purified by fluorescent-activated cell sorting, using an anti-N-CAM antibody), were injected through 55 perpendicular tracks into one biceps of each patient. The other biceps was injected with buffer as control. The patients, parents, injector and evaluators were blinded as to the experimental and control sides. The patients were immunosuppressed with cyclophosphamide for either 6 or 12 months. During the experimental period of one year, maximum voluntary force generation of each biceps was measured regularly and dystrophin content of the muscle was examined by microscopic immunocytochemistry and by Western blot analysis in 2 different biopsies taken at 8 - 12 weeks and 12 months post-HMT. Of the 5 patients who completed the one year experimental period and in whom the code has been broken, one patient showed significantly better and one borderline better force generation in the injected biceps compared to the control biceps. A significant amount of dystrophin was not present only in the injected side at one year in any of the 5 patients, although in the 10 week biopsy, one patient showed about 5% of normal dystrophin on the injected side and at one

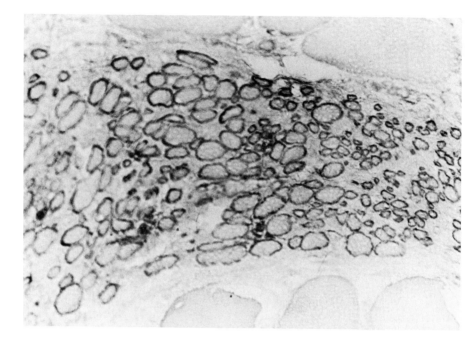

FIG. 2A. A large cluster of small- and medium-caliber dystrophin-positive regenerating muscle fibers are shown in the tibialis anterior muscle of an mdx mouse which received 20 Gray of gamma radiation 2 weeks prior to the experiment. This muscle was injected 8 days prior to obtaining this specimen at 3-5 sites with normal cultured mouse myoblasts in growth medium that also contained 0.75% bupivacaine and 0.05% collagenase. The area shown in this picture represents one such injection site where approximately 10 µl of injectate containing about 25,000 myoblasts was deposited. Since this was a previously gamma-irradiated muscle that inactivated most endogenous satellite cells, most of the dystrophin-positive regenerating fibers must have arisen by fusion of the donor myoblasts with each other within the old basal laminar tubes. Dystrophin was demonstrated with a polyclonal C-terminus antibody and the streptavidin-peroxidase technique. The section was faintly counterstained with eosin, X500.

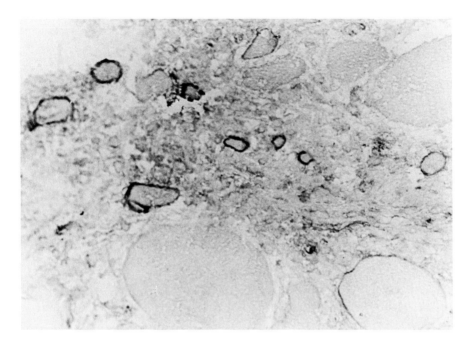

FIG. 2B. Another tibialis anterior muscle of an mdx muscle which was treated
in the same manner as described for panel (a) but the injectate did not
contain collagenase. The number of dystrophin-positive regenerating
fibers is much fewer, X500.

year another patient showed approximately 2% dystrophin in both biceps.

These preliminary findings indicate that HMT in DMD is feasible and relatively safe, but in its present form it is not (yet) sufficiently effective to consider it appropriate as a therapeutic measure.

Further studies are planned to modify the procedure along the lines described for the latest experimental HMT procedure in mdx mice that produced very encouraging results (see Fig. 2).

3B. GENE THERAPY

With the advent of modern molecular biology, it is possible to construct artificial genes and introduce them into living cells in the living organism. In DMD and mdx mice, the knowledge of the base sequence of most of the 75 exons and the muscle-specific promoter (22) permits the generation of either full length or partial cDNA. Even the cloning of the entire 2.5 megabase dystrophin gene in yeast artificial chromosomes (YAC) is close to completion (23).

In considering gene therapy, several important items require careful attention:

(1.)   What form of the gene to introduce?
(2.)   What promoter to use?
(3.)   Methods of targeting.
(4.)   What technique of introduction or dissemination to employ?
(5.)   Is integration of the introduced gene into the host genome necessary?

3B. (1.) What forms of gene to introduce?

The ideal choice is the entire dystrophin gene with its natural muscle-specific promoter. This way, some putative regulatory elements that could be residing in introns would also be present in the gene construct. However, the dystrophin gene's very large size makes such a goal rather difficult but not necessarily unattainable (23). An alternate possibility is to use the dystrophin cDNA which contains the entire coding sequence of the gene. Dystrophin cDNA is approximately 13.9 kb size and its efficient and mass cloning is within the present realm of feasibility (24). Full length murine dystrophin cDNA has, in fact, been successfully introduced into cultured cells (cos cells that normally do not express dystrophin) and this led to the expression of dystrophin in these cells (24). Alternatively, a construct containing only a part of the dystrophin cDNA ("minigene") may be chosen for gene therapy (22). The advantage of this approach is that by reducing the DNA size, the cloning efficiency can be considerably increased. The major drawback of the "minigene" approach is that a knowledge of the functionally indispensable domains of dystrophin and the corresponding coding sequence of the gene must be known if a significant therapeutic effect is to be expected. Since the precise functional role of the various domains of the dystrophin molecule is still not precisely known, such an approach to a functionally adequate "minigene" construction is difficult. A possible clue, in that respect, was the finding of a patient in whom a severely truncated dystrophin molecule, missing a large portion of the rod domain, permitted a relatively normal functioning of most skeletal muscles (25). Using such an artificial construct in preliminary direct gene transfer experiments (vide infra) in mdx mice is underway.

3B. (2.) What promoter to use?

The use of the natural promoter of the muscle-specific dystrophin gene assures that expression of the gene construct will only occur in skeletal muscle fibers. This could be an important point if the gene constructs are disseminated and become expressed in non-muscle cells, and if in some of these cells dystrophin could prove to be toxic. Other muscle-specific promoters, such as the one of the MM creatine kinase gene would also serve this purpose. Alternatively, constitutive (viral) promoters could be used which would probably be more efficient than the natural promoter but the expression of dystrophin constructs driven by such promoters would not be muscle-specific. It is possible to combine 2 promoters, i.e. use the muscle-specific dystrophin promoter, as well as a constitutive promoter to combine the advantages of both.

3B. (3.) Methods of targeting:

The ultimate aim of gene therapy is to land at least one copy of a functionally adequate dystrophin gene construct in as many myonuclei in as many muscle fibers as possible. Artificial genes must end up in nuclei to be transcribed by the RNA-polymerase. In order for a dystrophin gene construct, that are already in the interstitial space of skeletal muscles to reach the myonuclei it has to traverse the following potential barriers: a) basal lamina b) plasma membrane and c) the nuclear membrane.

Specific targeting of gene constructs can be achieved by linking them to another molecule which can be preferentially taken up by skeletal muscle cells. The most popular targeting molecules are replication defective viruses (26,27). In skeletal muscles adenoviruses have been used for this purpose and *in-vitro*, they considerably enhance the transfection of artificial genes into cultured myoblasts (27). However, most viral receptors on the muscle fiber surface appear to be scanty or absent and thus, *in-vivo* one must create abundant regeneration in order to contemplate this type of viral targeting of the dystrophin gene. Non-specific targeting of cells may be achieved by absorbing the gene construct to polycations (28) or loading the genes in microprojectile or *in-vivo* electroporation (29). Recently, Wolff et al. (30) reported the uptake and expression of bacterial genes in plasmids ("naked DNA") by some skeletal muscle fibers of mice after intramuscular injection of large amounts of DNA. This approach has been called direct gene transfer. While the simplicity of this technique is very attractive, its efficiency presently is extremely low considering the relatively few muscle fibers that show gene expression in relation to the amount of gene DNA that had been injected. Using a lac-Z gene coding for the bacterial β-galactosidase, we have been able to reproduce the results of Wolff et al. (30) in various muscles of mice and rats (Fig. 3). It is likely, that similar results can be obtained by using a full or partial dystrophin cDNA in mdx mice. However, the expected extremely low efficiency of dystrophin gene transfer by this method precludes its therapeutic use, even if the longevity of the artificial gene expression is favorable. We must first determine that the injected gene constructs are not rapidly degraded in the interstitial space before they had a chance to enter muscle fibers. If that is not the problem, we must assume that during direct gene transfer, that the supercoiled plasmids (containing the dystrophin construct) encounter considerable difficulty in negotiating the basal lamina in which the estimated pore size is 40 nm. We presume that relatively few copies of plasmids get through the basal lamina and are subsequently taken up into the cell across the plasma membrane by bulk endocytosis. It is not known how active bulk endocytosis is in DMD muscles. Of the relatively few plasmids, containing the construct, that eventually reach the

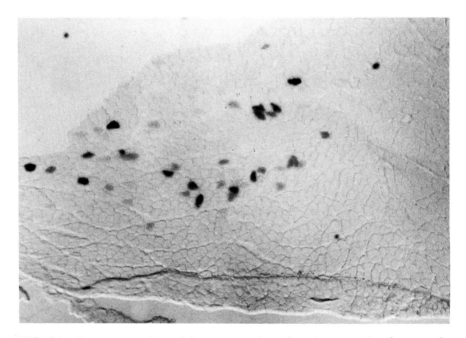

FIG. 3A. Low power view of the cross-section of a soleus muscle of a normal mouse into which a bacterial lac-Z gene construct was injected with a 25 gauge needle 7 days before (100 μl sucrose containing 100 mg DNA). Along the track of the injection many β-galactosidase-positive fibers are present. The staining ranges from very weak to very strong, presumably reflecting the number of lac-Z gene copies that were taken up by these muscle fiber segments, and became expressed. The β-galacto-sidase activity was developed by Bluo-gal staining technique (Bethesda Research Laboratories Life Technologies, Inc.), X80.

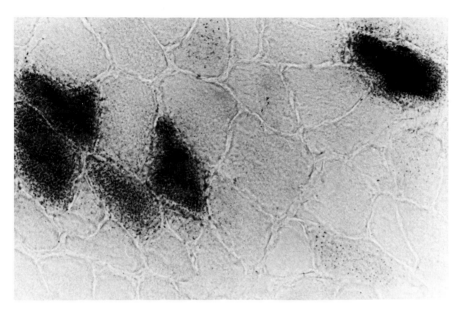

FIG. 3B. Higher power view of β-galactosidase-positive fibers from a muscle similar to the one described in panel 1, X500.

sarcoplasm, still fewer will randomly drift into the myonuclei through the nuclear pores. It appears that a major fenestration of the basal lamina and an enhancement of the bulk endocytosis may result in a sufficient upregulation of the efficiency of direct gene transfer. In such a case its use may be contemplated in the therapy of DMD in the not too distant future.

3B. (4.) Methods of introduction of gene constructs:

Direct gene transfer employs direct injection of the DNA into the muscle which is therapeutically cumbersome considering the large number of injectable muscles and the poor accessability of several important muscles (diaphragm, psoas, etc.). Intravascular dissemination would be a lot more efficient but it requires that whatever form of gene construct is used it must pass through the blood vessel walls. Vascular dissemination of gene constructs would be effective but would probably require the use of a muscle-specific promoter for reasons already discussed.

3B. (5.) Integration of the introduced gene constructs into the host genome:

In the direct gene transfer method employed by Wolff et al. (30) the bacterial genes appear to remain outside of the host genome ("episomal") and yet they remain transcriptionally active for at least 1 year. This suggests that for functional longevity of an introduced gene, integration into the host genome may not be essential. Furthermore, the skeletal myonuclei, being postmitotic, there is no chance of the introduced genes to be "diluted out" by repeated mitosis in skeletal muscle fibers. On the other hand, retroviral targeting could result in the integration of the introduced gene constructs into the host genome which, as discussed, may not be therapeutically essential. In fact, at least theoretically, it carries the danger of disrupting some tumor suppressor element which could result in cell transformation and possible tumor formation.

3C. Autologous myoblast transfer (AMT)

A combination of myoblast transfer and gene therapy can be achieved by obtaining myoblasts from a young DMD patient and transfecting these myoblasts with multiple copies of functional dystrophin gene constructs *in-vitro* and subsequently reinjecting them into the patients' muscles. The advantages of this approach include an elimination of the need for immunosuppression and the risk of immunorejection. Furthermore, multiple dystrophin genes in a myonucleus could augment the longitudinal cytoplasmic domain of dystrophin. The drawback of this approach is that myoblast transfer is still not an effective way of introducing normal genes into the host muscle fibers as discussed above. Furthermore, unless this procedure in done in very early DMD patients, in later years, many DMD satellite cells are close to senescence (31).

SUMMARY

Both HMT and direct gene transfer showed initial promise as a potential means of introducing functionally adequate genes into skeletal muscle fibers. Both procedures require major increases in efficiency before either of the two can be considered as a potential therapy in DMD and in other genetically determined muscle diseases. Only when this is achieved can one determine as to which of the two methods, (or perhaps also considering AMT) is more efficient, safer and has a better cost-benefit ratio.

ACKNOWLEDGEMENTS

Some of the myoblast transfer data briefly cited in this paper were generated by the collaborative efforts of the Myoblast Transfer Team, whose prinicipal investigators are: G. Ajdukovic, D. Arnold, R. Gledhill, R. Guttmann, P. Holland, G. Karpati, P. Koch, D. Spence, M. Vanasse, G. Watters and R. Worton. Drs. K. Hastings and E. Shoubridge prepared the lac-Z constructs to which reference has been made in relation to direct gene transfer.

This study was supported by the Muscular Dystrophy Associations of USA and Canada, and the Medical Research Council of Canada.

REFERENCES

1. Koenig, M., Hoffman, E.P., Bertelson, C.H., et al (1987): Complete cloning of Duchenne muscular dystrophy (DMD) cDNA and preliminary genomic organization of the DMD gene in normal and affected individuals. *Cell*, 50:509-517.
2. Hoffman, E.P., Brown, R.H. Jr., Kunkel L.M. (1987): Dystrophin: the protein product on the Duchenne muscular dystrophy locus. *Cell*, 51:919-928.
3. Mendell, J.R., Moxley, R.T., Griggs, R.C., et al (1989): Randomized double blind six months trial of prednisone in Duchenne's muscular dystrophy. *N. Eng. J. Med.*, 320:1592-1597.
4. Burrow, K.L., Coovert, D.D., Klein, C.J., et al (1991): Dystrophin expression and somatic reversion in prednisone-treated and untreated Duchenne dystrophy. *Neurology,* 41:661-666.
5. Love, D.R., Hill, D.F., Dickson, G., et al (1989): An autosomal transcript in skeletal muscle with homology to dystrophin. *Nature* 339:55-58.
6. Khurana, T.S., Hoffman, E.P., Kunkel, L.M. (1990): Identification of a chromosome 6-encoded dystrophin-related protein. *J. Biol. Chem.*, 265:16717-16720.
7. Pons, F., Augier, N., Leger, J.O.C., et al (1991): A homologue of dystrophin is expressed at the neuromuscular junctions of normal individuals and DMD patents, and of normal and mdx mice. *FEBS Letters,* 282:161-165.
8. Koenig, M., Monaco, A.B., Kunkel, L.M (1988): The complete sequence of dystrophin predicts a rod-shaped cytoskeletal protein. *Cell* 53:219-228.
9. Koenig, M., Kunkel, L.M. (1990): Detailed analysis of the repeat domain of dystrophin reveals four potential hinge segments. *J. Biol. Chem.*, 265:4560-4566.
10. Hammond, R.G., Jr. (1987): Protein sequence of DMD gene product is related to actin-binding domain of a-actinin. *Cell*, 51:1
11. Campbell, A.P., Kahl, S.D. (1989): Association of dystrophin and an integral membrane glycoprotein. *Nature*, 338:259-262.
12. Partridge, T.A. (1991): Invited Review: Myoblast Transfer: a possible therapy for inherited myopathies? *Muscle and Nerve,* 14:197-212.
13. Karpati, G. (1990): The principles and practice of myoblast transfer. *Adv. Exp. Med. Biol.*, 280:69-74.
14. Karpati, G: (1991) Myoblast transfer in Duchenne dystrophy: In Angelini, C., Danielli, G.A., and Fontanari, D. (eds) Muscular Dystrophy Research: From Molecular Diagnosis Toward Therapy. Excerpta Medica, Int. Congr.

Series 934, Amsterdam, pp 101-107.
15. Karpati, G., Pouliot, Y., Zubrzycka-Gaarn, E.E., et al (1989): Dystrophin is expressed in mdx skeletal muscle fibers after normal myoblast implantation. *Am. J. Pathol.*, 135:27-32.
16. Yurchenko, P.D. (1990): Assembly of basement membranes. *Ann. N.Y. Acad. Sci.*, 580:195-213.
17. Yurchenko, P., Schittny, J.C. (1990): Molecular architecture of basement membranes. *FASEB J.*, 4:1577-1590.
17a. Hughes, S.M., Blau, H.M. (1990): Migration of myoblasts across basal lamina during skeletal muscle development. *Nature*, 345:350-353.
18. Gulati, A.K., Reddi, A.H., Zalewski, A.A. (1983): Changes in the basement membrane components during skeletal muscle fiber degeneration and regeneration. *J. Cell Biol.*, 97:959-962.
19. Arahata, K., Ishiuwa, S., Ishiguro, T., et al (1988): Immunostaining of skeletal and cardiac muscle surface membrane with antibody against Duchenne muscular dystrophy peptide. *Nature,* 333:861-863.
20. Partridge, T.A., Morgan, J.E., Coulton, G.R., et al (1989): Conversion of mdx myofibers from dystrophin-negative to positive by injection of normal myoblasts. *Nature*, 337:176-179.
21. Morgan, J. (1990): Practical aspects of myoblast implantation: investigations on two inherited myopathies in animals. *Adv. Exp. Med. Biol.*, 280:89-96.
22. Ray, R.N., Klamut, H.J., Worton, R.G. (1990): The DMD gene promoter: A potential role in gene therapy. *Adv. Exp. Med. Biol.*, 280:107-112.
23. Monaco, A.P., Walker, A.P., Ishikawa-Brush, Y., et al (1991): Isolation of the complete human and mouse DMD gene in overlapping yeast artificial chromosomes. Presented at 4ieme Colloque National sur les Maladies Neuromusculaires, Montpellier, France.
24. Lee, C.C., Pearlman, J.A., Chamberlain, J.S., et al (1991): Expression of recombinant dystrophin and its localization to the cell membrane. *Nature,* 349:334-336.
25. England, S.B., Nicholson, L.V.B., Johnson, M.A., et al (1990): Very mild muscular dystrophy associated with the deletion of 46% of dystrophin. *Nature*, 343:180-182.
26. Price, J., Turner, D., Cepko, C. (1987): Lineage analysis of the vertebrate nervous system by retroviral-mediated gene transfer. *Proc. Natl. Acad. Sci.*, USA. 84:156-160.
27. Quantin, B., Stratford-Perricaudet, J-L., Mandel, J-L., et al (1991): Adenovirus as a vector for gene expression in muscle cells. In Angelini, C., Danielli, G.A., and Fontanari, D. (eds) Muscular Dystrophy Research: From Molecular Diagnosis Toward Therapy. Excerpta Medica, Int. Congr. Series 934, pp 157-162.
28. Kawai, S., Nishiwasa, M (1984): New procedure for DNA transfection with polycation and dimethylsulfoxide. *Mol. Cell Biol.*, 4:1172-1174.
29. Andreason, G.L., Evans, G.A. (1988): Introduction and expression of DNA into eukaryotic cells by electroporation. *Biotechniques*, 6:650-659.
30. Wolff, J.A., Malone, R.W., Williams, P., et al (1990): Direct gene transfer into muscle *in vivo*. Science, 247:1465-1468.
31. Blau, H.M., Webster, C., Pavlath, G. (1983): Defective myoblasts identified in Duchenne muscular dystrophy. *Proc. Natl. Acad. Sci. USA.,* 80:4856-4860.

DUCHENNE MUSCULAR DYSTROPHY: Animal Models and Genetic Manipulation, edited by Byron A. Kakulas, John McC. Howell, and Allen D. Roses.
Raven Press, Ltd., New York © 1992.

20

Skeletal Muscle Gene Control and Transgenic Mice

E. C. Hardeman, R. Arkell,
K. Brennan, S. Dunwoodie,V. Elsom*,
K. Esser*, M. Gordon, J. Joya, C. Shalhoub and C. Sutherland

Muscle Development Unit and Cell Biology Unit,
Children's Medical Research Foundation,
P. O. Box 61, Camperdown, NSW 2050, Australia

EVENTS DURING SKELETAL MYOGENESIS

Muscle development has been well characterized in a variety of species and myogenesis has successfully been observed *in vitro* in established cell lines and primary cultures. Skeletal myogenesis is characterized by the proliferation of mononucleated myoblasts which, as differentiation proceeds, withdraw from the cell cycle and fuse spontaneously to form multinucleated fibres. During avian and rodent development there are at least two distinct periods of myoblast fusion, termed primary and secondary fibre formation (13,18). Muscle maturation occurs immediately prior to and one week after birth following the onset of secondary fibre formation. During this time myofibres undergo significant biochemical and morphological changes (18). Mature motoneuron endplates are established and the sarcomeres come into register such that the distinct banding pattern which characterizes the adult myofibre is apparent (13). There are also marked transitions in the pattern of muscle gene expression (21).

Muscle Multigene Families

Concomitant with myoblast fusion is the expression of a variety of gene products characteristic of terminal skeletal muscle differentiation including the contractile proteins which comprise the sarcomere, acetylcholine receptors and key enzymes involved in the generation of energy for contraction, such as creatine kinase and glycogen phosphorylase. It is notable that most of the muscle gene products characteristic of terminal differentiation are members of multigene families (4,7). For example, multiple isoforms exist for each component of the thick and thin filaments of the sarcomere. Myosin heavy chain (MHC; isoforms include embryonic, perinatal, fast IIa, fast IIb, beta), alkali myosin light chain (MLC; 1 fast, 3 fast, 1 slow a, 1 slow b) and regulatory myosin light chain (2 fast, 2 slow, 2 nonmuscle) comprise the thick filaments. Sarcomeric actin (skeletal, cardiac), troponin C (Tn; fast, slow), troponin I (fast, slow), troponin T (fast, slow) and tropomyosin (Tm; beta, α-fast, α-slow) comprise the thin filaments.

Myoblast Predetermination
and the Emergence of the Adult Fibre Phenotype

Muscles are composed of three types of myofibres each of which is defined by the particular set of muscle contractile proteins utilised within the fibre. Myofibres are loosely characterised as to the relative rate of contraction and as such are designated fast, slow or of mixed composition, fast/slow. Within a given muscle type of an adult, the exact ratio of fast, slow and mixed fibres is determined (1,2). We examined the role of the myoblast and environmental stimuli in the determination of muscle fibre composition at the level of the expression of the contractile protein genes (21). Essentially, we wished to assess the relative contribution of muscle genetic and extracellular factors to myofibre determination. In order to undertake a comprehensive analysis of myofibre gene expression, we isolated cDNA probes which correspond to all members of the multigene families which encode the proteins of the contractile apparatus. We examined fast and slow contractile gene expression in RNA isolated from a detailed timecourse of rat hindlimb development.

If genetic programming of myoblasts plays a predominant role in the establishment of the composition of adult fibres, then this should be reflected in the coordinated expression of the fast and of the slow isoform genes as distinct subsets throughout fibre formation in the rat hindlimb. When plotted as a percent contribution of the total transcript output from the respective gene family with time during rat hindlimb development, all slow isoform graphs should be superimposable as would all fast isoform graphs. We found this not to be the case. Instead, each gene encoding a contractile protein is regulated independently throughout development and only in late skeletal muscle development, at the initation of the maturation period as defined by morphological changes, do we see the emergence of the adult pattern of contractile gene expression (FIG. 1). For example, in the two extreme cases, the MLC2 gene family contributes almost exclusively the fast isoform throughout hindlimb development. In contrast, the TnT gene family contributes the slow and/or cardiac isoforms exclusively until E18 when transcripts from the fast isoform gene are first observed. These results strongly suggest that a cue extrinsic to the muscle cells regulates the coordination of contractile protein gene expression at a time concomitant with the appearance of the mature sarcomere. This study points to this period of time as a critical decision-making stage in the contractile protein gene expression.

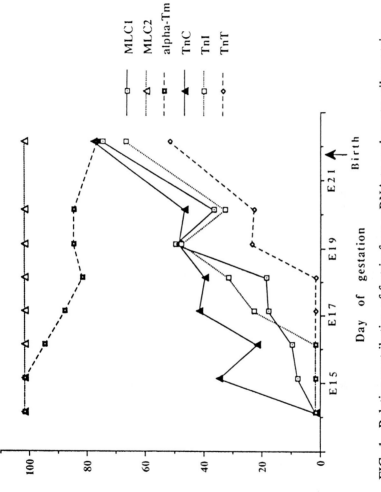

FIG. 1. Relative contribution of fast isoform mRNA to each contractile protein gene family in developing rat hindlimbs. Taken from Sutherland et al. (21).

MOLECULAR ANALYSIS OF SKELETAL MUSCLE MATURATION

Contractile Protein Gene Markers of Muscle Maturation

At different stages of skeletal muscle development, different combinations of contractile isoforms are expressed (4,16,20,22,26). For example, an 'embryonic' pattern of muscle gene expression is observed when skeletal muscle is composed exclusively of primary fibres. This period is characterized in part by the predominance of embryonic over perinatal myosin heavy chain (2.5 emb.:1 peri.) and cardiac over skeletal actin (19 c.:1 sk.). At the onset of maturation, transitions occur in MHC and sarcomeric actin isoform expression such that the ratio of embryonic to perinatal MHC is 1:5 and cardiac to skeletal actin is 1:2 (16,26). This trend continues until some time after birth at which time the 'adult' pattern of isoform expression is established (21). The adult MHC isoforms (IIa and IIb) replace both embryonic and perinatal; the ratio of cardiac to skeletal actin is 1:19. Indeed, a particular ratio of isoforms is accepted as a marker of a particular stage in skeletal muscle development.

Regulatory Elements in the Human Sarcomeric Actin Genes

In order to identify the regions of the human cardiac and skeletal actin genes which are necessary for their correct expression during skeletal muscle maturation, we introduced the constructs listed in FIG. 2 into the germlines of mice. Essentially, we found that the sequence necessary for the correct downregulation of the cardiac actin gene resided in the 3' flanking region. Expression of the transgene in lines carrying the #165BX construct failed to decrease in skeletal muscle from birth to the adult in contrast to the correct pattern of expression in lines containing constructs #165 and #174. The difference between these two lines of mice is a 1100bp fragment which is absent from the 3' portion of the gene in the #165BX construct. On the other hand, the expression of the human skeletal actin gene is regulated by the 5' portion of the gene during skeletal muscle maturation. The expression of the transgene in #480 mice increases appropriately during hindlimb development. Clearly, the regions of the two sarcomeric actin genes which respond to agents which bring about the mature striated muscle phenotype are located in different portions of the two genes. It remains to be determined whether or not these regulatory sequences in the two genes are related.

Autoregulation and the Expression of Multigene Families

There is a growing body of data which suggests that the total output from certain contractile protein multigene families is regulated both at the mRNA and protein levels. The evidence is most compelling for a number of multigene families which encode cytoarchitectural components (12). The observations imply that co-expressed isoforms from a given family "communicate" with one another to ensure that a constant contribution from the family is maintained within a cell. Perhaps this is not surprising if in mammals, as in the fly *Drosphila M.*, a strict ratio between the number of actin and MHC transcripts must be maintained in order to ensure the integrity of the sarcomere (5). In general, much of the

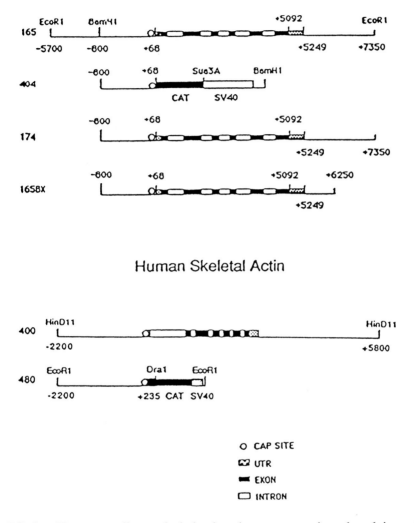

FIG. 2. Human cardiac and skeletal actin constructs introduced into the germline of mice. CAT denotes the coding region for the bacterial chloramphenicol acetyltransferase. SV40 designates the last intron, polyadenylation and termination signal from the SV40 early region.

supporting evidence for such a mechanism has been gleaned from reports for which the perturbation of isoform expression is coincidental to the main thrust of the studies. The body of data which supports such a mechanism can be grouped into three categories of observations.

First, muscle multigene families which undergo isoform switching or replacement during development exhibit a maximum level of transcript accumulation. This transcript ceiling is maintained during the transition periods such that mRNA levels of the isoforms involved display a reciprocal relationship. For example, using a MHC cDNA probe which recognizes all species of MHC transcripts, we have unambiguously demonstrated that both in cell culture and in human fetal and adult skeletal muscle the cumulative MHC transcript level remains constant (24). A similar observation was made with the sarcomeric actins (R. Arkell, unpublished observation).

Second, if the expression of one member of a multigene family is perturbed via a naturally-arising mutation or diseased state, then another isoform is called into play to compensate. The sarcomeric actins provide a good example in both instances. Garner et al. (9,10) observed that Balb/c mice carry a mutation in the cardiac actin locus which results in partial transcriptional suppression of the gene in the heart. In an apparent effort to compensate, cellular skeletal actin levels increase an order of magnitude. During cardiac hypertrophy in the rat many embryonic and perinatal muscle isoforms are re-expressed (3,6,14,15,19). Skeletal actin transcript levels, for example, increase approximately ten-fold, albeit transiently The most obvious explanation for the re-activation of transcription of early developmental isoforms is as follows. The demand for more contractile proteins due to increased cell size leads the cell to reactivate dormant genes presumably because the currently active genes are working at capacity.

Finally, in two cases where contractile protein genes have been introduced into the germline of mice, the transcriptionally active transgene has impacted upon the expression of the endogenous isoform. Shani et al. (20) reported that a transgenic mouse carrying the rat MLC2 gene expressed the transgene in a pattern reciprocal to that of the endogenous gene. Indeed, as development progressed, transcription from the transgene was dominant over that from the mouse gene, to the extent that a gene replacement of sorts was achieved. The introduction of a quail TnIfast gene into mice elicited a similar downregulation of the endogenous gene (12; H Bradshaw, P Hallauer and K. Hastings, personal communication).

Autoregulation and the Sarcomeric Actins

We have observed a similar phenomenon at the transcript level in our transgenic mouse lines carrying both the human cardiac and skeletal actin genes. In those lines in which the transgene is expressed at a level 50% or greater than that of the corresponding endogeneous mouse sarcomeric actin gene, a compensatory decrease in the transcript level of the corresponding mouse gene occurs. The observed decrease in the endogenous mouse cardiac actin in these transgenic lines is not due to the depletion of, or competition for transcription factors between the mouse sarcomeric actin and transgene promoter elements. If this were the case, then we would observe a correlation between the transgene copy number and the extent of downregulation of the endogenous mouse gene. Instead, we observe a strict correlation between the extent of expression of the transgene, which is irrespective of gene copy number, and a decline in the transcript level of the mouse gene.

CONCLUSIONS

Clearly, these findings argue for the existence of a cellular mechanism whereby the concentration of cytoskeletal mRNA/protein within a skeletal muscle cell is both finely sensed and tightly controlled. Although the results so far only speak to the fine control over the output from each isoform gene, it is conceivable that a similar type of mechanism which utilises autoregulation is in play to communicate levels of gene expression between members of a contractile protein multigene family. For example, at a particular time in development or in response to a physiological cue, there may be a demand for one isoform over the other(s) from a gene family. The subsequent increased expression of the desired isoform must be balanced with a compensatory decrease in the expression of the remaining isoforms. Since these gene families display a tight regulation on the output from each family and extensive changes in isoform expression during skeletal muscle maturation, it is possible that the mechanisms underlaying these two aspects of contractile gene regulation are the same. After all, the desired endpoint in both cases is the same, that the correct ratios of contractile proteins are expressed which meet the physiological demand on the muscle.

REFERENCES

1. Ariano, M.A., Armstrong, R.B., Edgerton, V.R. (1973): Hindlimb muscle fiber populations of five mammals. *J. Histochem. Cytochem.*, 21:51-55.
2. Armstrong, R.B. Phelps R.O. (1984): Muscle fiber type composition of the rat hindlimb. *Am. J. Anat.*, 171:259-272.
3. Bakerman, P.R., Stenmark, K.R. Fisher, J.H. (1990): α-Skeletal actin messenger RNA increases in acute ventricular hypertrophy. *Am. J. Physiol.,* 258:173-178.
4. Bandman, E. (1985): Myosin isoenzyme transitions in muscle development, maturation, and disease. *Int. Rev. Cytol.*, 97:97-131.
5. Beall, C.J., Sepanski, M.A. Fyrberg, E.A. (1989): Genetic dissection of Drosophila myofibril formation: effects of actin and myosin heavy chain null elleles. *Genes & Dev.*, 3:131-140.
6. Bishopric, N.B., Simpson, P.C. Ordahl, C.P. (1987): Induction of the skeletal α-actin in a α1-adrenoreceptor-mediated hypertrophy of rat cardiac myocytes. *J. Clin. Invest.*, 80:1194-1199.
7. Buckingham, M.E. Minty, A.J. (1983): In: *Eukaryotic Genes: Their Structure, Activity and Regulation.* edited by N. Maclean, S. P. Gregory and R. A. Flavell, pp. 365-395. Butterworth, London.
8. Bulinski, J.C., Kumar, S., Titani, K. Hauschka, S.D. (1983): Peptide antibody specific for the amino terminus of skeletal muscle α-actin. *Proc. Natl. Acad. Sci. USA*, 80:1506-1510.
9. Garner, I., Minty, A.J., Alonso, S., Barton, P.J. Buckingham, M.E. (1986): A 5' duplication of the α-cardiac actin gene in BALB/c mice is associated with abnormal levels of a-cardiac and α-skeletal mRNAs in adult cardiac tissue. *EMBO J.*, 5:2559-2567.
10. Garner, I., Sassoon, D., Vandekerckhove, J., Alonso, S. Buckingham, M.E. (1989): A developmental study of the abnormal expression of α-cardiac and α-skeletal actins in the striated muscle of a mutant mouse. *Dev. Biol.*, 134:236-245.
11. Gunning, P., Mohun, T., Ng, S.-Y., Ponte, P. Kedes, L. (1984): Evolution of the human sarcomeric-actin genes: evidence for units of

selection within the 3' untranslated regions of the mRNAs. *J. Mol. Evol.*, 20:202-214.

12. Hallauer, P.L., Hastings, K.E. Peterson, A.C. (1988): Fast skeletal muscle-specific expression of a quail troponin I gene in transgenic mice. *Mol. Cell. Biol.*, 8:5072-5079.

13. Harris, A.J. (1981): Embryonic growth and innervation of rat skeletal muscle. I. Neural regulation of muscle fibre numbers. *Phil. Trans. Roy. Soc.* Lond., B 293:257-277.

14. Hirzel, H.O., Tuchschmid, C.R., Schneider, J., Krayenbuehl, H.P. Schaub, M.C. (1985): Relationship between myosin isoenzyme composition, hemodynamics, and myocardial structure in various forms of human cardiac hypertrophy. *Circ. Res.*, 57:729-740.

15. Kennedy, J.M., Kamel, S., Tambone, W.W., Vrbova, G. Zak, R. (1986): The expression of myosin heavy chain isoforms in normal and hypertrophied chicken slow muscle. *J. Cell. Biol.*, 103:977-983.

16. Minty, A.J., Alonso, S., Caravatti, M. Buckingham, M. (1982): A fetal skeletal muscle actin mRNA in the mouse and its identity with cardiac actin mRNA. *Cell*, 30:185-192.

17. Ontell, M. Kozeka, K. (1984): The organogenesis of murine striated muscle: A cytoarchitectural study. *Am. J. Anat.*, 171:133-148.

18. Ross, J.J., Duxson, M.J. Harris, A.J. (1987): Formation of primary and secondary myotubes in rat lumbrical muscle. *Development,* 100:383-394.

19. Schwartz, K., De La Bastie, D., Olivero, P., Alonso, S. Buckingham, M. (1986): α-Skeletal muscle actin mRNAs accumulate in hypertrophied adult rat hearts. *Circ. Res.*, 59:551-555.

20. Shani, M., Dekel, I., Yoffe, O. (1988): Expression of the rat myosin light-chain 2 gene in transgenic mice: Stage specificity, developmental regulation, and interrelation with the endogenous gene. *Mol. Cell. Biol.*, 8:1006-1009.

21 Sutherland, C., Gordon, M., Elsom, V., Dunwoodie, S. Hardeman, E. (1991): Coordination of skeletal muscle gene expression occurs late in mammalian development. *Dev. Biol.*, 146:167-178.

22. Vivarelli, E., Brown, W.E., Whalen, R.G. Cossu, G. (1988): The expression of slow myosin during mammalian somitogenesis and limb bud differentiation. *J..Cell. Biol.*, 107:2191-2107.

23. Wade, R. Kedes, L. (1989): Developmental regulation of contractile protein genes. *Ann. Rev. Physiol.,* 51:179-188.

24. Wade, B., Sutherland, C., Gahlmann, R., Kedes, L., Hardeman, E. Gunning, P. (1990): Regulation of contractile protein gene family mRNA pool sizes during myogenesis. *Dev. Bio.*, 142:270-282.

25. Whalen, R.G. (1985): Myosin isoenzymes as molecular markers for muscle physiology. *J. Exp. Biol.*, 115:43-53.

26. Weydert, A., Barton, P., Harris, A.J., Pinset, C. Buckingham, M. (1987): Developmental pattern of mouse skeletal myosin heavy chain gene transcripts *in vivo* and *in vitro. Cell*, 49:121-129.

DISCUSSION

Dr. Manfred W. Beilharz:
I have one question and then I would like you to comment on tissue specificity. The question is that you showed that there was integration and at the level of expression of RNA the transgenes have been examined. I am just wondering if

you have done any research to confirm that the protein is also expressed appropriately.

Dr. Edna C. Hardeman:
We do not have any data present concerning the expression of the sarcomeric actin proteins in our mice. However, there is strong evidence from the cytoplasmic actins, that the protein is necessary to mediate the autoregulatory response. We are assuming that during evolution this mechanism was carried over when the sarcomeric actin genes arose from the cytoplasmic actin genes. However, we definitely need to address the issue directly.

Dr. Manfred W. Beilharz:
You were saying that the tissue specificity is not limited?

Dr. Edna C. Hardeman:
When we initiated our studies in mice, the current dogma predicted that the sarcomeric actins were only expressed in the striated tissues, heart and skeletal muscle. We observed that our largest fragment of the cardiac actin gene was expressed in nonmuscle tissues, lung, stomach, intestine and testis in the extreme case. This made us take a harder look at the expression of the cardiac actin transcript in nontransgenic mouse tissues. We found that the transcript was present at a low level in the lung in one strain of mouse. Interestingly, two other groups have observed inappropriate expression of a transgene in certain tissues: lung, brain and spleen for the troponin I fast gene (Hallauer et al. (1988). Mol. Cell. Biol. 8:5072-5079) and in brain, kidney and skeletal muscle for the immunoglobulin μ gene (Jenuwein and Grosschedl (1991). Genes and Dev. 5:932-943). Perhaps a pattern is emerging which indicates that a transgene is somewhat promiscuously expressed in certain tissues.

Dr. Miranda D. Grounds:
Is there any interaction between gene regulation of members of the different structural protein families. Does a change in expression of one family influence the expression of other gene products?

Dr. Edna C. Hardeman:
We would hope that the means of communication which we have observed between the sarcomeric actins are utilised by other muscle contractile gene families. Furthermore, these mechanisms could also be utilised to communicate preferred isoform associations between contractile protein multigene families. One could imagine that at a particular time in development, in response to a given cue, an isoform gene of one family is activated transcriptionally and that this elicits the subsequent activation of an isoform from another gene family. Perhaps in this manner, the most physiologically advantageous sarcomere is established.

Dr. Miranda D. Grounds:
About dystrophin. Is it possible that the presence or absence of dystrophin might influence the expression of other structural genes?

Dr. Edna C. Hardeman:
It is very possible that the lack of functional dystrophin in Duchenne dystrophy disrupts the regulation of associated proteins. Perhaps a somewhat related protein can substitute for dystrophin to some extent, but its ultimate physiological success

is dependent on parameters which differ between different species. This could explain why the lack of dystrophin is not deleterious in the mdx mouse. The point that I am trying to make with our studies is that you cannot think of structural protein genes as being regulated in isolation. In addition, you probably have to take into consideration the possibility that the regulation of associated, non-structural proteins, such as enzymes, may be influenced by the transcriptional activity of the associated structural genes.

Dr. Miranda D. Grounds:
Again that may be associated with maturation or a particular growth phase where something may be regulated.

Dr. Edna C. Hardeman:
Yes very possibly.

Professor Allen D. Roses:
Since the gene families are interspersed throughout the genome, do you have any idea about the mechanism for the coordinated expression would be.

Dr. Edna C. Hardeman:
At this time, I cannot propose a mechanism which would account for communication between, and coordination of genes located on different chromosomes. Our first step toward addressing this question will be to examine the region of the cardiac actin gene which we believe is involved in this communcation mechanism. We need to determine whether or not other muscle contractile protein genes carry this sequence and if so, how frequently this sequence is shared between members of the different multigene families.

Professor Allen D. Roses:
And multiple sites.

Dr. Henry J. Klamut:
Do you think that there might be regulatory sequence elements which are common to these gene families which might be involved, for example, in binding a factor involved in stabilizing the transcript? If these binding sites had somewhat different affinities for this putative stabilizing factor you might see this type of effect upon induction of a new transcript with a binding site of higher affinity.

Dr. Edna C. Hardeman:
Yes, that is possible. Again I think the best way to tackle the issue is to examine the degree with which this sequence is common to members of different contractile gene families.

GENERAL DISCUSSION

Afternoon Session

Leaders: George Karpati and Terence A. Partridge

Professor Allen D. Roses:
George, is there any information about the other trials that were performed in the other States?

Professor George Karpati:
To my knowledge, three major human myoblast transfer experiments, using a single muscle, are in progress in the U.S. One is in San Francisco and the others in Boston and Memphis respectively. No publications or convincing communications have appeared concerning the functional efficacy of the procedure. In view of the seriousness of this matter, it would be very wrong to jump to conclusions based on the results of only 1 or 2 groups. I think, therefore, it is very important that several competent groups perform this experimentation to see what would be their findings.

Dr. Terence A. Partridge:
There were a couple of things which interested me about your myoblast transfer work. The appearance of the Major Histocompatibility Complex (MHC) antigens on muscle fibres on the myoblast inject side. Do you know whose haplotype they were, the patient's or the donor's?

Professor George Karpati:
I suspect that it was host-derived, but we did not determine this precisely. We think that it is a non-specific reaction of the muscle to foreign protein (s). In other words, what we say is that some of the myoblasts you inject will disintegrate and these may well evoke a multiple antimuscle antibody response. However, these antibodies will not be harmful to host muscle fibres.

Dr. Terence A. Partridge:
The second point is about the whole myoblast transfer programme. All of the studies involve quite old children, 6-8 year olds in your case, but older in some of the other studies.

Professor George Karpati:
The experiment was for older people initially.

Dr. Terence A. Partridge:
Yes, and I can understand why this was done in terms of getting permission for these experiments. But was the inclusion of functional testing a purely ritual exercise, it seems to me that there is little reason to expect functional improvement in muscles at this age.

Professor George Karpati:

Functional improvement could have occurred primarily because if we had created enough dystrophin-positive muscle fibres in the injected muscle, those fibres would not have been destroyed and the natural growth would have allowed creation of larger fibres and hence greater muscle mass. Within a year we hoped that, on the injected side, the force generation would have been better than on the sham-injected side, but not necessarily improved from the original baseline. On the other hand, actual improvement still could have occurred because the natural growth would have allowed those fibres to grow in length and girth, producing an absolute increase in strength.

Dr. Terence A. Partridge:

For that to happen would have involved a contribution of myoblasts to growth of fibres as well as into regenerating fibres.

It seems to me that the questions you can reasonably ask in older children are: can you get expression of dystrophin in their muscles, can you avoid rejection and do you get tumours. These are answers you really need to know and which can only be answered for man by experiments in man. If you are going to ask for improvement in muscle function or for a stabilization against decline in function, you should ask that in younger children where the muscles have not been too badly damaged.

Professor George Karpati:

We are very much in favour of trying to do experimental myoblast transfer as early as possible. In young children, the muscles are small so much fewer myoblasts are necessary and fibrosis is much less. However, picking out Duchenne boys during the first year of life is not easy. It requires some sort of screening system. Secondly, it is difficult to tell a parent that you have a boy who looks to all practical purposes normal, but that this boy is going to become a cripple unless you do an experimental procedure, and on top of which, you cannot promise any success. Many of these parents will be disinclined to participate.

Dr. Terence A. Partridge:

Mayana Zatz might be a good person to find such children because she looks after large dystrophic families in Brazil where the parents have already seen the effects of the disease on their older children and would be prepared to cooperate in experiments involving their younger children.

Professor George Karpati:

We are in constant touch with her and as soon as we have the efficiency of myoblast transfer upgraded to a decent level, we will certainly involve her.

Professor Allen D. Roses:

It sounds to me that you have done the quick, emotionally laden try and you have identified problems which are making a perfect case for animal experimentation. I would think that the types of interventions that you are talking about like hologenetics and various other things could be tried in an authentic experimental model before you even applied to an Ethics Committee to perform the techniques on a child aged 1-3.

Professor George Karpati:
I could not agree more.

Dr. Terence A. Partridge:
As a minor protagonist of autologous transplantation of genetically rectified cells, I feel that I should defend the principle. The model you criticise is one whereby all myoblasts are equivalent, within a Gaussian distribution and go through a given number of divisions before senescing as they approach their "Hayflick limit". An alternative model, on which I gave evidence in my presentation, involves the concept of the self-replacing stem cell, giving rise to lines of myogenic cells which can pass through a limited number of divisions. These two models cannot be distinguished on the basis of present evidence. If there are myogenic stem cells, which might be expected to proliferate slowly, they would be lost by dilution in the type of serial passage experiment that is used to determine the maximal number of divisions. So this type of experiment would bias against finding stem cells even if they were present. If they do exist, the autologous myoblast transfer is a possibility. The other way in which autologous transfer might be achieved is by transfection with a tightly controlled oncogene, like that present in the H-2ts6 mouse but with extra safeguards. Such cells can be transfected with dystrophin genes, cloned and pushed through many division in tissue culture prior to being implanted into the patient's muscle.

Professor George Karpati:
Yes, I agree with everything you said in relation to the stem cell story. Some people brought up the possibility of injecting dissociated satellite cells without culturing. In such a case we must be sacrificing cell numbers because from a one gram muscle sample you could only generate about 10,000 myogenic cells.

Dr. Terence A. Partridge:
The only normal myogenic cells we have been able to inject into muscle and then rescue out into tissue culture as myogenic clones were in fact satellite cells derived from adult muscle. These cells were not as myogenic in vivo as cells derived from neonatal muscle.

Professor Allen D. Roses:
We theoretically think of a probe. In some viral infections, ie. viral myositis you can identify the PCR and immunological presence of viral enzymes and viral problems, many years after the infection has directly taken place. It seems to me if we are going to do anything for a Duchenne boy, his heart is going to be under considerable strain. I don't really see how directional grafting injected in the heart would be successful. No one can really try viral vectors. It is certainly not a thing that can be done in a human trial.

Professor George Karpati:
My answer to the heart problem in Duchenne is that perhaps it is more easily done by organ transplants, because organ transplants are relatively "easy". Now what you are suggesting, of course, is possible. However, it appears that organ transplants are still easier than generating replication-defective non-pathogenic cardio-myopathic viral vectors for dystrophin gene therapy.

Dr. Nicholas J.H. Sharp:
Dr. Karpati would you be a supporter for equal funding for canine and human

experimentation on these sort of topic?

Professor George Karpati:
I would say experimentation is necessary in all relevant animal models to sort out all the problems before human experimentation.

Dr. Terence A. Partridge:
You made the suggestion that one reason for the lack of success with myoblast injection in humans is that the external lamina in human dystrophic muscle prevents the passage of myoblasts into the damaged muscle fibres. Since this does not seem to be a problem in mice, is there any direct evidence that there might be differences in the coposition between the external laminas of muscle fibres in mouse and in man?

Professor George Karpati:
I do not know if anybody has made a very precise estimate of that. The chances are that if there are differences they are not really something that you would see with the transmission electron microscope or something like that. But even in the mouse you see as I have shown before, that if you fenestrate the basal lamina of host fibres and employ a myonecrotic agent, you have a far superior take of myoblasts in those areas.

Dr. Terence A. Partridge:
Have you injected these into biopsies of human tissue?

Professor George Karpati:
No this is a quantum jump. This will require a lot more animal experimentation and then a very thorough scrutiny by the appropriate people.

Dr. Miranda D. Grounds:
When you are speaking about experimental animals, are you talking about dogs?

Professor George Karpati:
No, mice.

Professor Joe N. Kornegay:
I have taken a few notes with regard to several comments that followed my presentation on the notexin injury model this morning. I think these studies take on greater significance, given the fact that Dr. Karpati has proposed to potentially conduct somewhat similar studies in Duchenne boys, as least with regard to using a "cocktail" including myoblasts, a myotoxin, and collagenase 4. Subsequent to my presentation, there initially appeared to be concern regarding the basic model itself, which is to say whether it would be appropriate to concomitantly inject notexin and myoblasts. There is obviously potential for the notexin to injure the myoblasts or to inhibit either fusion or perhaps migration. Our own results would suggest that these effects probably vary with the concentration of the notexin used. The optimal concentration of notexin, or for that matter any myotoxin, needs to be established. Manfred raised the question as to whether radiation might actually impede chimeric fiber formation and therefore be deleterious. However interestingly, studies reported by Terry Partridge showed myoblast migration actually was apparently enhanced in pre-irradiated mdx mice. The question of the use of surgical markers to identify the site of transplantation is

also valid. At least with regard to our own studies where we have the opportunity to evaluate an entire muscle, it is advantageous to identify the injection sites. Although methylene blue has been used as a surgical marker, it might be that tatoo dye would be preferable, as Terry suggested. The method of labelling cells to be transplanted is problematic. It is not clear whether fluorescent microspheres impair the function of labelled myoblasts. They have obvious limitations with regard to identifying chimeric fibers. Finally, Dr. Karpati has raised the question of the potential value of concomitant treatment with collagenase 4 to perhaps fenestrate the basal lamina. This might promote greater implantation. As luck would have it, slides illustrating muscle 21 days after concomitant myoblast transfer and notexin injury arrived by Federal Express 5 minutes after my presentation. With the Chairman's permission I would like to show these slides. They may raise additional questions but I believe they could be beneficial.

Professor George Karpati:
Just a brief comment on the possible applicability of x-irradiation in humans to prepare the host muscle for myoblast transfer. I think it is almost impossible to conceive that any ethics committee would approve that transplantable muscles of children be pre-irradiated.

Professor Joe N. Kornegay:
This initial slide again reviews the pattern of regeneration normally seen in non-irradiated notexin-injured canine muscle. Regeneration is essentailly complete by 21 days. This slide illustrates muscle 7 days after concomitant myoblast transfer and notexin injury. As I indicated earlier, transplanted cells are identified by the fluorescent microspheres. I was impressed that although large aggregates of labelled mononuclear cells are seen, there is little evidence of myotube formation. Again, recall that regeneration is normally quite advanced by 7 days after notexin injury in non-irradiated muscle. As we have discussed, this could indicate that the notexin is in some way impairing fusion or myoblasts migration. These slides are of muscle at 21 days after concomitant myoblast transplantation and notexin injury. There is again a distinct fascicular arrangement of the injected cells. The dark staining material is methylene blue.

Professor Byron A. Kakulas:
The last slide could pass for a centronuclear myopathy or myotubular myopathy. Or it just looks like about a 6 month human foetal muscle ie central nuclei or myotubes.

Professor Joe N. Kornegay:
So what you are saying Byron is that in your opinion these cells in your mind would pass for myogenic cells.

Professor Byron A. Kakulas:
It looks like foetal muscle. Quite well developed but still at the myotubular stage and it looks like some human myopathies where there is arrested development.

Professor Allen D. Roses:
It looks like in Duchenne studies with the muscle and associated lesions.

Professor Byron A. Kakulas:
Yes, it looks very much like it.

Professor Joe N. Kornegay:
This is the Toluidine blue stain viewed with the fluorescent microscope. The fluorescence and corresponding bright field microscopic sections taken at 21 days show apparent myotube fusion. Relatively mature myofibers at 21 days show apparent myotube fusion. Relatively mature myofibers are labelled with multiple fluorescent microspheres suggesting that fusion, with resultant incoporation of additional microspheres has occurred. We again see that the injected cells remain apart from the pre-existing muscle, either as a function of the irradiation or perhaps because of the methylene blue. Alternatively, factors such as fibrous connective tissue might impede migration of the injected cells.

Dr. Nicholas J.H. Sharp:
Joe, is methylene blue still there?

Professor Joe N. Kornegay:
Yes, this is methylene blue. Again, the methylene blue often appears to outline the fascicles formed by the injected cells. I mentioned yesterday briefly that we have used the 5.1H11 NCAM monoclonal antibody provided by Dickson and Walsh both with magnetic affinity and fluorescence-activated cell sorting, and in both cases, have been able to enrich our cultures for presumptive myoblasts. With regard to the fluorescence-activated studies, our data mirrors closely that published earlier by Webster. Others have of course used clonal cultures to enrich or purify cultures. George referred yesterday to this methodology and some of the potential problems of clonal cultures in terms of adequacy of cell numbers.

Part III

Gene Therapy

DUCHENNE MUSCULAR DYSTROPHY: Animal Models and Genetic Manipulation, edited by Byron A. Kakulas, John McC. Howell, and Allen D. Roses. Raven Press, Ltd., New York © 1992.

21

Expression of a Human Dystrophin Minigene in Myogenic Cell Cultures

Henry J. Klamut, Lucine O. Bosnoyan, Ronald G. Worton, Peter N. Ray

Department of Genetics and Research Institute, The Hospital for Sick Children, 555 University Avenue, Toronto, Ontario, M5G 1X8.

INTRODUCTION

The Duchenne muscular dystrophy (DMD) gene locus occupies over 2500 kb or approximately 1.5% of the entire length of the human X chromosome (9). Mutations within the Duchenne muscular dystrophy (DMD) gene which disrupt the abundance and/or integrity of the 427 kDa protein product dystrophin result in progressive degeneration of skeletal muscle which may be severe (DMD) or relatively mild (Becker muscular dystrophy, BMD) (21). Dystrophin is believed to be a member of a novel family of cytoskeletal proteins and is localized primarily to the inner surface of the skeletal muscle sarcolemma (2,7,31). Evidence has been presented which suggests that dystrophin does not interact directly with the surface membrane but rather is one component of an oligomeric glycoprotein complex of unknown function (11). These results are consistent with biochemical studies that have implicated the muscle surface membrane as the site of the primary defect in this disease (24). A precise definition of the role of dystrophin in the maintenance of skeletal muscle membrane integrity has not as yet been determined.

In the absence of dystrophin, skeletal muscle appears to develop normally but is susceptible to multiple rounds of segmental necrosis and regeneration leading to permanent muscle loss and its replacement with fibrotic tissue. A potential therapeutic approach to this disease lies in techniques which would allow for a functional dystrophin gene to be introduced into DMD patient muscle. Methods currently being considered include donor myoblast transfer, direct gene transfer, and patient myoblast-mediated gene transfer. In donor myoblast transfer, myoblasts carrying a normal DMD gene are isolated from donor muscle biopsies and expanded *in vitro* prior to implantation into DMD patient muscle. As normal myoblasts are incorporated into regenerating patient muscle, chimeric muscle fibers containing donor nuclei would be expected to produce dystrophin and be resistant to further rounds of necrosis. This approach has some advantages over direct gene transfer in that no provisions need to be made for the extremely large size of the DMD gene and injected myoblasts are targetted specifically to muscle tissue. Although initial trials have met with some success (12, 23), problems involving histocompatibility, the production of large numbers of myoblasts for injection, and the efficiency with which injected myoblasts are incorporated into patient muscle still need to be addressed.

The potential for direct and patient myoblast-mediated gene transfer of a DMD minigene construct has recently been enhanced by reports of sustained expression of a reporter gene in whole tissue directly injected with plasmid DNA (30) and the demonstration that retroviral vectors may be used to achieve high efficiency gene transfer into primary rat myoblasts (27). Also, Lee et al. (18) have recently described the construction of a full length 14 kb mouse dystrophin minigene under the control of a constitutive SV40 viral promoter which, when introduced into COS monkey kidney cells *in vitro*, produces a recombinant dystrophin molecule that is indistinguishable by Western blot analysis from mouse muscle dystrophin and is localized to the surface membrane of this cell line. In patient myoblast-mediated gene transfer, a recombinant DMD minigene would first be introduced into patient myoblasts *in vitro*. Recombinant patient myoblasts expressing a functional recombinant dystrophin molecule would then be re-introduced into patient muscle tissues. This technique may have some advantages over donor myoblast-mediated gene transfer in that problems with immunological incompatibility are circumvented and levels of recombinant dystrophin provided by each cell could be increased through the introduction of multiple copies or overexpression of the recombinant DMD minigene. This approach has recently been tested with some success in an experiment in which the human multidrug transporter (MDR1) gene has been introduced into rat L6 and primary myocytes prior to implantation into the tibialis anterior muscle of Wistar rats (26). As DMD patient myoblasts have proven difficult to grow in large numbers *in vitro* due to the high levels of regenerative activity early in this disease (28), efficient methods for patient cell transfection and recombinant myoblast implantation would be needed for this approach to be feasible. In addition, although retroviral vectors provide high efficiencies of recombinant gene transfer into a variety of cell types (3,8,20,22,27,29), problems have been encountered in achieving appropriate and sustained levels of transcription of the recombinant gene (22). Special attention would therefore have to be paid to the inclusion of appropriate transcriptional regulatory elements which would serve to optimize recombinant dystrophin expression in patient muscle fibers.

In addition to the technical problems associated with donor myoblast and direct gene transfer techniques, several fundamental questions relating to the pathogenesis of DMD must also be addressed prior to the establishment of these techniques as viable protocols for the treatment of this disease. For example, very little is known about the mechanism by which dystrophin acts to prevent the necrotic process in affected tissues, and no direct assay of dystrophin function is available by which to judge the effectiveness of a particular minigene construct in restoring normal phenotype. Other questions, such as the need for appropriate patterns of recombinant dystrophin expression with muscle development to allow for proper assembly of the submembraneous cytoskeleton, and the potential toxic effects of dystrophin overexpression in muscle and non-muscle cells must also be addressed.

Our approach has been to address these concerns in myogenic and non-myogenic cultures grown *in vitro*, and to then apply these findings to the optimization of DMD minigene expression and function in transgenic animals. Myogenic cell lines being used in this study include normal clonal human myoblasts, which display normal patterns of endogenous DMD gene expression (14, 15, 19) and support the expression of chimeric DMD promoter-reporter gene constructs (14), and DMD patient myoblasts, mdx mouse myoblasts, cmd canine myoblasts, and rodent muscle-derived myogenic cell lines such as H9C2(2-1) and L6 which are defective in the expression of dystrophin from their endogenous genes. Initially, two problems are being addressed which will impact directly on the design of DMD minigene constructs; 1) the identification of important functional domains within the dystrophin molecule and the development of assays which could be used to evaluate the degree with which recombinant dystrophin expressed in affected cells functions to restore normal phenotype; and 2) the identification of transcriptional regulatory elements within the DMD gene locus and an assessment of the requirement for appropriate tissue- and developmental stage-specific expression of recombinant dystrophin in muscle tissues.

CONSTRUCTION OF A HUMAN DMD MINIGENE AND ITS EXPRESSION IN MYOGENIC CELL CULTURES

The prototypic DMD minigene utilized in these studies was designed to determine whether; a) the muscle-specific DMD promoter can be used to express a DMD minigene construct in a developmental stage-specific manner similar to that observed from the endogenous DMD gene; b) expression of a recombinant dystrophin molecule in myogenic cell lines defective in the expression of their endogenous DMD gene restores surface membrane antigenicity to dystrophin antibodies; and c) a DMD minigene that is significantly reduced in size to fascilitate accessibility to as wide a range of vector systems as possible still retains function. In this regard, substantial deletions and duplications have been identified within the spectrin repeat domain in mild BMD cases with detectable dystrophin at the sarcolemma (1,10). Working under the assumption that mild phenotype reflects minimal disruption of dystrophin function in these patients, we have prepared a human DMD minigene that carries a 5.3 kb deletion of exons 16 to 48 corresponding to repeats 3 to 19 of the spectrin repeat domain (16,17). The minigene was assembled by splicing cDNAs 1-2a, 10.69, 8, and 9-14 (5,16) at unique restriction sites within each of these regions of the gene. A PCR-generated splicing adapter spanning unique Cla1 and Kpn1 sites near the splice junction and containing an exon 15-49 in-frame junction was used to complete the construction of the coding region. Incorporation of a unique Mlu1 site at the exon 15-49 junction introduces 6 nucleotides coding for two amino acids (arginine, threonine) not normally present in this region of dystrophin, but affords the opportunity to modify the minigene at the splice junction through the insertion of one or more repeat units to assess the biological importance of the spacing between the amino and carboxy terminal domains. The resulting minigene is deleted for exons 16 to 48 corresponding to spectrin-like repeats 4 to 18 and codes for a recombinant protein with a predicted molecular weight of 230 kD. No significant deviations in pI or percent amino acid composition (compared to full length dystrophin) result from this deletion. The 7.1 kb DMD minigene construct also contains 850 bp of sequence corresponding to the human muscle-specific DMD gene promoter (14), 244 bp corresponding to the complete 5' untranslated region, and 248 bp corresponding to a portion of the 3' untranslated region. Polyadenylation is provided by SV40 splice and polyadenylation sequences provided by the expression vector.

The H9C2(2-1) rat myoblast cell line (13) has been shown to produce reduced levels of endogenous DMD gene transcripts as compared to clonal human myotubes (14) and does not produce detectable levels of dystrophin as judged by Western blot analysis and indirect immunofluorescence. These properties, in conjunction with its capacity to direct high levels of expression of transiently-transfected chimeric muscle-specific DMD promoter-reporter gene constructs (14), has made this the cell line of choice for our initial evaluations of DMD minigene expression. Cells were transfected (6) with the DMD minigene construct in combination with a neomycin phosphotransferase gene expression plasmid and selected for resistance to the aminoglycoside G418. G418-resistant H9C2(2-1) clonal isolates were expanded and analyzed for DMD minigene expression upon differentiation into multinucleated myotubes. DNA isolated from several clonal isolates was analyzed for stable integration of the DMD minigene by PCR amplification (25) of the unique exon 15-49 splice adapter. Clones positive for the adapter at the genomic level were further analyzed for expression and surface membrane localization of recombinant dystrophin by Western blotting (4,31) and indirect immunofluorescence (15). The results demonstrate that:

1. Stable integration of a human DMD minigene into H9C2(2-1) myoblasts results in the expression of a recombinant dystrophin molecule of predicted molecular weight. Approximately 80% of G418-resistant clones testing positive for minigene integration by PCR also tested positive for recombinant dystrophin on Western blots. The levels of recombinant dystrophin expressed in different clonal isolates were somewhat variable, probably owing to differences in the sites of minigene integration, but in general levels of recombinant dystrophin expressed were equal to or greater than the levels of normal dystrophin synthesized in normal clonal human myotubes. Extracts prepared from untransfected H9C2(2-1) myotubes and G418-resistant clones which tested negative for minigene integration also tested negative for both full-length and recombinant dystrophin on Western blots.

2. All G418-resistant H9C2(2-1) clones testing positive for recombinant dystrophin on Western blots displayed surface membrane antigenicity to dystrophin antibodies. The patterns and levels of surface membrane staining observed upon differentiation of DMD minigene-transfected H9C2(2-1) myoblasts were qualitatively similar to those observed in clonal human myotubes expressing dystrophin from their endogenous gene (15). Untransfected and G418-resistant H9C2(2-1) myoblasts testing negative for recombinant dystrophin on Western blots did not display detectable levels of surface membrane antigenicity to dystrophin antibodies. The 850 bp muscle-specific DMD promoter therefore appears to contain the necessary regulatory signals to provide appropriate developmental stage-specific expression of recombinant dystrophin as myoblasts differentiate into multinucleated myotubes *in vitro*.

3. Consistent with the observation of apparently normal surface staining of muscle fibers in patients with large in-frame intragenic rearrangements, an in-frame deletion of 5.3 kb within the spectrin repeat region does not affect the ability of the recombinant dystrophin molecule to localize to the surface membrane. In addition, removal of a large portion of the 3' untranslated region of the DMD gene does not appear to be have a significant effect on the production of appropriate levels of recombinant DMD gene mRNA transcripts. Removal of these intragenic and 3' UTR sequences reduces the size of the DMD minigene such that it may be accomodated by most conventional plasmid and retroviral expression vectors.

These experiments were subsequently extended to several other cell lines. DMD minigene constructs under the control of the muscle-specific DMD promoter or viral LTRs in combination with the muscle-specific DMD promoter were introduced into fetal DMD patient myoblasts, cos-1 monkey kidney cells, and 3T3 fibroblasts. Similar patterns of recombinant dystrophin expression and surface membrane staining were observed in both DMD patient myotubes and cos cells. No surface membrane staining was observed in 3T3 fibroblasts. Recent reports of reduced concentrations in DMD patient muscle of components of the dystrophin-associated glycoprotein complex (11) has raised concerns about the availability of membrane binding sites for recombinant dystrophin in non-expressing muscle cells. Lee et al. (18) have suggested, based on their observation of surface membrane localization of recombinant dystrophin in cos cells, that the signals for membrane association may be contained within the dystrophin molecule itself. The essentially normal pattern of surface staining observed in transfected DMD myocytes suggests that sufficient levels of the dystrophin-associated glycoprotein complex are expressed at this early stage of muscle development in the absence of endogenous dystrophin expression, or that expression of recombinant dystrophin in these cells acts to trans-activate or stabilize components of the glycoprotein complex. The absence of surface membrane staining in recombinant fibroblasts suggests that these cells do not express the necessary surface membrane glycoprotein components required for dystrophin localization, and that dystrophin does not have the capacity to target to the surface membrane in the absence of these glycoprotein components.

SUMMARY

A human DMD minigene containing a large deletion within the central spectrin-like repeat domain and under the control of the muscle-specific DMD promoter has been introduced into rat H9C2(2-1) and fetal DMD patient myoblasts grown *in vitro*. Stable integration of the DMD minigene results in the expression of a recombinant dystrophin molecule of predicted molecular weight and the restoration of surface membrane antigenicity to dystrophin antibodies. These results provide the first demonstration that direct gene transfer of a DMD minigene into patient myoblasts may result in the restoration of normal phenotype, and establish an experimental system for the optimization of gene transfer protocols into muscle cells, for assessments of the utility of a variety of expression vector systems, for the refinement of DMD minigene design, and for determining the role of dystrophin in the maintenance of muscle membrane integrity.

REFERENCES

1. Angelini, C., Beggs, A.H., Hoffman, E.P., Fanin, M., Kunkel, L.M. (1990): Enormous dystrophin in a patient with Becker muscular dystrophy. *Neurology*, 40:808-812.
2. Arahata, K., Ishiura, S., Ishiguro, T., Tsukahara, T., Suhara, Y., Eguchi, C., Ishihara, T., Nonaka, I., Ozawa, E., Sugita, H. (1988): Immunostaining of skeletal and cardiac muscle cell surface membrane with antibody against Duchenne muscular dystrophy peptide. *Nature*, 333:861-863.
3. Bennet, V.J., Chang, P.L. (1990): Suppression of immunological response against a novel gene product delivered by implants of genetically modified fibroblasts. *Mol. Biol. Med.*, 7:471-477.
4. Bulman, D.E., Gangopadhyay, S.B., Bebchuck, K.G., Worton, R.G., Ray, P.N. (1991): Point mutation in the human dystrophin gene: identification through Western blot analysis. *Genomics*, 10:457-460.
5. Burghes, A.H.M., Logan, C., Hu, X., Belfall, B., Worton, R.G., Ray, P.N. (1987): A cDNA clone from the Duchenne/Becker muscular dystrophy gene. *Nature*, 328: 434-437.
6. Chen, C., Okayama, H. (1987): High efficiency transformation of mammalian cells by plasmid DNA. *Mol. Cell. Biol.*, 7:2745-2752.
7. Cullen, M.J., Walsh, J., Nicholson, L.V.B., Harris, J.B. (1990): Ultrastructural localization of dystrophin in human muscle by using gold immunolabelling. *Proc. R. Soc. Lond.*, 240: 197-210.
8. Culver, K., Cornetta, K., Morgan, R., Morecki, S., Abersold, P., Kasid, A., Lotze, M., Rosenberg, S.A., Anderson, W.F., Blaese, R.M. (1991): Lymphocytes as cellular vehicles for gene therapy in mouse and man. *Proc. Natl. Acad. Sci. USA*, 88:3155-3159.
9. Den Dunnen, J.T., Grootscholten, P.M., Bakker, E., Blonden, L.A.J., Ginjaar, H.B., Wapenaar, M.C., van Paassen, H.M.B., van Broeckhoven, C., Pearson, P.L., van Ommen, G.J.B. (1989): Topography of the Duchenne muscular dystrophy (DMD) gene: FIGE and cDNA analysis of 194 cases reveals 115 deletions and 13 duplications. *Am. J. Hum. Genet.*, 45:835-847.
10. England, S.B., Nicholson, L.V.B., Johnson, M.A., Forrest, S.M., Love, D.R., Zubrzycka-Gaarn, E.E., Harris, J.B., and Davies, K.E. (1990): Very mild muscular dystrophy associated with the deletion of 46% of dystrophin. *Nature*, 343:180-182.
11. Ervasti, J.M., Ohlendieck, K., Kahl, S.D., Gaver, M.G., Campbell, K.P. (1990): Deficiency of a glycoprotein component of the dystrophin complex in dystrophic muscle. *Nature*, 345:315-319.
12. Karpati, G., Pouliot, Y., Zubrzycka-Gaarn, E.E., Carpenter, S., Ray, P.N., Worton, R.G., Holland, P. (1989): Dystrophin is expressed in mdx skeletal muscle fibers after normal myoblast implantation. *Am. J. Pathol.*, 134:27-32.
13. Kimes, B.W., Brandt, B.L. (1976): Properties of a clonal muscle cell line from rat heart. *Exptl. Cell Res.*, 98: 367-381.
14. Klamut, H.J., Gangopadhyay, S.B., Worton, R.G., Ray, P.N. (1990): Molecular and functional analysis of the muscle-specific promoter region of the Duchenne muscular dystrophy gene. *Mol. Cell. Biol.*, 10:193-205.

15. Klamut, H.J., Zubrzycka-Gaarn, E.E., Bulman, D.E., Malhotra, S.B., Bodrug, S.E., Worton, R.G., Ray, P.N. (1989): Myogenic regulation of dystrophin gene expression. *Br. Med. Bull.*, 45:681-702.

16. Koenig, M., Hoffman, E.P., Bertelson, C.J., Monaco, A.P., Feener, C., Kunkel, L.M. (1987): Complete cloning of the Duchenne muscular dystrophy (DMD) cDNA and preliminary genomic organization of the DMD gene in normal and affected individuals. *Cell*, 50:509-517.

17. Koenig, M., Kunkel, L.M. (1990): Detailed analysis of the repeat domain of dystrophin reveals four potential hinge segments that may confer flexibility. *J. Biol. Chem.*, 265:4560-4566.

18. Lee, C.C, Pearlman, J.A., Chamberlain, J.S., Caskey, C.T. (1991): Expression of recombinant dystrophin and its localization to the cell membrane. *Nature,* 349:334-336.

19. Lev, A.A., Feener, C.C., Kunkel, L.M., Brown, R.H. (1987): Expression of the Duchenne muscular dystrophy gene in cultured muscle cells. *J. Biol. Chem.*, 262:15817-15820.

20. Luskey, B.D., Lim, B., Apperley, J.F., Orkin, S.H., William, D.A. (1990): Gene transfer into murine hematopoietic stem cells and bone marrow stromal cells. *Ann. N.Y. Acad. Sci.*, 612: 398-406.

21. Monaco, A.P., Bertelson, C.J., Liechti-Gallati, S., Moser, H., and Kunkel, L.M. (1988): *Genomics*, 2:901

22. Palmer T.D., Rosman G.J., Osborne W.R.A., Miller A.D. (1991): An explanation for the phenotypic differences between patients bearing partial deletions of the DMD gene locus. *Proc. Natl. Acad. Sci. USA*, 88:1330-1334.

23. Partridge, T.A., Morgan, J.E., Coulton, J.R., Hoffman, E.P., Kunkel, L.M. (1989): Conversion of mdx myofibers from dystrophin-negative to - positive by injection of normal myoblasts. *Nature,* 337:176-179.

24. Rowland, L.P. (1980): Biochemistry of muscle membranes in Duchenne muscular dystrophy. *Muscle and Nerve*, 3:3-20.

25. Saiki, R.K., Gelfand, D.H., Stoffel, S., Scharf, S.J., Higuchi, R., Horn, G.T., Mullis, K.B., Erlich, H.A. (1988): Primer-directed enzymatic amplification of DNA with a thermostabile DNA polymerase. *Science*, 239:487-491.

26. Salminen, A., Elson, H.F., Mickley, L.A., et. al. (1991): Implantation of recombinant rat myocytes into adult skeletal muscle: a potential gene therapy. *Human Gene Therapy* 2:15-26.

27. Smith, B.F., Hoffman, R.K., Giger, U., Wolfe, J.H. (1990): Genes transferred by retroviral vectors into normal and mutant myoblasts in primary cultures are expressed in myotubes. *Mol. Cell. Biol.*, 10:3268-3271.

28. Webster, C., Blau, H.M. (1990): Accelerated age-related decline in replicative life-span of Duchenne muscular dystrophy myoblasts: implications for cell and gene therapy. *Somat. Cell. Mol. Genet.*, 16:557-565.

29. Williams, D.A. (1990): Expression of introduced genetic sequences in hematopoietic cells following retroviral-mediated gene transfer. *Hum. Gene Ther.*, 1:229-239.

30. Wolff, J.A., Malone, R.W., Williams, P., Chong, W., Acsadi, G., Jani, A., Felgner, P.L. (1990): Direct gene transfer into mouse muscle in vivo. *Science*, 247:1465-1468.

31. Zubrzycka-Gaarn, E.E., Bulman, D.E., Karpati, G., Burghes, A.H.M., Belfall, B., Klamut, H.J., Talbot, J., Hodges, R.S., Ray, P.N., Worton, R.G. (1988): The Duchenne muscular dystrophy gene product is localized in sarcolemma of human skeletal muscle. *Nature*, 333:466-469.

DISCUSSION

Assist. Professor Richard J. Bartlett:
Henry, which antibodies did you use for detecting dystrophin on the cell surface?

Dr. Henry J Klamut:
The Western blot data that I've presented represents cross-reactivity of recombinant dystrophin to an antibody against epitopes at the extreme carboxy-terminal end. An amino-terminal antibody was used in the indirect immuno-fluorescence experiments that I have presented. We have also used carboxy-terminal antibodies in these experiments and they have provided similar results.

Assist. Professor Richard J. Bartlett:
Have you used an antibody which specifically recognized the region detected from your construct?

Dr. Henry J Klamut:
That is an important point and we hope to have those results soon.

Dr. Terence A. Partridge:
Your staining, is nicely located at the edges of the cell. Did you take that picture with a confocal scanning microscope?

Dr. Henry J. Klamut:
No, we have not used confocal microscopy.

Dr. Terence A. Partridge:
Is there no staining on the top surface? Normally you get a low level of top surface staining and a concentration effect in surfaces running perpendicular to the plane it focuses on.

Dr. Henry J Klamut:
I believe that the pattern of surface staining that we see may have something to do with our fixation technique. We are using a rather harsh methanol fixation and it is possible that this may be contributing in some way to the concentration of dystrophin at cell-substratum attachment sites along the edge of a myotube. We have used milder fixation techniques and the pattern of staining is somewhat different - more uniformly distributed along the surface and oriented along the longitudinal plane of the myotube.

Dr. Edna C. Hardeman:
What do you think is the reason for the lack of expression of dystrophin in the C2 and L6 cell lines? Do you think that they express transcriptional repressors?

Dr. Henry J Klamut:
That is a good question and one that we don't have a complete answer for yet. The absence of expression in these cell lines of DMD gene promoter constructs in which the repressor domain has been deleted suggests that these cell lines fail to produce adequate levels of one or more trans-activating factors required for promoter activity. However, the low levels of activity of the tandem RSV-DMD promoter construct in L6 myotubes suggests that there may also be other repressor-type factors involved.

Professor George Karpati:
With the construct where the gene was driven by two promoters, you created expression in non-muscle cell types. Did the dystrophin in those cell types also localise to the surface membrane?

Dr. Henry J Klamut:
Yes, we do have preliminary evidence that this is the case. We have seen recombinant dystrophin localised to the surface membrane of COS cells but not in 3T3 fibroblasts. This suggests that dystrophin does not have the capacity to localise to the membrane on its own but rather requires some sort of receptor - perhaps a glycoprotein complex like that described by Ervasti et al. (11). It is not clear, however, what this complex would be doing in COS cells, or whether it's components are the same as those described in muscle tissues.

DUCHENNE MUSCULAR DYSTROPHY: Animal Models
and Genetic Manipulation, edited by Byron A. Kakulas,
John McC. Howell, and Allen D. Roses.
Raven Press, Ltd., New York © 1992.

22

Potential Strategies for Gene Therapy in Golden Retriever Muscular Dystrophy

Richard J. Bartlett

*Department of Medicine, Neurology Division,
Duke University Medical Center, Durham, NC 27710
#Department of Companion Animals and Special Species Medicine,
College of Veterinary Medicine, North Carolina State University,
Raleigh, NC 27606

Through evidence presented for a molecular defect, the golden retriever muscular dystrophy model has been confirmed as a homologue of Duchenne muscular dystrophy (See Sharp, et al, this volume). The next logical step will be the utilization of this model for testing therapeutic strategies. Two of the major categories of strategies would include gene replacement through cell therapy (myoblast transplantation) or gene therapy. Dr. Kornegay has presented his initial studies using heterologous myoblast transplantation (See Kornegay, et al, this volume). Significant interest has been generated in the myoblast transplantation therapy approach to correcting muscle disease (4). Since muscle has the unique capacity to regenerate by incorporation of myoblast or satellite cells into the myofibers, the strategy of providing a cell with a normal gene through an injection route is predicted to be capable of correcting the defect in muscle diseases such as those caused by dystrophin deficiency. This has proven partially successful in the case of the *mdx* mouse (11). One potential drawback to this approach would be immunological problems caused by injecting heterologous cells into affected animals (5). To overcome this problem, we propose to study means of delivering dystrophin cDNA mini-genes into cultured myoblasts with the eventual goal to re-inject reverted myoblasts into autologous hosts. In addition, the study of mini-gene constructs proposed here would lay the basis for testing direct injection of cDNA mini-genes into muscle tissue in affected animals.

Since little is known about the capacity of cultured myoblasts to uptake and express a dystrophin cDNA minigene (See Klamut et al, this volume), we propose to study the effect of the transition in culture from actively growing cells to those that are undergoing fusion to form myotubes. Cultures will be seeded at densities and serum concentrations which will lead to continued active growth or to fusion. Transfection experiments would then be performed to optimize the capacity of cells to take up and express the dystrophin cDNA mini-genes. The initial experiments will utilize a cDNA mini-gene provided by Dr. George Dickson (See Figure 1) to test the conditions for transfection. This construct requires a co-transfection with a neomycin resistance gene construct. We are presently using pMAM.NEO.LUC from Clontech*. In addition to the immunocytochemical localization of dystrophin products, we will test for the expression of luciferase provided by the latter vector using a commercially available kit (Promega#) to confirm that cells have been transfected.

There are numerous methods whereby a minigene construct may be introduced into cells. Three very different modes, calcium phosphate co-precipitation,10 electroporation,(12) and biolystic wand (13) offer a wide variety for testing optimal uptake and expression of different cDNA minigene constructs. Each may have advantages, but our knowledge of the capacity of muscle precursor cells to take up and express a cDNA mini-gene the size of the dystrophin gene is limited and requires detailed study.

1.   Calcium phosphate co-precipitation

This procedure capitalizes on the capacity of a small number of cells to uptake and express DNA introduced into culture medium as a co-precipitate with calcium. (Calcium salts and phosphate salts do not mix well). The protocol for DNA preparation and transfection of cells has seen significant changes over the last 15 years to the point that commercial kits for co-precipitation are available (Promega#). Briefly, cells are split and freshly seeded at a density which will permit adherence and brief growth within 40 hrs. DNA from the gene construct of interest is precipitated with $CaPO_4$ solution to form microfine granules(10). These are maintained under aseptic conditions prior to overlaying on cells. To overlay, medium is decanted and replaced with fresh media containing the DNA co-precipitate at a relative concentration of 0.1 ugs/ml. Cells are maintained with and allowed to take in the DNA co-precipitates for 3 or 20 hrs. Then, cultures are rinsed with phosphate buffered saline (PBS) and gentimicin (200 ug/ml of G418) administered to select for the neomycin resistance conferred by the pMAM.NEO.LUC vector in the co-precipitate. Cells are maintained in antibiotic until confluency and myotube formation begins. Immunohistochemical analysis of dystrophin protein is assayed as described,(8) and luciferase according to the methods from a commercially available kit. The major drawback of this system is the low efficiency of transfection (from 1 to 10 x 10^{-6}/ ug DNA)

2.   Electroporation

The basic difference between the co-precipitation methodology and the electroporation methodology is the mode of delivery of the DNA mini-gene constructs. Electroporation relies on the use of high impedence fields to "punch" holes in the cell membrane and allow the charged DNA molecules to penetrate into the cells. Initial experiments will monitor for survivability. The optimal rate of uptake of DNA via electroporation varies slightly with each cell-line. Usually,

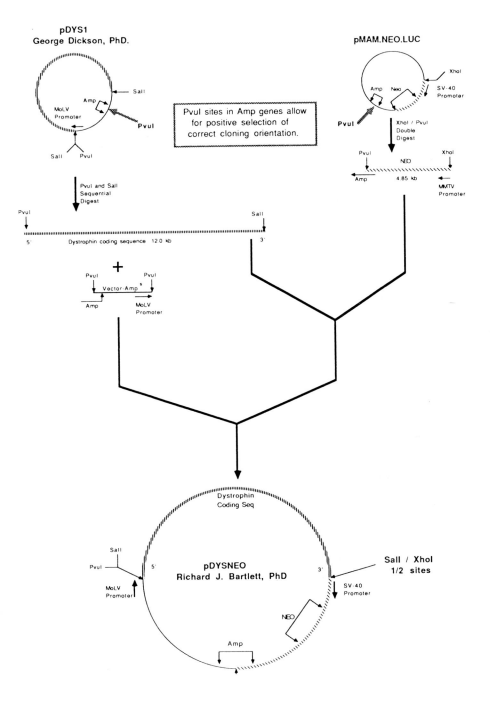

FIG. 1.   Expressing dystrophin cDNA clones.

this is reached at a 10-15% survivability ratio.(12) Thus, kill-curves will be determined for each of the fused and unfused cells. To compare the fused vs. unfused cells, cultures of each will be briefly scraped from flasks, rinsed once with sterile PBS, then suspended in the DNA containing solution prior to transfer to the electroporation cell. Cells will then be submitted to electric current based on the kill-curves and then replated at a 5-7 fold higher density based on the optimum range of survivability. Non-viablie cells will be removed by decanting media after 6 hrs and by providing fresh medium. This will provide live cells at a similar density to that found in the culture before treatment. Growth and selection in the presence of gentimicin will be as above.

Finally, trypsinization will also be tested as a means of providing good cell suspensions for electroporation. Since fused cells have a poor viability after replating from trypsinization,(1) it is believed that this method may work better for the actively growning myoblasts instead of the myotubes. Cultures will be tested for transfection using both the lucifierase assay and dystrophin assay as described above.

3. Biolystic Wand (13)

Another method for delivering a cDNA minigene into cells utilizes microspheres of either gold or tungsten which are coated with the DNA to be transfected. Recent evidence for the capacity of myoblasts to express DNA via this proceedure used cultures of chick muscle cells.(13) A high level of transfection was accomplished using this biolystic protocol (10-20%) and holds great promise for the proposed studies. In this proceedure, cultured cells would be exposed to microsphere injection under aseptic conditions *in situ* thereby eliminating the need to remove cells from culture as in the electroporation proceedure. This proceedure has also been used on live animals, and if proven useful in *ex vivo* studies, would herald *in vivo* studies of gene delivery in intact muscle.

The methods to be used are those described recently by co-developers of the most helium charge form of the instrument.(13) Briefly, gold particles (Alfa, Ward Hill, MA) having a range of diameters from 1 to 3 um or from 2 to 5 um, or tungsten particles (Sylvania) having an average diameter of 3.9 um are used for the bombardment of tissues. Microparticles are coated with DNA by mixing sequentially 25 ul of gold or tungsten particles in an aqueous slurry, 2.5 ul of DNA (1ug/ul), 25 ul of $CaCl_2$ (2.5 M) and 5 ul of free-base spermidine (1.0 M). After 10 min. of incubation, the microspheres were pelleted and the supernatant removed. The pellet is washed with 70% ethanol, centrifuged and resuspended in 25 ul of 100% ethanol. The DNA coated microspheres are then spread onto macro-carrier discs and allowed to dry in a desiccator prior to firing at cells. The biolystic wand is available from duPont and can be adapted for use with cultured cells or live animals.(2) Thus, *ex vivo* experiments aimed at optimal delivery of minigene constructs will be excellant as forerunners for *in vivo* experiments with intact muscles exposed under aseptic surgery.

In summary, if one were to diagram the relative efficiency of these three methods it would look something like this:

Biolistics >> Electroporation > Co-precipitation

One area of study which will be emphasized will be to determine what improvements can be made in the expression of a dystrophin cDNA minigene construct *ex vivo* ? More precisely, what will be the consequences of substituting various available promoters and untranslated regions of cloned genes into dystrophin cDNA constructs and introducing these into cultured GRMD muscle cells?

To attempt to reproduce normal transcriptional control, we have cloned the human and canine DYS promotors using PCR primers derived from the human sequence (See Figure 2) and will use these in some mini-gene constructs. These sequences will be positioned upstream from the DYS coding sequence. In addition, other promotors such as hormone responsive or viral promotors may be utilized to increase the expression of the cDNA mini-gene construct and therefore minimize the number of successfully transplanted cells required to restore normal function to the transplanted muscle. Experimental constructs will be first tested *ex vivo* in cultured affected myoblast and myotube cells prior to the long-range goal of direct injection into donor animals. While the initial experiments above will utilize a cDNA mini-gene construct with a modified murine leukemia virus LTR provided by Dr. Dickson from Guys and St. Thomas's in London, subsequent experiments will be used to select an optimal promoter for the minigene constructs. These experiments will rely on the development of testing gene delivery above as well as the same methodology for analysis for luciferase and dystrophin detection. The insertion of the various promoter cartridges will be facilitated by a SalI site which is upstream from the coding region of the dystrophin mini-gene as constructed by Dr. Dickson and as modified here through the inclusion of a neo resistance gene from the pMAM.NEO.LUC vector (See Figure 1). Each of the promoter constructs described below will first be assessed for relative expression of dystrophin by quantitative Western blots using constant amounts of cellular protein from each culture. The following is a short list of potential promoters. Others may be tested as they become available.

1. Human or canine dystrophin promoters.
2. Creatine kinase promoter.
3. Retrovirus LTR (Moloney MULV presently attached to cDNA construct, while MMTV LTR in pMAM.NEO.LUC would provide a hormone responsive promoter).

One concern about therapy in this disease will be whether a single transplanted cell or cDNA construct will be sufficient to provide any significant compensation for the dystrophin defects expressed by neighboring nuclei.(6) These questions will most certainly need to be addressed *in vivo* for an absolute answer. But, through the following experimental, approach some of these questions might also be preliminarily addressed *ex vivo*. Myoblasts from an affected male animal, which have been proven to express any of the above developed mini-gene constructs, will be allowed to take up fluorescent microspheres as intra-cellular markers(1). Then, these transgenic, marked cells will be co-cultured with myoblasts from a homozygous affected female which have not received a transgene. Cells will be permitted to fuse and form chimeric fibers, and then analyzed by immunocytochemistry for the presence of dystrophin and luciferase in the female cells. Antibodies to luciferase are available and this gene product will serve as an internal control. Those cells which do not have fluorescent microspheres and which do have dystrophin reactivity will provide evidence for the compensitory capacity of a particular experimental transgene. In

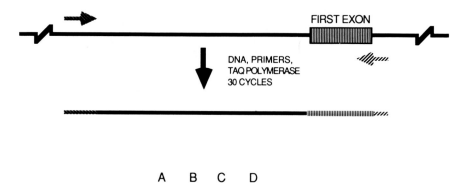

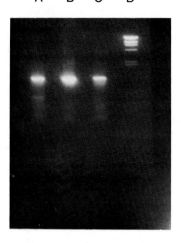

FIG. 2.   PCR Isolation of dystrophin promoters from human (a), normal canine female (b) and GRMD male (c).

collaboration with Manfred Beilharz, canine y-specific DNA probes will be used to confirm the male nuclei marked with the fluorescent microspheres (See Beilharz et al, this volume). Finally, exon seven-specifc assymetric PCR transcripts (see Sharp et al, this volume) can be prepared and used as *in situ* probes for the normal cDNA minigene transcripts in the cytoplasm of all cells. Luciferase transcripts may also be monitored in like manner. In summary, the relative success of the transfection will assessed by the following:

1. Fluorescent immunohistochemistry using dystrophin antibodies.
2. Y-specific repeat markers to mark male nuclei.
3. *In situ* localization of mRNA (exon 7 probe).

The full-length DYS cDNA has 13,976 base-pairs. Only 11,052 bases are required for coded protein (7). Thus, approximately 3400 bases of 3' untranslated may be tested to determine minimal requirements for expression of functional peptide. In fact, this region has been conserved through evolution from chickens, mice and dogs through humans (9). It could be possible to speculate that this region may have a functional domain required for compartmentalized expression of the dystrophin mRNA. This may be true when one considers that transplantation studies in *mdx* mice suggest that the expression of the normal dystrophin is compartmentalized around the normal nuclei contained in the chimeric syncitia (6). We will test this by substituting the 3' and/or 5' untranslated region from other muscle-specific mRNAs - creatine kinase, human beta-actin, and from human beta-globin. These genes have altogether different patterns of expression and sub-cellular localization of product and might represent potentially useful sequences to investigate this possible function in the dystrophin mRNA sequence. These segments will be substituted using key unique restriction sites in the human dystrophin sequence at the 5' end at position 351, and at the 3' untranslated region at position 11,316. Adapters will be synthesized to join any segments that do not have compatable cohesive ends. Analysis of dystrophin production will be the same as that in sections above. Thus, the following untranslated regions are in the process of inclusion into constructs.

1. CKM-M 3' and 5' untranslated regions.
2. Human skeletal actin 3' and 5' untranslated regions.
3. Globin 3' and 5' untranslated regions.

One bonus to doing studies of transfection of GRMD affected muscle cells in culture is the ability to combine the gene and cell therapeutic studies. In this, reverted GRMD cells expressing human dystrophin cDNA minigenes would be transplanted back into the autologous host. Thus, potential problems associated with heterologous transplantation would be by-passed. In addition, using the appropriate proven construct, the cells that would be injected would already be proven to producing enough dystrophin to complement a significant proportion of the chimeric fibers with which they might fuse. For this reason, biopsies will be taken from each affected animal by three months of age to be used for *ex vivo* transformation studies.

The demonstration of the direct injection of and expression of DNA constructs into living muscle tissue by Wolfe and co-workers (14) has provided an intriguing potential for gene therapy. This may now be tested in GRMD. Constructs which have demonstrated utility in culture would be readily testable in intact animal muscle. It is therefore critical to do the *ex vivo* studies to optimize the expression of dystrophin from a particular cDNA construct.

Finally, the original application and purpose of the design of the biolistic wand was to deliver DNA directly to living organisms. Some of these experiments have been successful in intact mouse liver surgically exposed.(13) Therefore, through surgical exposure, certain muscles in GRMD affected animals could be tested for expression of dystrophin produced by constructs shot into the muscle with the wand. Theoretically, the efficiency of the Biolistic delivery should be significantly higher than the direct injection methodology. But, these questions remain to be answered. Fortunately, we have a most appropriate model in the GRMD dog to test all of these approaches before going to human patients.

REFERENCES

1. Alameddine, H.S., Dehaupas, M., Fardeau, M.(1989): Regeneration of skeletal muscle fibers from autologous satellite cells multiplied in vitro. An experimental model for testing cultured cell myogenicity. *Muscle and Nerve,* 12:544-555.

2. Arahata, K., Ishiuri, S., Ishiguro, T., Tsukahara, T., Suhara, Y., Eguchi, C., Ishihara, T., Nonaka, I., Ozawa, E., Sugita, H. (1988): Immunostaining of skeletal and cardiac muscle surface membrane with antibody against Duchenne muscular dystrophy peptide. *Nature,* 333:861-866.

3. Dickson, G., Davies, K.E., Love, D., Walsh, F.S. (1991): Journal of Cellular Biochemistry (Supplement 15C): 37.

4. Myoblast Transfer Therapy, Advances in Experimental Medicine and Biology Volume 280, R.C. Griggs and G Karpati, eds. (1990): Plenum Press New York, N.Y.

5. Karpati, G. (1990): Immunological Aspects of Histoincompatible Myoblast Transfer into Non-tolerant Hosts, in Myoblast Transfer Therapy, Advances in Experimental Medicine and Biology Volume 280, R.C. Griggs and G Karpati, eds., Plenum Press, New York, N.Y., 31-34.

6. Karpati, G. (1990): The Principles and Practice of Myoblast transfer in Myoblast Transfer Therapy, Advances in Experimental Medicine and Biology Volume 280, R.C. Griggs and G Karpati, eds., Plenum Press, New York, N.Y., 69-74.

7. Koenig, M., Monaco, A.P., Kunkel, L.M. (1988): The complete sequence of dystrophin predicts a rod-shaped cytoskeletal protein. *Cell,* 53: 219-228.

8. Kornegay, J.N., Sharp, N.J.H., Bartlett, R.B., Van Camp, S.D., Burt, C.T., Hung, W.Y., Kwock, L., and Roses, A.D.(1990): Golden retriever muscular dystrophy: Monitoring for success. In Advances in Experimental Medicine and Biology, Eastwood, A.B., Griggs, R.C., Karpati, G., eds. (Plenum Publishing Corporation, NY) 280: 267-272.

9. Lewaire, C., Heilig, R. and Mandel, J.L. (1988): Nucleotide sequence of the chicken dystrophin cDNA. *Nucleic Acids Research,* 16:11815-11816.

10. Maniatis, T. (1990): Molecular Cloning 16.32-16.36, Cold Springs Harbor Press.

11. Partridge, T.A., Morgan, J.E., Coulton, G.R., Hoffman, E.P., Kunkel, L.M. (1989): Conversion of mdx myofibres from dystrophin-negative to - positive by injection of normal myoblasts. *Nature,* 337:176-179.

12. Sollazo, M., Zanetti, M. (1989): Simple and efficient electroporation of myeloma cells. *Focus,* 10;4:64-67.

13. Williams, R. S., Johnston, S.A., Riedy, M., DeVit, M.J., McElligott, S.G., Sanford, J.C. (1991): Introduction of foreign gees into tissues of living mice by DNA-coated microprojectiles. Proceedings of the National Academy of Sciences (USA) 88:2726-2730.
14. Wolff, J.A., Malone, R.W., Williams, P., Chong, W., Acsadi, G., Jani, A., Felgner, P.L. (1990): Direct gene transfer into mouse muscle *in vivo*. *Science*, 247:1465-1468.

DISCUSSION

Professor George Karpati:
Perhaps at this time it would be worthwhile to put on record as to what has so far been published in terms of in vitro transfection of a dystrophin construct. In that regard, we have to mention that in Tom Caskey's laboratory, Lee has successfully transfected COS cells with a full length mouse cDNA using a viral promoter and found expression, not a great expression but an acceptable expression, and the protein seemed to be localised to the surface membrane. This is now published. The second item is again from Caskey's laboratory and this concerns the creation of a transgenic mouse where the full length mouse dystrophin cDNA driven by a human MM creatine kinase promoter was introduced and dystrophin protein expressed in many muscle fibres but curiously in a checkerboard distribution instead of an equal expression in all muscle fibres. This work, to my knowledge, has not been published. Apparently a paper is coming out soon concerning direct gene transfer of dystrophin gene constructs in mdx mice showing expression of the protein in a relatively small number of muscle fibres comparable to the direct gene transfer of bacterial reporter genes reported earlier by Wolfe's group in Madison, Wisconsin.

Dr. Manfred W. Beilharz:
Richard, can you could comment on what the state of play is in terms of the isolation and culturing of the cells which you are going to attempt to manipulate.

Assist. Professor Richard J. Bartlett:
The source of material we are presently using is skeletal muscle in a biopsy at a young age. After we get over the crisis period of 10 days to 2 weeks which Dr Kornegay has described with these animals, the time period is usually about 2-3 months. These biopsies are cultured and frozen early so that we can have them as a resource for further transfection experiments. We are focusing on this primarily because we find that we should be able to do homologous transplantation at the same time as doing studies in the expression in these genes in muscle cells in culture.

Dr. Manfred W. Beilharz:
Are these cells now purified with a monoclonal antibody or are they still mixed cultures?

Professor Joe N. Kornegay:
I might be able to give you a bit of update on what I mentioned yesterday briefly. We have used the Walsh/Weston/Encam myomodel of the 5.18.11, we have used it both with magnetic affinity cells spores and fluorescent activated cell spores and in both cases we have been able to show that we get an enrichment of more or less the same log value as what was originally published by Webster. So, I

think, those two methods are the ones we are currently pursuing, obviously others have used clonal culture. George referred yesterday somewhat to their methodology, some of the problems that one would encounter with clonal culture in terms of adequacy of numbers of cells. That is why we have pursued the magnetic affinity cells sorting method and that's why the guy working with Terry Partridge is pursuing this.

Dr. Edna C. Hardeman:

I would like to insert a word of caution about juxtaposing cis-acting elements which normally would not be located in close proximity. An inexplicable and possible aberrant pattern of expression may result in transgenic mice. This has implications for the 'checkerboard' pattern of expression of a dystrophin construct observed in transgenics. A publication in Nature in 1985 (Swanson et al., 317: 363-366) demonstrated that a construct bearing the 5' portion of the metallothionein gene and the 3' portion of the growth hormone gene was expressed consistently in the brain. This represented a novel tissue-specific expression pattern which neither reflected normal metallothionein expression (liver) or growth hormone expression (pituitary). The point is that when genes are carved up and inserted into the mouse genome, the potential exists for an unexpected pattern of expression based on the unnatural proximity of sequences both within the introduced gene and with sequences near the site of insertion in the mouse DNA.

Assist. Professor Richard J. Bartlett:

To follow up on that, we are not going to try to create a transgene, we are trying to create something that is going to express in the target tissue. A tissue that likes to take up DNA anyway. We are trying experiments.utilizing episomal vectors for this We are not going to try to create something that is going to integrate, but be passed on to the syncitia in the muscles of affected dogs. We have less of a concern in the muscle grafts about trans-acting clonal problems as you describe because we are not trying to create a heritable change.

Professor George Karpati:

On the other hand, there is still this promising approach by Tony Monaco with the cloning of practically the entire 2.5 megabase mouse dystrophin gene and human as well. Thus, there is a possiblity of going for the whole thing.

Assist. Professor Richard J. Bartlett:

Yes, I still would refer back to the problems that Gert Son Van has had with that one high frequency deletion segment, I wonder if that intron is present. If you could eliminate that one intron in the construct you may have less problems because the yeast artifical chromosomes are unstable themselves. Just to propagate the constructs would create tremendous problems. Does he have one continuous construct or are they multiple pieces?

Professor George Karpati:

One, it was created from several pieces but it now is in one piece.

Assist. Professor Richard J. Bartlett:

The question you have to ask is how do you wish to go about introducing this large segment into cells? Do you want to try to create a lot of recombinational situations or do you want to just keep this as an episome to express freely. Then you have problems with the method of delivery of such a large segment. There is a lot of questions to be asked in view of the size of this 2.2 million base pair gene.

Dr. Terence A. Partridge:
Can I ask a question of the molecular biologists about the experiments of John Wolff on genes directly transfected into skeletal muscle fibres? How firm is the evidence that the genes being expressed in the fibres are episomal and not integrated. I know that the only copies of the construct detectable in the muscle were circular and therefore thought to be episomal, but are these the genes which are responsible for the very low level of patchy expression of protein.

Assist. Professor Richard J. Bartlett:
There are a number of viral vectors that we could select which have a strong promotor but do not integrate and remain episomal. Numerous laboratories have shown that anything inserted in these is expressed. These episomal elements are just as reactive to RNA polymerase as an integrated sequence, possibly more so.

Dr. Terence A. Partridge:
Yes, but the curious thing about the expressed constructs in Wolff's experiments is their persistence.

Assist. Professor Richard J. Bartlett:
This is not an actively dividing system. We have a muscle fibre which is differentiated. We can deliver something that's going to express the gene. We don't really have to have an integration event since these cells are not dividing.

Dr. Terence A. Partridge:
No, I was wondering whether there is any evidence that the genes that are expressed after direct transfection are those which can be detected as non-integrated copies or whether there is a low level of genomic integration.

Assist. Professor Richard J. Bartlett:
I do not have any evidence, I have no idea.

Professor George Karpati:
Henry, can you comment on the strength of the evidence for the claimed episomal transcription of the reporter genes after direct gene transfer into muscle by J Wolff's group?

Dr. Henry J Klamut:
It is my understanding that the evidence points to the conclusion that the bulk of the transfected DNA is not integrated but remains extra-chromosomal. The presence of plasmid DNA in Hirt supernates prepared from transfected muscle suggested that at least some of the transfected DNA is maintained extra-chromosomally for quite a long period of time. It is difficult, however, to estimate what proportion of the transfected DNA is maintained in plasmid form, and I don't think that they were able to absolutely discount the possibility of a low level of plasmid integration. My impression, however, is that most of the reporter gene activity was attributed to the persistence of extra-chromosomal plasmid DNA.

Dr. Terence A. Partridge:
I think that the experiments John McGeachie described yesterday show that turnover of normal muscle nuclei is very slow if it occurs at all.

Dr. Manfred W. Beilharz:
I would just like to add a point. At the Colorado meeting, there was some discussion of this work and the ability to reproduce this work in laboratories was raised.

Professor George Karpati:
Yes, I've shown pictures yesterday to indicate that it works to a very low efficiency. The maximum percent of fibres that expressed the reporter gene lacZ, in our case, the maximum number of b-galactosidase + cells was 4% in a rat soleus. It is quite variable; some animals don't get anything, some animals get 4% and the degree of expression is quite variable: Some fibres were extremely blue, others were barely blue.

Dr. Manfred W. Beilharz:
Maybe I misrepresented my question. I was not questioning the validity of the work as such, but what I was particularly referring to was the sustained episomal expression which was found out to 12 months.

Professor George Karpati:
Henry Klamut and Ron Worton were kind enough to let us have their dystrophin minigene construct which is being introduced into mdx mouse muscle by direct transfer. We do not have many results but I can tell you that it is promising to the same extent as the bacterial reporter genes. That is to say, there is a dismally low efficiency of expression but it is still there.

Assist. Professor Richard J. Bartlett:
I would like to follow up on Terry's question. Mitochondrial DNA should separate from analytical centrifuge.

Dr. Terence A. Partridge:
Yes, they did demonstrate that they could only extract the constructs in an episomal form, but given that expression is very low anyway. I am not sure that it has been demonstrated that the expressed gene is this episomal form.

Assist. Professor Richard J. Bartlett:
If you do the Hurt supernatant procedure you should isolate super coiled episomes similar to isolation of mitochondrial DNA.

Dr. Terence A. Partridge:
In the initial paper their conclusion was that they could not exclude integration at a low level and as expression occurs at a low level, it is possible that the expressed sequences are rare integrated copies.

Assist. Professor Richard J. Bartlett:
You certainly would not see a neomyosin resistance gene normally in the genome of the dogs. If that shows up in the genomic sequences as tested by PCR, you can prove that the clone has integrated.

Dr. Terence A. Partridge:
So you would use PCR?

Assist. Professor Richard J. Bartlett:
Yes.

Professor Allen D. Roses:
I would like to just switch here a second and maybe put some attention to the three prime region that seems to be a large unique region with no apparent purpose. It is my understanding that in some of the other muscles with specific genes like C-1T, this type of 3 prime sequence also exists and potential function for such a sequence might be the coordinated expression, similar to the question that I asked Dr. Hardeman yesterday, how does this thing happen of several of these genes in a coordinated manner. If that is the case then the inclusion of such a sequence in the construct may be critical to us.

Dr. Henry J Klamut:
I would like to expand a little on Dr Roses' comment about including non-coding regulatory domains within a minigene construct. We have identified a muscle-specific enhancer within muscle intron 1 and also have some preliminary evidence of the presence of muscle-specific regulatory sequences within the 3' untranslated region. While it is not as yet clear what the precise role of these regions is in regulating DMD gene transcription, it may prove to be advantageous and/or necessary to include these and potentially other as yet unidentified transcriptional regulatory domains in order to achieve appropriate patterns of tissue and development stage-specific expression of a DMD minigene in vivo. Tight controls on the expression of a DMD minigene may also allow for more systemic approaches to the introduction of a minigene construct to patient tissues.

DUCHENNE MUSCULAR DYSTROPHY: Animal Models
and Genetic Manipulation, edited by Byron A. Kakulas,
John McC. Howell, and Allen D. Roses.
Raven Press, Ltd., New York © 1992.

23

The Interaction Between Sperm Cells and Exogenous DNA: Factors Controlling DNA Uptake

M. Lavitrano[#], V. Lulli[*], B. Maione[#], S. Sperandio[*], D. French[#],
L. Frati[#*], M. Francolini[§], C. Lora Lamia [§], F. Cotelli [§], C. Spadafora[#*]

[#] Department of Experimental Medicine, Institute of General Pathology,
University "La Sapienza", Rome, Italy.
[*] Institute of Biomedical Technology, CNR. Via G.B. Morgagni 30/E
Rome, Italy.
[§] Department of Biology, University of Milan, Milan, Italy.

INTRODUCTION

The finding that epididymal mouse sperm cells spontaneously take up exogenous DNA, prompted the use of spermatozoa as vectors for transferring foreign DNA into eggs at fertilization. Such fertilization generated transgenic mice (1). Recent results of other groups have now shown that permeability to foreign DNA is not restricted to mice spermatozoa but is a general feature of many different species as for instance echinoid (2), insect (3), fish (4), bird (4) and several mammals (5-7). Moreover preliminary reports have appeared of successful experiments of sperm mediated gene transfer conducted by ourselves in pigs (8) and by others in mice at embryonic (9) and adult (10,11) stages, in bovine (11,12), sea urchin (2), insect (13) and bird (14), confirming and extending our earlier results.

However several groups have made unsuccessful attempts to obtain sperm mediated DNA transfer into mouse embryos (15). It was pointed out that unidentified parameters may play key roles in the sperm mediated DNA transfer process.

The interaction between sperm cells and exogenous DNA is the first, and probably most critical step of the whole process leading to the generation of transgenic animals. Nothing is known about the unexpected, spontaneous capacity of spermatozoa to bind nucleic acids; the molecular basis of such mechanism have been studied. We believe that the understanding of such mechanisms is of paramount importance.

Here we report that exogenous DNA specifically binds to the posterior half of the sperm heads, corresponding to the nuclear area, both in mouse and bovine spermatozoa. Autoradiographic ultrastructural analysis would suggest that exogenous DNA is localized at two preferential levels in this area: i) underneath the plasma membrane, between the plasma and the nuclear membrane (about 80% of the labelled cells) and ii) within the nucleus (about 20% of the labelled cells). Association between sperm cells and exogenous DNA occurs through interactions with DNA binding proteins of 35KD located at the nuclear level. Moreover, we have identified in the ejaculated semen a second factor, a glycoprotein, with a very high binding affinity for the 35KD "receptor", which virtually abolish any DNA binding to spermatozoa. A mechanism modulating, through specific proteins factors, sperm permeability to exogenous DNA is now emerging from our results.

PREPARATION OF SPERM CELLS, UPTAKE OF DNA AND AUTORADIOGRAPHY

Sperm cells were prepared from mouse cauda epididymis as described (1). Sperm cells were routinely suspended at a concentration of about 5×10^6/ml in fertilization medium (FM) (1), mixed with about 500 ng/ml of linearized end-labelled DNA plasmid and incubated at 37°C in 5% CO_2 in air. Bovine sperms cells were obtained from ejaculates and diluted in Talp Medium (16) at a concentration of 10^7 cells/ml. Routinely 10^6 sperm cells, incubated with end-labelled DNA, were centrifuged at 9000 rpm for 4 min, suspended and smeared on glass slides. A portion of the labelled cells were counted to determine the amount of labelled DNA that was taken up, others were treated for autoradiography in the following way: sperm cells were smeared on glass slides and fixed for 10 min at room temperature in a 3:1 (vol/vol) mixture of ethanol/acetic acid and then air dried. Autoradiography were performed using Ilford K5 emulsion (17). The slides were developed after three days of exposure. Each slide contained about 5×10^5 sperm cells. Specific activity of H^3 end-labelled DNA was about 10^6 cpm/μg. All experiments were performed using the 7 Kb pCH110 plasmid DNA linearized with Hind III.

ULTRASTRUCTURAL AUTORADIOGRAPHY

After the incubation with labelled DNA, sperm were fixed in 3% glutaraldehyde buffered with 0,1M cacodylate buffer pH 7.4. After at least three hours at 4°C the spermatozoa were centrifuged at 9,000 rpm for 4 min, rinsed in cacodylate buffer, postfixed in 1% OsO_4 and dehydrated in a series of ethanol. Epon embedded material was sectioned using a Reichart Ultracut E. Ultrathin sections mounted on gold grids previously coated with a formvar film backed by a thin carbon layer, were stained with uranyl acetate and lead citrate, coated with a carbon film and covered with Ilford L4 emulsion (18). Grids were exposed in the dark at 4°C for 8 days, autoradiographs were then developed with Microdol X, fixed with Unifix (Kodak) and examined in a JEOL 100 SX electron microscope.

PREPARATION OF SEMINAL FLUID AND DNA UPTAKE INHIBITION

Seminal fluid was prepared by subsequent centrifugations of human semen. Sperm cells were sedimented at 700 g for 10 min. Supernatant was further centrifuged for 1 min at 12,000 g in a microfuge. Increasing volumes of seminal fluid were mixed with epididymal sperm cells to give a volume of 200 µl containing 10^6 sperm cells and incubated for 30 min at 37°C. Labelled DNA (100 ng/200 µl) was then added for an additional 30 min. Washing and counting were as already described.

SPERM CELLS FRACTIONATION, EXTRACTION OF TOTAL PROTEINS, SOUTH/WESTERN ANALYSIS AND FILTER HYBRIDIZATION

Sperm heads were separated from tails by homogenizing sperm cells in a buffer containing 0.25M sucrose, 50mM Tris pH 7.5, 5mM $MgCl_2$, 3% Triton and washed twice by subsequent centrifugations with the same buffer without Triton. The final pellet was suspended in the same buffer without Triton, loaded in a cushion containing 2M sucrose, 50mM Tris pH 7.5, 5 mM $MgCl_2$ and centrifuged for 10 min at 14,000 g. Sperm heads were pelleted and tails were retained at the interface. Sperm cells were suspended in Laemmli buffer and viscosity was reduced by short sonication pulses.

Proteins were routinely fractioned in 8x6 cm Acrylamide SDS minigel (19). South/Western analysis were performed by electroblotting SDS Acrylamide gel for 12-16 hours on nitrocellulose filters (Hybond-C, Amersham) in a buffer containing 20% Methanol, 0.3% Tris and 1.44% Glycine. Filters were then incubated for at least 1 hour at room temperature in 10mM Tris HCl pH8, 15mM $Mg(CH_3COOH)_2$, 7mM KCl, 10 mM ßmercaptoethanol, 0.1mM EDTA and 1x Denhardt's solution. Filters were then individually sealed in plastic bags and pre-hybridized at 25°C for 2 hours in 3 to 5 ml of 50mM Tris HCl pH 8, 2mM ßmercaptoethanol, 25mM NaCl, 1mM EDTA.

When required, seminal fluid was added to the pre-hybridization medium. Plastic bags were then opened and about 10^5 cpm/ml of the end-labelled pCH110 plasmid DNA probe were added. Hybridization was allowed for 2 additional hours at 25°C. After hybridization, filters were washed for 15 min at room temperature in hybridization buffer, air dried and exposed.

ASSOCIATION OF EXOGENOUS DNA WITH SPERM CELLS

Mature, intact and mobile sperm cells incubated with DNA rapidly took up the nucleic acid molecules. Autoradiographic analysis under light microscope of mouse epididymal sperm cells and of ejaculated, washed bull spermatozoa showed that, in both cases, the DNA was specifically concentrated in the posterior part of the sperm head in correspondence to the nuclear area. No

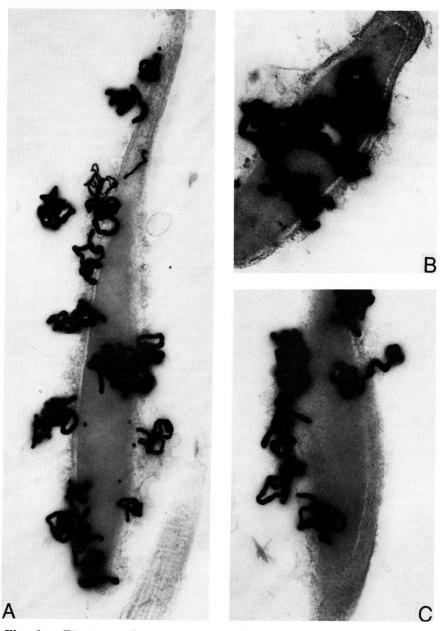

Fig. 1.   Electron microscope autoradiography:

2×10^6 mouse spermatozoa were incubated with 100ng of H3 end-labelled plasmid DNA for 30 min at 37°C and then fixed with 3% glutaraldehyde buffered with cacodylate 0.1 M pH 7.4.   (A) Longitudinal ultrathin section (x19800). (B) Tangential section (x20250). (C) Tangential section (x24750).

appreciable amounts of labelled DNA were interacting with the acrosoma nor with the tail, and this distribution of DNA was particularly sharp in bovine spermatozoa (B). It has to be stressed that ejaculated spermatozoa were only accessible to foreign DNA, if thoroughly washed and deprived of seminal fluid.

In order to answer the question is the DNA internalized inside the spermatozoa or doesit remain on the outside, ultrastructural autoradiographic analysis was performed on thin sections of sperm cells using the electron microscope. Fig. 1, panels A, B and C shows examples representative of the distribution of exogenous DNA in the sperm head. Exogenous DNA seems to have two preferential localizations: a predominant one, accounting for about 80% of the incorporated labelling, is underneath the plasma membrane, more specifically between the plasma and the nuclear membrane (Fig. 1 panels A, C) and a minor one, accounting for about 15-20%, is totally within the nucleus and tracks are found inside the nucleus (Fig. 1 panel B). The two localizations can coexist in the same sperm cell, as in panel. Regardless of the fact that the labelled DNA is within the nucleus or peripherally distributed, the tracks are always in the post acrosomal region of the sperm head. These results show that nuclear internalization of exogenous DNA can spontaneously occur.

A 35 KD PROTEIN OF THE SPERM HEAD IS A POTENTIAL SUBSTRATE FOR THE BINDING WITH EXOGENOUS DNA

Sperm cells have been observed to interact not only with the DNA but also with other negatively charged macromolecules (20,21). The relevant role of the ionic charge suggested that a key step may be the interaction of such molecules with a "substrate" located on the sperm head. The existence of a substrate, probably a protein, on the sperm heads where negative charged molecules may bind, is therefore an obvious implication. South\Western blot analysis was used to search for such a substrate. Total proteins were extracted from sperm heads, fractionated on SDS polyacrylamide gels, electroblotted on nitrocellulose filters and finally hybridized with P^{32} end-labelled plasmid DNA probes. Our aim was to detect one or more proteins, electrophoretically distinguishable from protamines, able to bind DNA.

Fig. 2 lanes 1,2 and 3, shows two distinct hybridization signals: a signal below 20 KD corresponding, as expected, to the hybridization with the protamines and a second one corresponding to a protein of approximately 35 KD. Curiously, these proteins have a very sharp dose response since DNA hybridization occured only above a threshold concentration (lanes 1-3) but not below (lanes 4-7). In contrast keeping constant the amount of proteins of the filters, and varying the amount of the DNA probe, the intensity of the hybridization signal increased linearly (Fig. 3). Binding of exogenous DNA with the 35 KD proteins may explain its interaction with sperm heads.

PERMEABILITY OF SPERM CELLS TO FOREIGN DNA IS BLOCKED BY A FACTOR PRESENT IN THE SEMINAL FLUID

Fig. 1, panel B, shows that ejaculated, washed mouse spermatozoa was able to take up very efficiently exogenous DNA. However if sperm cells are challenged with DNA in the presence of the seminal fluid the ability to capture

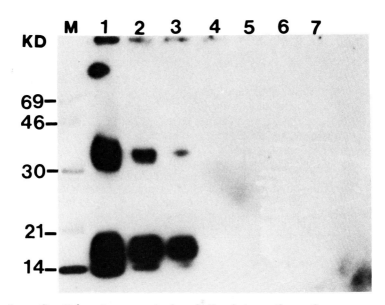

Fig 2. South/western analysis of the interaction of mouse sperm head proteins with end-labelled pCH110 DNA:

Increasing amounts of sperm head proteins were fractionated by electrophoresis 15% polyacrylamide gel and electroblotted on nitrocellulose filter as described. The filter was pre-hybridized at 25°C for two hours with P^{32} end-labelled pCH110 (10^5 cpm/ml) at 25°C. Lane 1: 3.3 µg, 2: 1.65 µg, 3: 1 µg, 4: 0.65 µg, 5: 0.5 µg, 6: 0.33 µg, 7: 0.165 µg. Lane M contains protein size markers and numbers on the left indicate kilo Daltons.

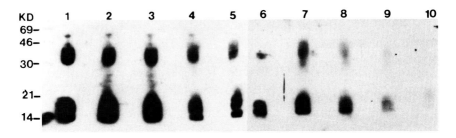

Fig. 3. South/Western blots hybridization with increasing amounts of DNA probe:

Each lane contains 3 µg of proteins. Filters were hybridized, under identical experimental conditions, with increasing amounts of P^{32} end-labelled DNA. Lane 1: 166000 cpm/ml, 2: 133000, 3: 100000, 4: 66000, 5: 33000, 6: 33000, 7: 25000, 8: 16000, 9: 8000, 10: 3500.

foreign DNA molecules was lost. Removal of seminal plasma restored sperm permeability (not shown).

The presence of a factor blocking sperm permeability in seminal fluid was confirmed in the experiment shown in Fig. 4. Aliquots of 10^6 mouse spermatozoa were first incubated with increasing volumes of seminal fluid (from human or bovine origin) and then with end-labelled DNA. The increased amount of seminal fluids paralleled the decrease ability of sperm cells to take up the DNA. 25-30 µl of seminal fluids virtually blocked 10^6 sperm cells to bind exogenous DNA in a heterologous system. This factor present in the seminal fluid interfered with the binding of the 35 KD protein with the DNA.

Fig. 5 shows that small amounts of seminal fluid added in the hybridization mixture, abolished the hybridization of the 35 KD protein with labelled DNA. Also the interaction with protamines was considerably reduced although with a lower efficiency. We have identified and purified the blocking factor and its characterization is in progress (see Discussion).

DISCUSSION

In good agreement with the pioneering observation of Brackett et al. (22) on rabbit spermatozoa is our finding that mouse sperm cells can act as vectors transferring exogenous DNA into eggs at fertilization thereby causing a genetic transformation of the resulting offsprings which is then stably inherited by the progeny (1).

The importance of such a process leading to the generation of transgenic animals is obvious, both for biotechnological purposes and also for its evolutionary implications, provided that a similar event may occur spontaneously in nature.

A full understanding of the molecular basis of the interaction between exogenous DNA and sperm cells, of the internalization pathway inside the sperm head and the identification of factors playing a role in such process is imperative. Autoradiographic analysis using light and electron microscopy revealed that the interaction with the DNA specifically restricted to the post-acrosomal region of the sperm head. No appreciable amounts of labelled DNA were detected on the acrosome area nor on the tail. No difference in the pattern of DNA distribution was observed comparing mouse and bovine or epididymal and ejaculated spermatozoa. A qualitative removal of the seminal fluid was however an essential step in order to obtain sperm permeability to foreign DNA. Autoradiographic ultrastructural analysis on thin sections showed two preferential distributions of exogenous DNA: i) underneath the plasma membrane, namely between the plasma and the nuclear membrane, and ii) inside the nucleus. The first localization was the most frequent and abundant, accounting for about 80% of the sperm incorporated labelled DNA while about 15-20% of the DNA was found inside the nucleus.

These results prove that part of the sperm cells allowed free access to exogenous DNA through the plasma and nuclear membranes. This confirms our earlier observation (17) which showed that pancreatic DNase mixed with intact, motile spermatozoa penetrated into the nucleus degrading the sperm chromosomal DNA. We are, so far, not able to explain why all the DNA easily passes through the plasma membrane, while only 15-20% passes the nuclear one reaching the inside of the nucleus.

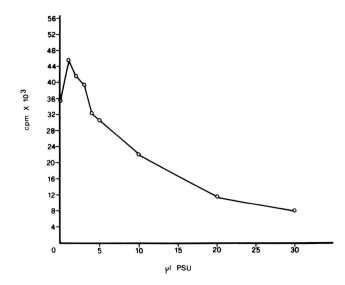

Fig. 4. Inhibition of DNA uptake by mouse sperm cells with increasing amounts of human seminal fluids:

Epididymal mouse sperm cells at a concentration of 10^6/ml, were incubated with increasing volumes of human seminal fluid depleted of its own cells for 30 min at 37°C in 5%CO_2 in air. 100 ng. of end-labelled plasmid DNA were then added for an additional 30 min to each sample. Sperm cells were then washed and counted as described.

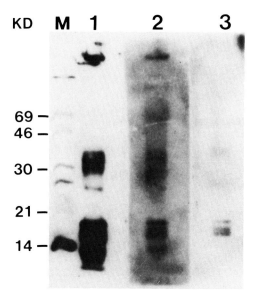

We believe that only spermatozoa carrying exogenous DNA which has been internalized into the nucleus is potentially able to generate transgenic offspring. The DNA excluded from the nucleus is most probably carried into the zygote but is not integrated into the genome and is progressively diluted during the embryonic differentiation. On these grounds we can explain the results by Hochi et al.(9) who reported the achievement of 80-100% transgenic mouse embryos, while no transgenic adults were obtained. Possibly, under their experimental condition most of the exogenous DNA was not internalized into the nucleus.

The existance on the sperm head of a 35 KD DNA binding protein could be the reason of the spontaneous capacity of sperm cells to capture foreign DNA. This protein has been purified and its characterization is in progress. Preliminary data show that electrophoretically similar proteins can be extracted in the same manner from human, bovine and echinoid spermatozoa (not shown). The function of this protein *in vivo* is not clear, but the high affinity of sperm heads for exogenous DNA make each fertilization a potentially risky event for the genetic identity of the progeny. Such danger is abolished, or very much reduced, when fertilization occurs naturally under normal conditions, because the seminal plasma contains a factor that protects spermatozoa, virtually avoiding undesired intrusions. Preincubation of mouse epididymal sperm cells with small volumes of seminal fluid of heterologous origin abolished sperm permeability blocking penetration of foreign DNA (Fig. 4). The factor present in the seminal fluid may exert the inhibitory effect by interfering in the interaction between the 35 KD protein on the sperm head and the exogenous DNA (Fig.5). This factor from echinoid spermatozoa has been purified and partially characterized (23). It is a glycoprotein of about 37 KD, present in the seminal fluid of mammals and on spermatozoa of invertebrates. It exerts a very powerful inhibitory effect on sperm permeability.

Sperm/DNA interaction is the first event and probably the most critical step of the process leading to the generation of transgenic animals. This phenomenon is not simply due to a passive internalization of DNA through membrane "pores" but is a rather complex mechanism controlled by specific protein factors. A full understanding of this mechanism is extremely important not only for biotechnological purposes but also for possible evolutionary implications.

Fig. 5.   **Effect of human seminal fluid on sperm protein/ DNA interaction:**

South/Western blotted filter was prehybridized in 3 ml hybridization buffer containing increasing volume of human seminal fluid for two hours at 25°C, then 10^5 cpm/ml of P^{32} end-labelled pCH110 were added and the hybridization allowed for an additional two hours at 25°C. Filters were then washed at room temperature and exposed. Lane 1, filter prehybridized without seminal fluid; lane 2 and 3, filters prehybridized with 20 µl and 50 µl, respectively of human seminal fluid. Slot M contains protein size marker.

ACKNOWLEDGEMENTS

We thank Dr. Ignacio J. Ansotegui for helpful cooperation and Ms. Clara Valli and Mr. Graziano Bonelli for skilful technical assistance.

This work was supported by the Associazione Italiana Allevatori in the frame of the Project Nuove Biotecnologie Riproduttive of the Ministry of Agriculature D.M. No. 15262 and by a grant to C.S. Prof. CNR Progetto Finalizzato Ingegneria Genetica.

REFERENCES

1. Lavitrano, M., Camaioni, A., Fazio,V., Dolci, S., Farace, M.G., Spadafora, C. (1989): Sperm cells as vectors for introducing foreign DNA into eggs: genetic transformation of mice. *Cell*, 57: 717-723.
2. Arezzo, F. (1989): Sea urchin sperm as vector for foreign genetic information. *Cell. Biol. Int. Rep.*, 13:391-404.
3. Atkinson, P.W., Hines, E.R., Beaton, S., Matthaei, K.I., Reed, K.C., Bradley, M.P. (1991): Association of exogenous DNA with cattle and insect spermatozoa in vitro. *Molec. Reprod. and Develop.*, 29:1-5.
4. Castro, F.O., Hernandez, O., De Armas, R., Herrera, L., de la Fuente, J.(1991): Introduction of foreign DNA into the spermatozoa of farm animals. *Theriogenology*, 34:1099-1110.
5. Horan, R., Powell, R., McQuaid, S., Gannon, F. Houghton, J.A. (1991): The association of foreign DNA with porcine spermatozoa. *Arch of Andr.*, 26:83-92.
6. Gagnè, M.P., Pothier, F., Sirard, M.A. (1991): Electroporation of bovine spermatozoa to carry foreign DNA in oocytes. *Molec. Reprod. and Develop.*, 29:6-15.
7. Clausen, P.A., Iyer, A.P., Zaneveld, L.J.D., Polakoski, K.L., Waller, D.P, Drisdell, R. (1991): DNA uptake by mammalian spermatozoa. 16th Annal Meeting An. Soc. Andrology, J. of Andrology Suppl. to Vol. 12, ab 1.
8. Gandolfi, F., Lavitrano, M., Camaioni, A., Spadafora, C., Siracusa, G. Lauria, A. (1989): The use of sperm mediated gene transfer for the generation of transgenic pigs. *J. Reprod. Fert.*, Abstract Ser No 4, p. 21.
9. Hochi, S., Ninomiya, T., Mizuno, A., Honma, M., Yuki, A. (1990): Fate of exogenous DNA carried into mouse eggs by spermatozoa. *Animal Biotechnology*, 1:25-30.
10. Bachiller, D., Dotti, C., Schellander, K., Rutheur, U. (1990): Investigation of the use of sperm as vehicle for the introduction of exogenous DNA into oocytes. Cold Spring Harbor Symposium 178.
11. De La Fuente, J., Castro, F.O., Hernandez, O., Guillen, I., Ullver, C., Solano, R., Milanes, C., Aguilar, A., Cleonart, R., Martinez, R., Perez, A., De Armas, R., Herrera, L., Limonta, J., Cabrera, E., Herrera, F.(1991): Sperm mediated foreign DNA experiments in different species. *Biotech. USA*, in press.
12. Perez, A., Solano, R., Castro, R., Leonart, R., De Armas, R., Martinez, R., Aguilar, A., Herrera, L., De La Fuente, J.(1991): Sperm cells mediated gene transfer in cattle. *Biotecnologia Aplicada*, 8:90-94.

13. Milne, C.P., Elschen, F.A., Collis, J.E., Jensen, T.L. (1989): Preliminary evidence for honey bee sperm mediated DNA tranfer. International Symposium on Molecular Insects Science

14. Feinsod, A., Frumkin, A., Rangini, Z., Revel, E., Yarus, S., Ben-Yehuda, A., Gruenbaum, Y.(1990): Chicken homeogenes expressed during gastrulation and the generation of trangenic chicken. EMBO-EMBL Symposium 1990, "The Molecular Biology of Vertebrate development".

15. Brinster, R.L., Sandgren, E.P., Behringer, R.R., Palmiter, R.D. (1989): No simple solution for making trangenic mice. *Cell,* 59: 239.

16. Ball, G.D., Leibfried, M.L., Lenz, R.W., Ax, R.L., Bavister, B.D., First, N.L. (1983): Factors affecting successful *in vitro* fertilization of bovine follicular oocytes. *Biol. Reprod.,* 28: 717-725.

17. Lavitrano, M., French, D., Camaioni, A., Zani, M., Mariani-Costantini, R., Frati, L., Spadafora, C. (1991): Uptake of foreign DNA by sperm cells. Factors affecting sperm permeability. VI International Congress on Spermatology. Comparative Spermatology 20 years after. In press.

18. Fakan, S. Fakan, J. (1987): Autoradiography of spread molecular complexes. in "Electron microscopy in molecular biology, a practical approach" p. 201-214. J. Sommerville and U. Scheer Eds. IRL Press.

19. Laemmli, U.K. (1970): Cleavage of structural proteins during assembly at the head of bacteriophage T4. *Nature,* (Lond.). 227:680-682.

20. Lavitrano, M., French, D,. Zani, M., Frati, L. Spadafora, C. (1991): Uptake of exogenous DNA by mammalian spermatozoa. Interaction between sperm cells and foreign DNA. International Symposium on Biotechnology of cell regulation. In press.

21. Lavitrano, M., French, D., Camaioni, A., Zani, M., Frati, L. Spadafora, C.(1991): The interaction between exogenous DNA and sperm cells. *Molec. Reprod. and Devel.*

22. Brackett, B.G., Baranskza, W., Sawiicki, W., Koprosky, H.(1971): Uptake of heterologous genome by mammalian spermatozoa and its tranfer to ova through fertilization. *Proc. Nat. Acad. Sci. USA.,* 68: 353-357.

23. Lavitrano, M., Frati, L., Spadafora, C., Poltronieri, P., Nfuien, L., Mariotto, S., Suzuki, H., Libonati, M. (1991): The interaction of sperm cells with exogenous DNA. Partial purification and characterization of a protein factor controlling sperm permeability. Proteine '91; VI Congresso Nazionale. P3/106,141.

GENERAL DISCUSSION

All Participants

Leaders: Allen D. Roses and Nigel G. Laing

Professor Allen D. Roses:
Nigel and I talked about this three days ago and I asked him if he would try to be eloquent to perhaps summarise some of the points that came up. A few things that happened in discussions which have been somewhat private and off the beaten track. The most recent during the last coffee break about the risk benefit ratios and how do you stop the onslaught of patients asking for minigenes and things like that. Some scientific issues I think that are important to consider and there is one that really bothers me and that is the notion of a revertent fibre. Stepping back from it I find the idea that there is a genetically revertant fibre using the gene that is suppose to be there when it isn't in the animal, somewhat strange to say the least and wonder in the course of some of the discussion that comes up whether or not Prof. Sugita's antibody really does answer that question in that what we might see early on these so called revertant fibres in the expression of a different gene that is only seen during an embryological period or a short period of time. I'd like somebody if possible in the course of this discussion to perhaps speak to what a revertant fibre really is and what they expect in the mechanism of such a fibre, it existing seems to be something like immunology when you can't explain something that you created, a new cell type or a new type of antibody and then its clear to everybody and that the revertant is a nice word and it implies function, but I don't understand it and I wonder if anybody has a better insight. I'm going to ask Nigel to go over some of his things then we can really get into a general discussion about some of these issues.

Dr. Nigel G. Laing:
I too wish to raise the subject of revertant fibres later, but I thought perhaps we should first consider the reason that we are here. The aim of the meeting as far as I am concerned is to reduce the burden of Duchenne and Becker dystrophy on society. That means the burden on the patients themselves, their families and society as a whole. I state my own position clearly here. I believe that prevention is better than cure and prevention in these terms means making sure that as few boys as possible are going to require the cure, whatever the cure turns out to be. The way of doing that at present is ascertaining families, providing accurate carrier status determination and prenatal diagnosis; allowing couples the opportunity to have normal boys, allowing them to make the decision as to whether they want affected boys or not. The best therapy for Duchenne muscular dystrophy may well be prevention. One way of reducing the number of affected boys is to perform infant screening and this was mentioned in passing by Professor Karpati but it is not something that is widely discussed. I know that there are ethical problems involved with infant screening, but I think that at least some effort needs to be put towards coping with those ethical problems and I believe that the West German model of voluntary infant screening is a model that other societies around the world could well take up. At the meeting two and a half years ago I said that it was a pity that you have to have an affected boy before

you realize that you have a family. In many cases one or two previous opportunities of identifying a family were missed. These opportunities were the mother and perhaps the grandmother of the affected boy who frequently now are recognised as carriers and could perhaps have been detected by screening. I think that some effort, if we are serious about reducing the burden of these diseases, should be put towards identifying ways of detecting those mothers and grandmothers. The advantage of this work is that it is known technology, it is not inventing new techniques.

Professor Byron A. Kakulas:

Jack Goldblatt is a medical geneticist for the metropolitan region in Western Australia and perhaps, as this seems to be a question more in line with counselling and prevention through those efforts, Jack might like to respond to Nigel's question?

Dr. Jack Goldblatt

There is no question that we have reached an era where we can do carrier screening and primary prevention. Certainly its almost technically possible in the one disease where it will probably be done first at a DNA level which will be cystic fibrosis. The major problems to be overcome are not the technical ones, as Nigel said. Really with Health Departments prioritizing this and society accepting it and the education side of it which has always been the problem with a classic example being sickle cell anaemia carrier screen in America. If it is done properly it works very well and is a very good screen, it is voluntary and confidential and people accept. But you do need a tremendous amount of public education and costs before you can jump in and do the technical side of it. The technical side is routine. It is not a problem. In parts of the world at the moment where there are great constraints on spending on health, it is a difficult area to get into and I really can't say more about looking at it from the Duchenne side, but as you said it has been shown to work in parts of the world, but we certainly have not thought of that as a priority to get up here, I don't know what other views are from other parts of the world.

Professor Byron A. Kakulas:

Is there some aspect of this also which is relevant to the eventual curative therapy? That is the identification of the sporadic case very early on in infancy.

Dr. Nigel G. Laing:

Professor Karpati also talked about that, but again it is an area where perhaps the ethical questions are unanswered. The other question I asked two years ago was when and if we would stop performing prenatal diagnosis, because we could say to the parents "we can cure the boys". This meeting is about providing a cure for Duchenne and Becker dystrophy. At the meeting two years ago, people were daunted by the logistics of producing enough myoblasts to attempt the therapy in boys. Perhaps at this point we should express our congratulations to Professor Karpati, and the other MDA sponsored labs who are investigating myoblast transfer in humans, on what has been achieved in such a relatively short period. The question of how many years or decades you work with animal models, how many Duchenne boys you are going to wait through while working with animal models before trying again in humans, is problematical. If human trials are stopped now, is their any consensus of how long animal trials will proceed before work is recommenced in humans?

Professor Allen D. Roses:
I don't think that we make that policy. George, in his experiments with the boys has uncovered some technical problems. Some of these technical problems can be worked out in animals. Other things are going to be done in animals. As soon as something appears to work it isn't going to be scientists sitting around the room deciding about how it is going to be administered. The AIDS story and the current situation with Duchenne dystrophy boys flocking to centres for myoblast transfer in the United States without good knowledge how it works, that type of public pressure for doing something fast will be there and I think then you are talking about essentially risks and benefits and those things go together when we talk about these things. We can wax poetic about the risks of putting a minigene in some sort of factor into a dog and then into a human or through a mouse, dog then a human, but the risks are relative to the benefit and I would say to you that a threat of cancer causing problems that appears to be a risk may not actually be a risk that exceeds the benefit that a child might have in getting up and walking around. That might be an acceptable risk by some people in some circumstances. So we talk about risks of doing human experiments. It is a risk/benefit ratio that is important. Now the risk of doing any human experiment where the benefit is zero is infinity. On the other hand even the slightest benefit then changes that ratio and makes the risk relative and I think its really too early to say, but I don't think anybody in this room or any other room of professionals is going to hold back the tide of people wanting treatment if you can show that it works.

Dr. Terence A. Partridge:
I would like to make the comment that there is a good example of how this sort of thing works and that is bone marrow transplantation. There has not been a sudden jump or a cut off of work on animals and a start of human experiments. Progress has been made by initial work on experimental animals and the lessons have been transferred to the human situation. I suspect that if myoblast transfer or gene therapy is to be made to work it will follow the same sort of course.

Dr. Nigel G. Laing:
Now perhaps is the point to discuss the "revertant" fibres. Some of the Duchenne muscular dystrophy fibres appear to have cured themselves and those are the revertant fibres. I think studying the molecular biology of those revertant fibres is something that should be going ahead. I think in the past few days that we have discussed it, as Allen says, out of the meeting room. There are various ways in which revertant fibre molecular biology could be studied. Two ways are: 1) examining clones of myoblasts grown from Duchenne boys, picking dystrophin positive clones and looking at their molecular biology; 2) trying to scrape the positive fibres off slides and examining them by polymerase chain reaction. I would be interested to know how much has been done on these fibres already.

Professor George Karpati:
Eric Shoubridge in our group has been interested in this issue and we thought that the mdx mouse was the best model to approach it because it has a rather simple single base mutation. His approach has been to dissect these "revertants" from thick frozen sections and look for the wild-type allele and the mutated allele using PCR products of the exon where the mutation is. The main aim is to establish if the stop codon has been converted into a translatable codon (and there are 9 possibilities of that) or deleted if the stop codon persists, but it is still translated by

a suppressor tRNA. The limiting factor in this approach is that in a "revertant" segment there are probably both mutated and "reverted" copies.

Dr. Barry J. Cooper:
I might add that the clonal growth of myoblasts in the dog would be possible. We have been able to clone pure populations of canine myoblasts and I do not think that has been done in the mouse. It has also been done in humans so that approach would be possible. The problem is, in the dog, that the incidence of revertant fibres is only probably one in a thousand or not much more than that in most cases, so you would have to screen a lot of clones before you had something to work with. There is another aspect of revertant fibres I think that we need to be concerned about. That is that it's clear if you look at muscles of dystrophic dogs, and I think that its the same in the mouse and probably the same in the human, as the animals become older you can find more of these fibres usually accounted for by the fact that they occur in small clusters which one assumes are clones. The thing that bothers me about it is that they never seem to migrate away from the site at which they occur, so they always remain very localised in one spot. I think a similar phenomenon occurs in manifesting human carriers, where one can see populations of myofibres that express dystrophin adjacent to what are almost fascicles that lack dystrophin, and there seems to be no re-population of the dystrophic population by the functional population. This, I think, is something that we need to be concerned about and need to address to try to increase our chances of being able to carry out therapy by myoblast transfer,or by the transfer of cells that have been treated by gene therapeutic methods or whatever.

Professor John B Harris:
I dislike the term revertant fibre intensely. It pre-supposes that these fibres were at one time abnormal and have somehow reverted to become completely normal. I think it is a misleading term because I don't know that this is the case. All we know is that they are now capable of reacting with an anti-dystrophin antibody. We think that it is a form of "normal muscle dystrophin that is being expressed in these cells in the majority of human biopsies because of our experience with a panel of monoclonal antibodies of varying degrees of specificity. The point is that we don't know that those unusual cells in human biopsies that are dystrophin competent have derived any physiological benefit from the presence of "dystrophin" Until we know something more of the function of dystrophin we won't be able to answer that point.

Dr. Terence A. Partridge:
As Barry Cooper said earlier. I am sure that one of the ways of approaching this problem is to clone the myoblasts and to examine the clones responsible for these "revertant" fibres in isolation from the normal mdx myogenic clones. In the mouse it is possible to clone efficiently using the H2ts6 background which can be cross-bred onto the mdx. This makes cloning easy but leaves the problem of selection; of getting the needle out of the haystack. I think that there are a couple of ways of doing this.

Dr. Nigel G. Laing:
One of the things that strikes me about the pictures that people show of the revertant fibres is that they don't look like Becker fibres with patchy staining; they look like normal fibres. Is this just selection of the best-looking fibres for slides

or is this the way they are?

Professor John B Harris:
They do look "normally active" but they are rare.

Dr. Terence A. Partridge:
In the mdx mouse the "revertant" fibres form what appear to be clusters. The fibers are usually centrally nucleated, I think George Karpati showed this too. On serial sectioning, many of these apparent clusters turn out to be branched fibres. What is particularly interesting about them is that sometimes two branches both become dystrophin-negative before they join up. This means that dystrophin is not travelling from one branch to another by diffusing along their connecting surface. The whole picture suggests a clonal somatically-inherited event of some sort.
We found that these groups in the mdx mouse to be more numerous and possibly bigger as the mice got older. (It is difficult to distinguish between increase in number and increase in size without a great deal of work). This suggests that the myoblasts which are responsible for this abberrant expression of the defective dystrophin gene persists in the rgion and continue to proliferate.

Dr. Barry J. Cooper:
I just want to ask Terry a question because he worked with Eric Hoffman, whose mdx colony has a very high reversion rate. What do Western blots show on those?

Dr. Terence A. Partridge:
We have not done this. We cannot get a signal off of our mice on immunoblots and most people have found the dystrophin-immunoblots from the mdx mouse to be devoid of signal. Our mdx colony has only 1 dystrophin-positive fibre per 10,000-100,000 fibres. We are about 10 fold more common in Eric Hoffman's colony, it was because we started looking at his mice as controls that we picked up these fibres and perhaps these are the mice to look at more carefully by immunoblutting, but I do not know if it has been done.

Dr. Nigel G. Laing:
Perhaps it can be true reversion if a point mutation mutates back to normal and it is easier to envisage this than a true reversion in a Duchenne boy who has a huge deletion, where intuitively one might more reasonably expect an alteration of the mutation from a Duchenne mutation to a Becker mutation.

Dr. Barry J. Cooper:
We tried to address this in the dog too, because one would predict that the most common way for this to happen would be for secondary mutations to occur that clip off some number of nucleotides putting the gene back in frame, so the protein is generated. It seems to me that you should predict then that each of these clones that occurs throughout the muscle should be a little bit different. It is extremely unlikely that the same event occurs in every focus. Certainly with immunohistochemical analysis we were not able to distinguish any differences; they may have been just too subtle a difference to distinguish using antibodies, PCR and sequencing would be better obviously.

Assist. Professor Richard J. Bartlett:
I think in the case of the dog which we see in revertant fibres are alternate spliced products. The normal product would give you the frame-shift, but.there are about 3-4 possibilities, and people in Toronto have looked at a lot of patients in this same region where you see a lot of different possibilities for alternate splicing products which will give you a functional protein or partially functional protein.

Dr. Barry J. Cooper:
The question is, then, how different are the proteins, are they grossly different?

Assist. Professor Richard J. Bartlett:
There may be differences between each fibre. I don't know, it needs to be investigated.

Professor Allen D. Roses:
That would lead to a naturally occurring experiment. We have boys who have no large deletions and we have boys who do not know what they have but they seem to have the boy without having genomic deletions. Is the prevalence of quote "revertant fibres" higher or lower in one of the lower subgroups?

Professor George Karpati:
The event is so random that to base statistics on small pieces of muscle could be very misleading. You could find a muscle sample where you got 50% of the fibres "revertant" and in the next five neighbouring pieces there are none. You need an autopsy to get true percentages.

Professor Allen D. Roses:
Let me ask a question. Is it anybody's experience that they see large numbers of "revertant" fibres in patients with known large deletions?

Professor George Karpati:
Jerry Mandell of Columbus, Ohio, has looked at this and he has been unable to correlate it on single small specimens. No post-mortem has been examined for that purpose.

Dr. Barry J. Cooper:
Allen, the dog does not have a large deletion but certainly has several revertant fibres. John has me so concerned about using the term that I am reluctant to say revertant.

Professor John B Harris:
I think the terminology is misleading because it is open to too many interpretations. That's why I dislike it.

Dr. Barry J. Cooper:
Can you suggest an alternate term which we can switch to.

Professor Allen D. Roses:
Dystrophin positive?

Professor John B Harris:
Yes, that is what I would prefer. However our experience is that one is no more likely to pick up these dystrophin reactive fibres in non-deleting patients than in deleting patients which I think was the point of your question. I think that George Karpati's point is an extremely interesting one. We would very much like to do a wide screen at autopsy on a number of different muscle types in these patients to study the presence of dystrophin competent fibres but as everyone knows, getting autopsies performed on these boys is very difficult.

Professor Allen D. Roses:
There is enough diagnostic muscle fibres still being done with regards to dystrophin tests, so that sort of wipes that out. This could be done at least on the quadriceps or the deltoid, which are the two I guess are the most commonly biopsied. At a time when there are considerable fibres here, I would really be surprised, I would be shocked, I would be astounded if there were large numbers of revertant fibres which came from a Duchenne gene in a major deletion. My conclusion then is whatever we are looking at is not coming from that gene.

Professor J. McC. Howell:
How many fibres do you in fact find at the end stage of the disease.

Professor George Karpati:
Jacques Tremblay's team, of Quebec City, did myoblast transfer in rather late Duchenne cases in their teens and found islands of dystrophin-positive fibres that he believes to be the result of his myoblast injections. However, there is a possibility that what he actually has is what you are suggesting; that these dystrophin-positive fibres were the only ones that survived and formed these tiny little islands in a sea of fat. That, in some respect, answers John Harris' concern as to whether these "revertant" dystrophin-positive fibres are protected from destruction. It would appear so.

Professor Allen D. Roses:
What are the kinds of things that could come out of this group over the past 3 days, which we could do,that needs to be done to accelerate the time line of work. Together, interactive. We each think about our own experiments to do and all resources are not necessarily in one place and it may be very possible that there are certain aspects which could be coordinated as a result of this meeting.

Professor Joe N. Kornegay:
Going back to Nigel's comments regarding our time table for studies leading to a "cure" in either the mdx mouse or golden retriever model, clearly the problems with which we are dealing are complex. We have learned of many of the problems that need to be addressed from Dr. Karpati's presentation yesterday. Availability of models in which to address these questions is a critical problem. Speaking for our two groups, I think both Barry and I have from the onset been willing to make the golden retriever model available. However, there naturally is reluctance on the part of groups without necessary veterinary support to pursue studies in dogs. On the other hand, these same individuals often have expertise far in advance of ourselves in other fields, such as molecular biology. This calls for the collaborations that we developed over the years, in which veterinary expertise such as functional studies is integrated with expertise in cell biology and so forth. We have nonetheless fostered establishment of other colonies of the dog

model, as I outlined the day before yesterday. As more colonies become available and as we enlist the talents of more and more people in the areas in question, we will see a natural progression. The actual time table is, however, up in the air.

Dr. Nigel G. Laing:
We are entering the area of possible interventional therapies with two discussed routes forward. One is by transferring myoblasts and the other is by transfection with some sort of construct. Myoblast transfer is perhaps closer to realisation than the transfection models. The transfection constructs, we thought would have to be safe over the lifespan of a human being, but from what Allen was saying earlier it may not be entirely necessary that this is the case. Making the constructs work safely are perhaps new technologies which are not quite in existence yet. What you are trying to say Allen, is where do we go from here. Do any of those working with constructs wish to talk to this point?

Dr. Barry J. Cooper:
I tried to make a point this morning, I do not know how well I did it. You really do need to know a lot more about dystrophin. If we find something critical in the next week or tomorrow it is possible that all this gene therapy and myoblast therapy would not be necessary and all we would need is some sort of systemic introduction that will help us. So a lot of people are looking for a quick cure by introducing a recombinant gene, you have to also keep in mind that if we understand what dystrophin is doing better, there may be other approaches which are much more easily approachable.

Professor George Karpati:
I say the same thing. The only other immediate therapeutic prospect that would fall into this category is neither myoblast transfer nor gene therapy of any form. It is the use of glucocorticoids which are beneficial through a mechanism that is completely unknown. Of course, there are many problems, namely, the side-effects. But apparently there are good glucocorticoid analogues (ie. Deflazocort) that have much less side-efects and that is being tried now in several centres. So I guess the point is well taken that several therapeutic avenues must be pursued and these should not be lost in the glamour of gene therapy and myoblast transfer.

Professor Byron A. Kakulas:
Well we saw that very elegant model of Henry's this morning where the dystrophin antigen and the glycoprotein were deficient. We don't know the function of glycoprotein as yet and his matter may be relevant to what George said about the steroids which might be put forward as an effective treatment.

Professor George Karpati:
I listened to one of Kevin Campbell's presentations recently and the linkage system is actually a glycoprotein complex with five subunits; three of them are membrane spanning; one is fully on the inside and one is fully on the outside of the membrane. The precise interaction of this complex with the dystrophin molecule is still not know. It is even disputed if it is the C-terminal domain that is attached to it. Incidentally, in Duchenne dystrophy this glycoprotein does not disappear completely. It just goes down to 20-25% of the normal according to Campbell. I guess there are 2 ways of looking at this glycoprotein. You might say that this is simply an anchoring protein. In other words dystrophin is the main player and the glycoprotein is simply an anchoring protein just like vinculin is

anchoring for spectrin. The other way of looking at it is what Kevin Campbell likes to emphasize that it is dystrophin which is the anchoring protein and the glycoproteins are the functional molecules which may have a physiological function in the membrane. It is very difficult right now to make a definitive judgement on those two opposing positions.

Dr. Terence A. Partridge:
I also heard Kevin Campbell speak recently and one of the interesting findings was that, although the glycoprotein complex almost disappears from mdx skeletal muscle, it is present in the mdx heart at approximately normal levels although there is no dystrophin in the mdx heart muscle and the heart undergoes necrosis in these animals.

Dr. Barry J. Cooper:
It seems to me that the amount of glycoproteins could be 100% normal but 0% functional if the role of the dystrophin is to maintain that glycoprotein complex in the correct polarity, correct orientation or whatever, in the membrane. Quantitation of the amount of glycoprotein is not necessarily going to tell you these things. I think when the sequences become available and so on that we might find more out. I believe that the complex must have some important function in the muscle and I am very enthusiastic myself about understanding how that complex functions and how it behaves in dystrophic muscle. I happen to think that it is one of the things which is uniquely suitable to look at using the dog model because of the large quantities of muscle that you can get. You can actually make microsomes from dystrophic canine muscle, which is much more difficult in the mouse and nearly impossible in the human.

Professor Byron A. Kakulas:
If you look at the models of the cytoskeleton produced by Lazarides of Caltech, almost all of these are attached to a membrane glycoprotein.

Professor John B Harris:
One of the things which really intrigues me about the glycoproteins is that a patient deleted or missing a crucial part of the glycoprotein complex will almost certainly express a Duchenne type phenotype with normal dystrophin.

Professor George Karpati:
You had a patient who had a primary glycoprotein deficiency?

Dr. Barry J. Cooper:
Those glycoproteins are obviously important candidate genes for a variety or genetically transmitted muscle diseases. They may not, manifest exactly as a Duchenne patient. Depending on which one is defective and how it is defective.

Dr. Nigel G. Laing:
The aim of this meeting was to discuss the current state of therapy for Duchenne and Becker dystrophy and possibilities for the future. The difference it seems to me between the end of this meeting and the one two and a half years ago is that everyone seemed very positive then with the route forward through myoblast transfer mapped out. There seems to be a cold realisation now of how much is ahead.

Professor Allen D. Roses:

I interpret it just the opposite Nigel. I think what is happening here is that people are beginning to think beyond the simplistic, "let's put some dystrophin in and get it in any old way". These rare patients, they may not be so rare, these recognizable rare patients are not common knowledge now but will soon be reported, I think that they are going to be very important to the interpretation of what these sorts of things mean. What John just said about that patient astounds me, I did not know about that patient but it puts a whole bunch of things in a whole new light. To look at the potential up regulation of other known genes that are membrane associated, one close to my heart would be alpha or beta spectrin and to look at these in a different sort of light. What is actually happening around this. I really don't think the silence is lack of enthusiasm. It is more that things are beginning to settle, in at least my mind, that there is not going to be a quick fix. There are technical problems that can be approached. We have all talked about them and the different ways of approaching these matters. Gene therapy is marching on at whatever pace it will and that there is definitely a push forward. I received a fax today from my lab. which is sort of remarkable in putting in the context of this meeting, I hope the editors of science do not read this, but there is a news article in science which was published yesterday about the report card for the genome project and the major significant things which were brought out for the genome project was not what the genome projects specific aims are, but rather the unstable X was there. The fragile X sequences have been identified and chromosome 19 has had 67% of it mapped. There are a few things like that at a cost of mega billions and the progress that this area has made I think over the last 5 years, starting with the work of Worton and Kunkel, the people who got us to dystrophin in the first place, has been done at a phenomenally reasonable budget with striking results and I am just the opposite, I am very enthusiastic to see what starts incubating here and I think one of the main reasons to get together is that names which previously were on the top of the page, you really did not get a chance to talk to people and learn what they are really like and flash out ideas in this type of Workshop other than a Convention or a larger meeting has had some very subtle effects will in itself accelerate the fuel. I would like to thank Byron and the Institute on behalf of at least one frequent guest and on behalf of the other guests here for the hospitality that has been shown and the whole tenor of the meeting.

Professor Byron A. Kakulas:

I would like to thank everyone for contributing to this conference and I wish you all a safe trip home.

Subject Index